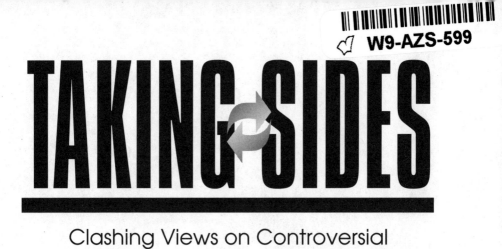

TAKING SIDES

Clashing Views on Controversial

Issues in Health and Society

SIXTH EDITION

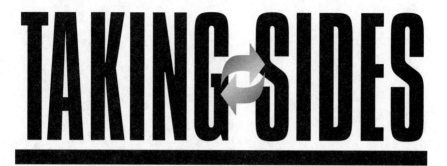

TAKING SIDES

Clashing Views on Controversial

Issues in Health and Society

SIXTH EDITION

Selected, Edited, and with Introductions by

Eileen L. Daniel
State University of New York College at Brockport

McGraw-Hill/Dushkin
A Division of The McGraw-Hill Companies

To Ann

Photo Acknowledgment
Cover image: © 2004 by PhotoDisc, Inc.

Cover Art Acknowledgment
Charles Vitelli

Manufactured in the United States of America

Sixth Edition

23456789BAHBAH7654

Library of Congress Cataloging-in-Publication Data
Main entry under title:
Taking sides: clashing views on controversial issues in health and society/selected, edited, and with introductions by Eileen L. Daniel.—6th ed.
Includes bibliographical references and index.
1. Health. 2. Medical care—United States. 3. Medical ethics. 4. Social medicine—United States.
I. Daniel, Eileen L., *comp.*
362.1
0-07-295330-6
ISSN: 1094-7531

Printed on Recycled Paper

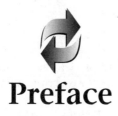

Preface

This book contains 42 selections arranged in 21 pro and con pairs. Each pair addresses a controversial issue in health and society, expressed in terms of a question in order to draw the lines of debate more clearly.

Most of the questions that are included here relate to health topics of modern concern, such as managed care, abortion, alternative medicine, and drug use and abuse. The authors of the selections take strong stands on specific issues and provide support for their positions. Although we may not agree with a particular point of view, each author clearly defines his or her stand on the issues.

This book is divided into six parts, each containing related issues. Each part opener provides a brief overview of the issues and offers several related sites on the World Wide Web, including Web addresses. Each issue is preceded by an *introduction,* which sets the stage for the debate, gives historical background on the subject, and provides a context for the controversy. Each issue concludes with a *postscript,* which offers a summary of the debate and some concluding observations and suggests further readings on the subject. The postscript also raises further points, since most of the issues have more than two sides. At the back of the book is a listing of all the *contributors to this volume,* which gives information on the physicians, professors, journalists, theologians, and scientists whose views are debated here.

Taking Sides: Clashing Views on Controversial Issues in Health and Society is a tool to encourage critical thought on important health issues. Readers should not feel confined to the views expressed in the selections. Some readers may see important points on both sides of an issue and may construct for themselves a new and creative approach, which may incorporate the best of both sides or provide an entirely new vantage point for understanding.

Changes to this edition The sixth edition of *Taking Sides: Clashing Views on Controversial Issues in Health and Society* includes some important changes from the fifth edition. Ten completely new issues have been added: *Is the Pharmaceutical Industry Responsible for the High Cost of Prescription Drugs?* (Issue 4); *Is Drug Testing Vital to the Workplace?* (Issue 5); *Should the Government Regulate the Sale, Advertisement, and Distribution of Junk Food?* (Issue 7); *Should Race Play a Role in the Treatment and Study of Disease?* (Issue 8); *Should Addiction to Drugs Be Labeled a Brain Disease?* (Issue 10); *Does Abortion Increase the Risk of Breast Cancer?* (Issue 13); *Does Anabolic Steroid Use Cause Serious Health Problems for Athletes?* (Issue 17); *Does Multiple-Chemical Sensitivity Pose a Serious Health Threat?* (Issue 19); *Is the Atkins Low-Carbohydrate Diet a Valid Weight-Loss Plan?* (Issue 20); *and Should Alternative Medicine Be Combined With Conventional Medicine?* (Issue 21). For other issues, I kept the issue question from the fifth edition but replaced one or both of the selections in order to make the issue more current or more clearly focused. As a result, there are a total of 10 new issues and 27 new articles. In addition, the issue introductions and postscripts have been revised and updated.

A word to the instructor   An *Instructor's Manual With Test Questions* (both multiple-choice and essay) is available through the publisher for instructors using *Taking Sides* in the classroom. Also available is a general guidebook, *Using Taking Sides in the Classroom,* which discusses teaching techniques and methods for integrating the pro-con approach of *Taking Sides* into any classroom setting. An online version of *Using Taking Sides in the Classroom* and a correspondence service for Taking Sides adopters can be found at http://www.dushkin.com/usingts/.

  Taking Sides: Clashing Views on Controversial Issues in Health and Society is only one title in the Taking Sides series. If you are interested in seeing the table of contents for any of the other titles, please visit the Taking Sides Web site at http://www.dushkin.com/takingsides/.

Acknowledgments   Special thanks go to John, Diana, and Jordan. Also thanks to my colleagues at the State University of New York College at Brockport for all of their helpful contributions. I was also assisted in preparing this edition by the valuable suggestions from the adopters who filled out comment cards and questionnaires. Many of their recommendations were incorporated into this edition. Finally, I appreciate the assistance of the staff at McGraw-Hill/Dushkin and thank them for all of their help.

Eileen L. Daniel
State University of New York
College at Brockport

Contents In Brief

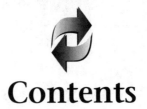

Contents

Christopher F. Koller, CEO of Neighborhood Health Plan of Rhode Island, a health plan serving Medicaid enrollees based in Providence, asserts that the pharmaceutical industry has achieved its rapid growth by political protection and by exploiting the vulnerabilities of patients. Ronald Bailey, science correspondent for *Reason* magazine, states that spending on prescriptions is rising rapidly because Americans are buying more drugs. Bailey maintains that the drug companies have actually enriched the quality of our lives.

PART 2   HEALTH AND SOCIETY   69

William F. Current, president of WFC & Associates, a national consulting firm specializing in drug-free workplace policies, states that pre-employment drug testing is accepted by employees, hassle free, and beneficial to employers. Jacob Sullum, senior editor of *Reason* magazine, argues that employment-based drug testing is insulting to employees and mostly irrelevant to future job performance.

Richard T. Hull, professor emeritus of philosophy at the State University of New York at Buffalo, asserts that physician-assisted suicide is the only re-source terminally ill patients have with which to communicate that their end-of-life care is inadequate. Margaret Somerville, Gale Professor of Law and professor in the faculty of medicine at the McGill University Cen-tre for Medicine, Ethics, and Law in Montreal, Canada, argues that basic reasons to oppose euthanasia include the sanctity of human life and the harms and risks to individuals and to society. Somerville contends that these reasons outweigh any possible benefits.

Alan I. Leshner, director of the National Institute on Drug Abuse at the National Institutes of Health, states that addiction to drugs and alcohol is not a behavioral condition but a treatable disease. Psychiatrist Sally L. Satel counters that labeling addiction as a chronic and relapsing brain disease is propaganda. Satel asserts that most addicts are the instigators of their own addiction.

The editors of the *Harvard Health Letter* maintain that there is evidence that individuals who are chronically stressed possess an increased risk of cancer and heart disease. Writer Christopher Caldwell argues that no one, including doctors, can come to an agreement on what stress is, so stress can not be blamed as the cause of disease.

Herbert Benson, an associate professor of medicine at Harvard Medical School, and journalist Marg Stark contend that faith and spirituality will enhance and prolong life. William B. Lindley, associate editor of *Truth Seeker*, counters that there is no scientific way to determine that spirituality can heal.

The American Association of ProLife Obstetricians and Gynecologists state that for any woman already pregnant, choosing abortion will leave her with a greater long-term risk of breast cancer than she would have if she were to complete her pregnancy. Joyce Arthur, editor of the Canadian newsletter Pro-Choice Press and abortion rights activist, contends that the assertion that having an abortion significantly increases a woman's risk of breast cancer is deceptive and false.

Clinical psychologist Steven Ungerleider asserts that anabolic steroids are dangerous to the health of athletes and should not be used. Freelance writer Dayn Perry states that the health risks of anabolic steroids are greatly exaggerated and that they pose limited harm to athletes.

Issue 18.   Is Marijuana Dangerous and Addictive?   292

Eric A. Voth, medical director of Chemical Dependency Services at St. Francis Hospital in Topeka, Kansas, argues that marijuana produces many adverse effects and that its effectiveness as a medicine is supported only by anecdotes. Ethan A. Nadelmann, director of the Lindesmith Center, a New York drug policy research institute, asserts that government officials continue to promote the myth that marijuana is harmful and leads to the use of hard drugs. He states that the war on marijuana is being fought for purely political, not health, reasons.

PART 6   CONSUMER HEALTH   309

Issue 19.   Does Multiple-Chemical Sensitivity Pose a Serious Health Threat?   *310*

Journalist Paul Yanick, Jr. states that a condition known as multiple-chemical sensitivity is becoming one of our greatest health challenges. Psychiatrist Stephen Barrett argues that multiple-chemical sensitivity is an ill-defined problem and that no scientific test has ever provided evidence that it has an organic basis.

Issue 20.   Is the Atkins Low-Carbohydrate Diet a Valid Weight-Loss Plan?   328

Journalist Gary Taubes asserts that eating fatty meats, cheeses, cream, and butter is the key to a long, healthy life. Michael Fumento, senior fellow at the Hudson Institute, argues that there are ample studies that dispute the benefits of a high-fat, low-carbohydrate diet.

Andrew Weil, director of the University of Arizona Program on Integrative Medicine, asserts that alternative medicine helps patients and should be incorporated into conventional medical practices. Physician and editor Arnold S. Relman argues that integrating alternative healing with conventional medicine would be a step backward and would not improve medical care.

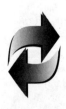

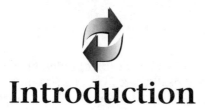

Introduction

Dimensions and Approaches to the Study of Health and Society

Eileen L. Daniel

What Is Health?

Traditionally, being healthy meant being absent of illness. If someone did not have a disease, then he or she was considered healthy. The overall health of a nation or specific population was determined by numbers measuring illness, disease, and death rates. Today this rather negative view of assessing individual health and health in general is changing. A healthy person is one who is not only free from disease but also fully well.

Being well, or wellness, involves the interrelationship of many dimensions of health: physical, emotional, social, mental, and spiritual. This multifaceted view of health reflects a holistic approach, which includes individuals taking responsibility for their own well-being.

Our health and longevity are affected by the many choices we make every day. Medical reports tell us that if we abstain from smoking, drugs, excessive alcohol consumption, fat, and cholesterol, and if we get regular exercise, our rate of disease and disability will significantly decrease. These reports, although not totally conclusive, have encouraged many people to make positive lifestyle changes. Millions of people have quit smoking, alcohol consumption is down, and more and more individuals are exercising regularly and eating low-fat diets. These changes are encouraging, but the many people who have been unable or unwilling to make them are left feeling worried and/or guilty over continuing their negative health behaviors.

Additionally, experts disagree about the exact nature of positive health behaviors, and this causes confusion. For example, some scientists maintain that overweight Americans should make efforts to lose weight, even if it takes many tries. Many Americans have tried unsuccessfully to lose weight by eating a low-fat diet. However, experts debate on whether a low-fat, high-carbohydrate diet or a low-carbohydrate diet, which includes ample protein and fat, is best. Other debatable issues include whether or not people should utilize only conventional medicines or if they should also seek out alternative therapies.

Health status is also affected by society and government. Societal pressures have helped pass smoking restrictions in public places, mandatory safety belt legislation, and laws permitting condom distribution in public schools.

The government plays a role in the health of individuals as well, although it has failed to provide minimal health care for many low-income Americans.

Unfortunately, there are no absolute answers to many questions regarding health and wellness issues. Moral questions, controversial concerns, and individual perceptions of health matters all can create opposing views. As you evaluate the issues in this book, you should keep an open mind toward both sides. You might not change your mind regarding the morality of abortion or the limitation of health care for the elderly or mentally handicapped, but you will still be able to learn from the opposing viewpoint.

The Health Care Industry

The issues in this book are divided into six parts. The first part deals with the health care industry. Issue 1 contains a debate on whether or not managed health care offers consumers an improvement over traditional care. In the United States approximately 40 million Americans have no health insurance. Furthermore, there has been a resurgence in diseases such as tuberculosis and antibiotic-resistant strains of bacterial infections, which threaten thousands of Americans and strain the current system. Those enrolled in government programs such as Medicaid often find few, if any, physicians who will accept them as patients because reimbursements are low and the paperwork is cumbersome. On the other hand, Americans continue to live longer and longer, and for most of us, the health care available is among the best in the world.

Issue 2 debates the wisdom of using expensive life-prolonging treatments on elderly patients. While many Americans agree that there are some situations in which health care should be rationed, many also find it difficult to decide exactly how it should be rationed and how this decision should be made.

Issue 3 introduces the question of how people obtain health insurance. The majority of the insured in this country receive their coverage through a group plan offered by their employer. They—and/or their employer—pay lower premiums than the self-employed, the unemployed, or those employed by a business that does not provide an insurance plan. Many of those without employment-based health insurance cannot afford adequate insurance, or, frequently, any insurance at all. Also, those who have employment-based health insurance often experience difficulty maintaining their coverage when they move from one employer to another. Should adequate health insurance be so closely tied to where and how a person is employed?

Issue 4 addresses the high cost of prescription drugs. Many lifesaving medications have been developed in recent years, but they come at a high price. Should consumers pay for the research and development of drugs?

Health and Society

Part 2 introduces current issues related to health from a societal perspective. Issue 5 discusses drug testing in the workplace. Many companies require their employees to undergo drug testing prior to employment. Some firms also engage in random testing for current workers. There is concern that this infringement of privacy may not provide benefits to employers. Does drug testing result in increased productivity and decreased costs? Do the benefits outweigh the potential invasion of privacy?

Issue 6 deals with whether or not physicians should intervene to hasten death for hopelessly ill persons. Many Americans agree that we cannot and should not prolong the lives of terminally ill patients, although others believe that physicians should not hasten the process of dying but rather should offer these individuals relief from pain and quality of life management strategies.

The topic of whether the government should regulate the sale, advertisement, and distribution of junk food is explored in Issue 7. This debate parallels discussions concerning governmental regulations of tobacco companies. The sale, distribution, and advertisement of tobacco is controlled by national, state, and local governments in an effort to generate tax revenues and to reduce smoking. Should nonnutritious foods that encourage obesity and other health problems be similarly treated?

The issue of combining health care, medical care, and race is addressed in Issue 8. As scientists develop the ability to genetically "map" the human body, the role of race has surfaced. Is race important when considering how to treat disease? Is it clear that more research is needed in determining how to treat disease? It is clear that more research is needed in determining how much of a role, if any, race should play in the study and care of disease. Could the inclusion of race as a factor in deciding how best to treat disease lead to abuse?

Issue 9 asks, Should human cloning ever be permitted? Cloning technology offers the *potential* to asexually produce a human child. While there are pros and cons to the ability to clone cells, ethical and moral questions also arise—especially when the issue involves the creation of a new human life.

Mind/Body Relationship

Part 3 discusses three important issues related to the relationship between mind and body. Issue 10 examines the relationship between drug addiction and brain disease. Millions of Americans use and abuse drugs that alter their minds and affect their bodies. Use of these substances can lead to physical and psychological addiction and the related problems of family dysfunction, reduced worker productivity, and crime. Are addictions within the control of those who abuse drugs? Issue 11 deals with stress and how it relates to disease. Over the past 10 years, both laypeople and the medical profession have placed an emphasis on the prevention of illness as a way to improve health. Not smoking, for instance, certainly reduces the risk of developing lung cancer. Unfortunately, the current U.S. health care system places an emphasis on treatment rather than on prevention, even though prevention is less expensive, less painful, and more humane. Stress management programs have arisen to prevent stress-related illness, which many believe is responsible for the majority of doctor visits. Does stress cause disease, and will managing stress actually prevent disease?

Issue 12 discusses the role of spirituality in the prevention of illness. Many studies have found that religion and spirituality play a role in recovery from sickness. Should health providers encourage their patients to seek spirituality?

Sexuality and Gender Issues

The first issue in this section contains a debate on whether or not abortion increases the risk of breast cancer. The abortion issue continues to cause major controversy. More restrictions have been placed on the right to abortion as a result of the political power wielded by the pro-life faction. Pro-choice followers, however, argue that making abortion illegal again will force many women to obtain dangerous "back-alley" abortions. One controversial issue relating to abortion is its relationship to breast cancer. Pro-life groups maintain that there is a connection and urge women to avoid abortion. Pro-choice factions disagree and state that data do not show any linkage between breast cancer and abortion.

The second issue in this section discusses whether or not our health care system favors men at the expense of women. Although they live longer than men, many women assert that they have been excluded from drug tests and other medical research and that they receive inferior care when they see doctors. Opponents of this view maintain that women see their doctors more frequently than men, are hospitalized more often, and continue to outlive men by several years.

Public Health Issues

The first controversy in this section is about the epidemic of homicide and the potential benefits of more stringent gun control. Doctors and public health officials state that homicides involving guns are increasing, which is driving health care costs up and diminishing quality of life. They maintain that gun control would help reduce the shooting and deaths. Opponents of gun control argue that under such a policy only criminals—not law-abiding citizens—would have access to guns. They also contend that doctors should leave the gun control issue to criminologists.

The threat of bioterrorism has resurrected the risk of smallpox, which was thought to be eradicated in the late 1970s. Issue 16 focuses on whether or not all parents should be forced to have their children immunized against smallpox.

At the turn of the twentieth century, millions of American children developed childhood diseases such as tetanus, polio, measles, and pertussis (whooping cough). Many of these children died or became permanently disabled because of these illnesses. Today vaccines can prevent all of these conditions; however, not all children receive their recommended immunizations. Some do not get vaccinated until the schools require them, and others are allowed exemptions. More and more, parents are requesting exemptions for some or all vaccinations based on fears over their safety and their effectiveness. The pertussis vaccination seems to generate the biggest fears. Reports of serious injury to children following the pertussis vaccination (usually given in a combination of diphtheria, pertussis, and tetanus, or DPT) have convinced many parents to forgo immunization. As a result, the incidence rates of measles and pertussis have been climbing after decades of decline. Is it safer to be vaccinated than to risk getting pertussis?

The final two issues in this part concern drug use and abuse in the United States. Millions of Americans use drugs that alter their minds and affect their bodies. Issue 17 asks, Does anabolic steriod use cause serious health problems for athletes? Some contend that assertions about health risks are greatly exaggerated. Short-term use is said to be harmless, and many athletes consider the benefits of steroid use to outweigh any possible side effects. However, others counter that steroid use can be linked to illness and death.

Because of drug-related crime, many experts have argued for the legalization of drugs, particularly marijuana. Issue 18 considers the argument that if currently illegal drugs were legalized, the enormous profits from illegal drug sales would no longer exist, which would reduce criminal behavior in this area and allow law enforcement officials to focus on other crime areas. The American drug crisis is often related to changes in or a breakdown of traditional values. The collapse of strong family and religious influences may affect drug usage, especially among young people. It has been argued, however, that some people, regardless of societal or familial influences, will use drugs based on need. For example, some people have testified that cancer patients can benefit from marijuana because it reduces the severity of the effects of chemotherapy. Although there is a movement to legalize this drug for its medicinal purposes, many experts want marijuana to remain illegal.

Consumer Health

Part 6 introduces questions about particular issues related to personal choices about health care: Issue 19 contains a debate concerning whether or not multiple-chemical sensitivity (MCS) is a legitimate condition or a psychosomatic illness. MCS begins with exposure to a certain environmental substance that eventually causes the sufferer to develop severe reactions to other ordinary chemicals. Some assert that test have failed to provide any evidence of this condition. However, those who suffer from MCS argue that this condition prevents them from participating in many daily activities.

As Americans grow increasingly overweight, many debate about what is the most effective means of weight control Some researchers believe that a Mediterranean-style diet, which includes ample amounts of olive oil along with a variety of fruits and vegetables, is the most effective way to maintain a healthy weight. Others argue that a low-fat or low-carbohydrate diet is best. Issue 20 explores the relationship between the Atkins diet, which includes low-carbohydrate foods, and weight loss.

Issue 21 deals with alternative medicines and conventional medicines. Many patients are choosing to combine the two, believing that they are uniting the best of both worlds. Are there risks associated with doing so? Some are concerned about potential side effects that will harm the patient when combining alternative medicines with conventional medicines. While some will testify to the benefits they have personally gained from alternative medicines, others will point out the lack of rigorous testing of alternative drugs. Are patients being done a disservice if their physicians do not make them aware of alternative medicines that may help them? Or will they find that alternative medicines that may help them? Or will they find that alternative medicines undermine the effectiveness of conventional medicines?

Will the 21 debates presented in this book ever be resolved? Some issues may resolve themselves because of the availability of resources. For instance, funding for health care for the elderly may become restricted in the United States, as it is in the United Kingdom, simply because there are increasingly limited resources to go around. As health costs continue to rise, an overhaul of the health care system to provide managed care for all while keeping costs down seems inevitable. Other controversies may require the test of time for resolution. Several more years may be required before it can be determined if certain diseases are caused by stress. The debates over the effectiveness of low-fat diets and the long-term benefits of drug testing may also take years to be fully resolved.

Other controversies may never resolve themselves. There may never be a consensus over the abortion issue, gun control, rationing health care or physician-assisted suicide. This book will introduce you to many ongoing controversies on a variety of sensitive and complex health-related topics. In order to have a good grasp of one's own viewpoint, it is necessary to be familiar with and understand the points made by the opposition.

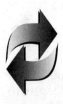

On the Internet . . .

The National Committee for Quality Assurance

The National Committee for Quality Assurance's Web page features an HMO accreditation status list that is updated monthly. It also provides accreditation summary reports on a number of HMO plans and other consumer information on managed care plans.

http://www.ncqa.org

Huffington Center on Aging

The Huffington Center on Aging, Baylor College of Medicine's home page, offers links to related sites on aging and Alzheimer's disease.

http://www.hcoa.org

United States Census Bureau Health Insurance Data

On this site are Census Bureau data on health insurance coverage status and type of coverage by age, sex, gender, race, Hispanic origin, state, and other characteristics.

http://www.census.gov/hhes/www/hlthins.html

Prescription Drugs: The Issue

This site contains a profile of prescription drugs, including a look at the interest groups behind the issue and the campaign contributions that are made based on records.

http://www.opensecrets.org/news/drug/

PART 1

The Health Care Industry

*T*he United States currently faces many challenging health problems, including an aging population and lack of universal health insurance for its citizens. Society must confront the enormous financial burden of providing health care to the elderly, including the increasing costs of prescription drugs. At the same time, millions of Americans have enrolled in health maintenance organizations, which attempt to control health care costs through managing care. Although many people are happy with managed care, others state that it restricts access to the health care they need. Also included in this part is a debate on whether health care insurance should be based on employment. Many employers do not provide health care benefits. The unemployed often have to rely on government programs that may not address their needs. Is some type of universal coverage a better alternative?

- Will Managed Care Improve Health Care in the United States?

- Should Health Care for the Elderly Be Rationed?

- Does Employer-Based Health Insurance Provide Adequate Coverage for Most Americans?

- Is the Pharmaceutical Industry Responsible for the High Cost of Prescription Drugs?

ISSUE 1

Will Managed Care Improve Health Care in the United States?

YES: David Jacobsen, from "Cost-Conscious Care," *Reason* (June 1996)

NO: Ronald J. Glasser, from "The Doctor Is Not In: On the Managed Failure of Managed Health Care," *Harper's Magazine* (March 1998)

ISSUE SUMMARY

YES: Surgeon David Jacobsen states that health maintenance organizations (HMOs) offer quality care and that high-quality medical care at an affordable price is not only possible under managed care, it is a reality.

NO: Pediatrician and author Ronald J. Glasser argues that managed care companies care more for profits than for people.

Many Americans have perceived serious wrongs with the current health care system. In general, these concerns are (1) increasing health care access to the uninsured, (2) gaining the ability to keep one's health insurance when one changes or loses a job, and (3) controlling the escalating costs of health care.

Health care in the United States is handled by various unrelated agencies and organizations and through a number of programs, including private insurance, government-supported Medicaid for the needy, and Medicare for the elderly. Currently there are between 35 and 40 million people—about 16 percent of the population—who do not have any health insurance and who do not qualify for government-sponsored programs. These people must often do without any medical care or suffer financial catastrophe if illness occurs. A *New York Times* article in 1992 claimed that 50 percent of personal bankruptcies in the United States have been attributed to medical costs.

In addition to the number of uninsured people, America's health care is the most expensive in the world. The United States spends more on health care than any other nation, about $2,600 per capita. The share of the national output of wealth, the gross domestic product (GDP), expended by the United States on health is 14 percent and rising. Yet the United States has a lower life expectancy, higher infant mortality, and higher percentage of low birth weight infants than Canada, Japan, or most western European nations. Ironically, the United States is the only industrialized nation other than South Africa that does not provide government-sponsored health care to all its citizens.

One solution to America's health care problems has been the shift to managing care through various plans, such as health maintenance organizations (HMOs). HMOs are organizations that provide health care in return for prefixed payments. Most HMOs provide care through a network of doctors and hospitals that their members must use in order to be covered. Currently, more than 50 million workers—70 percent of the nation's eligible employees—now have health care through some type of managed care. The rise in managed care is related to employer efforts to reduce health care benefit costs. There are cost savings, but consumer groups and physicians worry that managed care will move medical decisions from doctors to accountants. Proponents of the managed care industry argue that health care will actually improve under its care. They state that it makes good financial sense for managed care providers to intervene before patients get sicker. Unfortunately, seriously ill patients, who are the most expensive to treat, may lose out under managed care.

The underlying principle of managed health care is to maintain the health of a community by offering early detection tests and preventive care, such as cholesterol screenings, vaccinations, physical exams, and smoking cessation programs. These services are usually provided at a modest fee or co-payment. In exchange for these reduced fees, the consumer agrees to see a limited group of doctors and providers selected by the managed care plan. The plan keeps rates down by limiting the patient's access to costly specialists and procedures, using less expensive and lesser-trained providers, and reducing hospital stays. Some health care workers have complained that pressure has been put on them to discharge patients as quickly as possible. Managed care plans have also increasingly demanded that certain medical procedures that were once done only in a hospital now be done in a less costly outpatient setting.

Does managed care compromise quality? Studies comparing traditional fee-for-service and managed care have found that the quality of care is similar. Consumer satisfaction surveys do not necessarily agree. Managed care patients are less likely to be satisfied with their care than those in a traditional practice. The more seriously ill they are, the more dissatisfaction they report. A recent survey by the Harvard School of Public Health found that managed care patients reported longer waits to see a specialist. They were also more likely to report incorrect care by their primary care physicians. Most experts believe there is a wide range in quality among managed care plans. In cities where managed care is relatively new, managed care plans tend to offer the lowest possible premiums in order to attract new subscribers. Quality is often sacrificed. In communities where managed care has been well established, the quality tends to be higher.

In the following selections, David Jacobsen argues that HMOs offer quality care that is comparable with the traditional fee-for-service. Ronald J. Glasser counters that managed care companies are more concerned with profits than with patients.

3

David Jacobsen 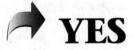 **YES**

Cost-Conscious Care

Torture by HMO" is the title of a March 18 [1996] column by Bob Herbert in *The New York Times*. Herbert tells the story of a North Carolina family with a baby suffering from leukemia. Their health maintenance organization insisted that the child undergo treatment in another state, at great cost and inconvenience. Herbert condemns the HMO's "inflexible and thoroughly inhumane" policies, adding that "humanitarian concerns are not what corporate care is about. In the competition with profits, patients must always lose."

This portrait of HMOs as soulless money-making machines has become increasingly popular in recent years, as skyrocketing health care costs have driven a shift from fee-for-service medicine to managed care. Critics such as Harvard Medical School professor David Himmelstein contend that HMOs reward doctors for providing less care, trapping them in a conflict between their incomes and their patients' welfare, and impose "gag clauses" that forbid them to discuss this conflict with patients. "The bottom line is superseding the Hippocratic oath," write Jeff Cohen and Norman Solomon in their syndicated column. "Cost-cutting edicts from HMO managements put doctors in a box. . . . Faced with directives to help maximize profits, many physicians are under constant pressure to shift their allegiance from patients to company stockholders."

From my perspective as both a physician and a patient in the same HMO, these charges do not ring true. I do not doubt that HMOs, like any other business, sometimes serve their customers poorly. But there is no reason to believe that managed care systematically undermines patient welfare because of the imperative to cut costs. To the contrary, I have found that efficiency is perfectly compatible with compassionate, effective health care. (Since this article was written, I have myself become a cancer patient. Thus far, my care has been unsurpassed. I have the option of being treated outside my HMO, but would not think of going anywhere else. I expect from my plan the same level of care as a patient that I have provided as a physician.)

My plan delivers care at several neighborhood health centers. Each member chooses a "home" center and a primary care physician at that center. Surgical, pediatric, obstetrical, and mental health services, as well as radiology, laboratory, pharmacy, and physical therapy, are all provided under one roof. While our "staff model" HMO does not offer as extensive a choice of physicians as many "network" HMOs, our arrangement does offer economies of scale and strict control of physician quality. Surveys consistently show that patients rate quality of care above greater choice of providers.

I am paid a straight salary and modest bonuses tied to both the plan's profitability and a patient satisfaction index. Frequent advisory audits help me and my patients sort out health care they *need* from health care they *want*. My goal is healthy, satisfied patients and a financially sound business. Every day, I put my professional reputation on the line. So does my HMO. Our challenge is to cut costs without cutting quality. Fortunately, there are many ways to do this.

෴

Changing the venue of medical care from hospital to out-patient center, office, or home is the most important factor driving health care costs down and quality up. Hospitals are very expensive pieces of architecture. They are also complex places and therefore potentially hazardous to your health. Despite rigorous safeguards, medication and treatment errors can and do occur. As many as 15 percent of hospitalized patients go home with a hospital-acquired infection, often caused by antibiotic-resistant organisms. Furthermore, most patients do not wish to be in a hospital. In the last three years, my HMO has reduced hospital use by 25 percent.

Inguinal hernia repair is one of the most frequently performed operations. Just a few years ago, the cost of this operation included a preoperative night in the hospital, one to two hours in the operating room under general anesthesia, and up to five postoperative days in the hospital. The patient had to take four to six weeks off work, and the recurrence rate was 10 percent. In 1996, at my HMO, this operation requires 40 minutes of surgery in a free-standing, outpatient surgical center under local anesthesia using a $100 plastic-mesh plug. Patients have less discomfort, return to unrestricted work in one week, and enjoy a recurrence rate of less than 1 per 1,000. This approach to hernia repair has been technically feasible for several years but was usually employed sporadically, at the discretion of the surgeon or the patient. In the era of cost containment, it has rapidly become the standard in the profession, regardless of reimbursement mode.

Thanks to the innovation of laparoscopic surgery, 80 percent of my patients who need their gallbladder removed can undergo the operation as outpatients and return to work in a week. The original inspiration for this procedure was the development of miniature video cameras, and the early reports were dismissed as mere technical wizardry. But as it became clear that laparoscopic gallbladder removal was not only safe but much less expensive than conventional surgery, surgeons quickly adopted the procedure as the standard approach, and patients demanded it.

The challenge of providing better care at lower cost has spurred not only the development of new procedures but the resurrection of old ones. Pilonidal abscess, a chronic and painful anorectal condition, used to be treated with radical surgery in the hospital. Recovery was frequently prolonged and painful. I now treat this problem with a 20-minute office procedure. Patients can return to work in two days, and the recurrence rate is less than 2 percent. This procedure was first described 15 years ago but languished until managed care created the incentive to implement it on a wider scale.

Open-heart surgery is expensive. Traditionally, the payer is billed separately by the hospital, the surgeon, and the anesthesiologist. My HMO recently negotiated a contract in which we pay a flat fee per operation that is about half our previous cost. As for concerns that surgeons might offer less surgery for less money, our studies show no change in mortality or morbidity since this contract went into effect. Beyond the question of ethics, no reputable provider group would risk a lucrative contract with a large HMO by delivering less than first-class care. Based on this experience, we are exploring package pricing for other high-cost procedures, such as organ transplantations.

Childhood asthma is a distressing and sometimes frightening problem for parents and children. Our studies showed that repeated visits to the emergency room were not only unnerving for families but accounted for a substantial portion of the cost of treating asthma. Through an aggressive program of family education, we are teaching our patients how to handle most asthma attacks at home, even how to give adrenaline injections. A nurse practitioner is available by telephone 24 hours a day to advise families whether a visit to the hospital may be necessary. Emergency room visits are down 40 percent in the last two years. So far, we have noted no adverse effects on patient care, and the response from families has been almost entirely positive.

Treatment of minor lacerations used to involve a trip to the hospital emergency room and frequently entailed a long wait. On nights and weekends our health centers are now staffed with specially trained physician assistants who repair 90 percent of all minor lacerations. In the first year this program has saved more than $100,000 in hospital emergency room charges while taking care of our patients better and more quickly.

For many of our patients with chronic wounds, such as bedsores and diabetic ulcers, treatment has often involved lengthy stays in rehabilitation hospitals or prolonged, expensive home visits by nurses. Under our wound-care program, most patients with chronic wounds can be treated directly at our health centers under the supervision of a physician. In most cases, patients and their families can be trained to do the daily wound care at home. In the first year, this program saved more than $70,000 in outside utilization costs.

Patients needing hip replacement surgery are often elderly and suffering from other medical problems. We now begin physical therapy evaluation in the patient's home *prior* to surgery. By knowing the level of family support and the location of stairs and bathrooms, we can much better prepare the patient for recuperation and rehabilitation. The new approach has cut the average hospital stay in half, eliminated the need for intermediate rehab hospital care in many cases, and accelerated recuperation.

For the past three years, my HMO has followed a policy of early discharge after childbirth. The childbirth program includes comprehensive prenatal education, post-partum home visits, and individual screening. A 16-year-old first-time mother with no family support and no telephone at home is not sent home in 24 hours. But 70 percent of women with uncomplicated vaginal deliveries are discharged in 24 to 36 hours. And despite the recent brouhaha over "drive-thru" deliveries, a recent survey documents that 90 percent of our patients are satisfied with their care—the same percentage as before the early discharge policy was adopted. There is no evidence that the health of mother or infant has been compromised. Most mothers and their babies belong at home with an attentive family, rather than in a potentially dangerous hospital.

Unnecessary diagnostic tests are probably the most familiar example of American medicine's spendthrift ways. Our computers are now set up so that every time a physician orders a laboratory test or X-ray procedure, a window on the screen displays the cost. Before managed care we neither knew nor asked. Preliminary analysis shows that this minor innovation has significantly reduced the ordering of routine laboratory and X-ray tests, especially among medical residents (physicians in training).

❧❦❧

Much criticism of HMO care focuses not on common procedures such as these but on rare, emotionally charged illnesses. The cover story in the January 22 [1996] issue of *Time,* for example, chronicles the experience of a woman with advanced breast cancer whose HMO refused to pay for bone marrow transplantation. In such desperate cases, everyone understandably feels that something ought to be done. But the truth is that bone marrow transplantation for advanced breast cancer is a dangerous and expensive treatment of *no* proven benefit. This kind of case must be handled on an individual basis with consummate compassion and understanding, but it should not divert our attention from the myriad ways in which good medical care can be delivered for less money.

The significance of the potential conflict between physician income and patient welfare has also been exaggerated. First of all, it is offensive to me and the overwhelming majority of my colleagues to suggest that we would pad our bank accounts by obstructing or denying *necessary* medical care to our patients. I hew to an ethical standard of care, and so does my HMO. I am first and foremost the advocate of my patients, but always within the constraints of appropriate care and limited resources. More care is not always better care, and wishing that medicine could be exempt from the laws of economics does not make it so.

While there are various arrangements by which physicians are compensated under managed care, the incentives are to provide neither too little care nor too much care but *optimal* care. Under managed care, the worst course I could follow is to provide less than optimal care. Delay in diagnosis or treatment would only invite more expensive diagnosis and treatment down the line (and probably a lawsuit as well). Denying needed care is not only bad ethics; it is bad business.

As for the highly publicized "gag clauses," which have been outlawed in Massachusetts and a number of other states, my HMO does not have one. HMOs are entitled to insist on the confidentiality of proprietary information, but my HMO and most others encourage physicians to discuss financial incentives, covered benefits, and care options with patients. Many physicians are understandably dispirited by what they view as the demise of traditional health care and by projections of a 150,000-physician glut by the year 2000. But grievances and frustrations should be discussed with management and peers. Discussing them with patients can only erode an already embattled doctor–patient relationship.

⋯◈⋯

Despite the charges of conflict and carnage, the evidence suggests that most physicians and patients are adjusting remarkably well to the managed care revolution and that the quality of care remains high. Studies have consistently shown that HMO patients are at least as satisfied with their care as patients receiving traditional fee-for-service care. A recent survey by CareData Reports, a New York health care information firm, revealed that, among members of 33 HMOs nationwide, nearly 80 percent were satisfied with their care. (The lowest ratings were not for quality of care but for administration and communication.) A 1994 study of 25,000 employees conducted by Xerox showed that HMO patients were significantly more satisfied with their overall care than were fee-for-service patients. In a 1994 Federal Employee Health Benefits Program survey of 90,000 federal employees, 86 percent of HMO members said they were satisfied with their plans, compared with 82 percent in fee-for-service plans. Interestingly, a 1994 survey by Towers Perrin revealed that patient satisfaction with HMO care rose with years of membership.

The results of research using objective measures have been similar. A 1996 study by KPMG Peat Marwick found that, in cities where most health care was provided by HMOs, costs were 11 percent lower, hospital stays 6 percent shorter, and death rates 5 percent lower than in cities where most care was provided under fee-for-service arrangements. A study recently published in the *Journal of the American Medical Association* looked at costs and outcomes of treatment for several chronic illnesses. Compared with fee-for-service specialists, HMO primary care physicians used 40 percent fewer hospital days and 12 percent less drugs. At four- and seven-year follow-ups, patient outcomes were the same.

A 1995 North Carolina study looked at the cost and outcome of treatment for lower-back pain. Costs for a single episode ranged from $169 in an HMO to $545 at a fee-for-service chiropractor, while outcomes were identical. As David Nash, an HMO expert at Jefferson Medical College in Philadelphia, told the *Chicago Sun-Times* last year [1995], "Overwhelmingly, the published evidence supports the notion that quality of care in the managed care arena equals, if not surpasses, the care in the private, fee-for-service sector."

The shift to managed care unquestionably imposes greater responsibility on patients. More information is becoming available to enable them to compare costs and benefits and make intelligent choices. We ought to disabuse ourselves of the notion that we can have a perfect health care system in which no one is ever misdiagnosed, mismanaged, or missed altogether. But high-quality medical care at an affordable price is not only possible under managed care; it is a reality.

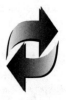

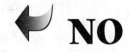

The Doctor Is Not In

We are born, we live, and then we die, but these days we do so with less and less help from a medical profession paid to discount our suffering and ignore our pain. Proofs of the bitter joke implicit in the phrase "managed care" show up in every morning's newspaper, in casual conversations with relatives or friends recently returned from a hospital or from what was once thought of as a doctor's office instead of an insurance company's waiting room, and in a country generously supplied with competent and compassionate doctors, 160.3 million of us now find ourselves held captive to corporate health-care systems that earn $952 billion a year but can't afford the luxury of a conscience or a heart.

Childless women in every city in America dread the simplest fertility workups because they know that the evaluation probably will serve as evidence denying them future payments for diseases of the vagina, uterus, or ovaries; the rest of us have had our co-payments increased, our use of prescription drugs curtailed or replaced by corporate-sanctioned medications, stays in the hospital reduced or eliminated, "pre-authorizations" required for necessary and routine tests. The broad removal of health-care benefits takes place at all points of the country's medical-industrial complex, and in line with the tone and temper of the times more than 2,300 Massachusetts physicians in December of last year signed a despairing manifesto in the *Journal of the American Medical Association:*

> The time we are allowed to spend with the sick shrinks under the pressure to increase throughput, as though we were dealing with industrial commodities rather than afflicted human beings. . . . Physicians and nurses are being prodded by threats and bribes to abdicate allegiance to patients, and to shun the sickest, who may be unprofitable. Some of us risk being fired or "delisted" for giving, or even discussing, expensive services, and many are offered bonuses for minimizing care.

Such forced denial of care occurs at a time when new medical and surgical technologies allow physicians to treat and often cure any number of conditions that only a few years ago barely could be diagnosed; organs now can be digitally reconstructed in three dimensions to locate previously inoperable tumors; heart attacks can be stopped with injections of a compound known as tPA; blind people may wake up and see with implanted plastic lenses; one-and-a-half-pound premature babies, once given up for lost, routinely are nursed to health; a new generation of medical research brings us genetically engineered tests and one nearly miraculous drug after the next. At the same moment, presumably well-insured women diagnosed with disseminated breast cancer must hire lawyers to have their health plans pay for life-saving bone-marrow transplants and managed-care companies can deny powered wheelchairs to handicapped children who pass a "utilization review" showing them able to stagger twenty-five feet with the help of a walker.

But although a good many of us suspect that somehow we are being swindled, and those of us who have fallen seriously ill know for a fact that the purveyors of managed care often wish we would go away or die—as quietly and quickly as possible—we're reluctant to draw the commercial moral of the tale. The system wasn't meant to care for sick people; it was meant to make and manage money.

≈◆≈

The theory of "managed care" first attracted attention in the 1940s in the coal regions of Kentucky and West Virginia. Labor unions hired doctors, constructed clinics and hospitals, and supplied prepaid medical services at a fixed monthly rate to their members and their families. The fixed rate per patient was unrelated to the patient's use of the service. By the 1950s, a few large companies had taken a similarly paternalistic stance and were offering contract health care to their own employees. The arrangement was not designed to profit anyone other than those who received care, which was why it worked.

But in the 1970s, the government and large corporate employers began to seek ways to reduce health-care costs, and the concept of contract medicine was injected with the virus of the profit motive. Cadres of systems managers, some of whom had planned the failed technowar in Vietnam, brought forth new corporate structures meant to introduce market forces into the industry and named by the several acronyms (HMO, PPO, POS, etc.) for preferred or managed medicine.[1] Not only were a lot of people going to get well, but some of them were going to get rich. First promoted by what is known as InterStudy (a health-policy think tank organized in 1972), the proposition relied on the idea that an HMO could make money if it provided medical care only to people who enjoyed the prior benefits of perfect health and a full-time job. Thus the practice known as "cherry picking," which virtually removed the burden of insuring people who were seriously ill. You simply cannot be employed full time if you suffer from the effects of a crippling disability or disease.

The full story of how and why, over the short span of twenty years, the concept of the HMO came to dominate nearly every phase of American medicine (directing the distribution of every operation, wheelchair, test, and pill) would embrace all the arts of financial chicanery made popular in the 1980s with appropriate reference to junk-bond financing, the prosperity of the drug companies, the general acceptance of the 401-K plan, the demographics of the baby boom, and probably a list of every fund-raiser attended by Presidents Ronald Reagan and George Bush. Here was but one scheme in an era of schemes, the HMO as a brilliant means of redistributing income from individual physicians to corporate executives and shareholders. The short-term profits were extraordinary: PacifiCare, for example, swelled from a $168,911 enterprise in 1986 to a $10 billion behemoth by 1997.

For corporations and small businesses burdened with rising medical costs, the HMO appeared as a gift from heaven. As recently as 1980 company health plans enrolled only a small percentage of the eligible employees; last year the plans enrolled 85 percent, up from 48 percent in 1993. The percentage of doctors practicing outside the HMOs meanwhile has dwindled to the present 19.9 percent.[2]

But the spectacular success of managed care proved to be the cause of its equally spectacular failures. Cherry picking is another name for a Ponzi scheme, and sooner or later it falls apart. Even a company blessed with tens of thousands of healthy subscribers eventually finds itself obliged to pay for the occasional premature birth at $1,500 a day, or the occasional employee who develops a brain tumor or whose wife is diagnosed with ovarian cancer. There are car accidents and near drownings. There are the late complications of diabetes, the forty-year-old struck down with a heart attack, the previously undiagnosed melanoma, the complications of hypertension. The odd executive may need a hip replacement because of an old football injury, or a chief financial officer a heart transplant after what should have been a routine viral illness. If the HMO acquires 400,000 or half a million new members (as it must if its stock price is to keep rising), the costs mount at an exponential rate. Now there may be as many as 20,000 claims a month—a metastasis of paperwork, a hemorrhage of cash. The co-payments coming in from new enrollees can no longer keep up with the money going out. New restrictions must be implemented, new administrators hired to guarantee compliance, more controls, more advertisements to attract new members. The whole operation begins to unravel.[3]

When a company finds itself hard-pressed for profit, then behind the closed doors of the executive suite what has been left unsaid becomes the loud and forthright voice of reason: *Yes, we are a company that cares about the well-being of the American people, but the free market is the free market, and so . . .* And so, among the middle managers and accountants of the nation's health plans the talk these days turns to ways of lowering what Wall Street calls an HMO's "medical-loss ratio"—i.e., that percentage of yearly revenues allotted to patient care. The term, in and of itself, repudiates every principle that undergirds the profession of medicine and flatly contradicts the Hippocratic oath, which pledges a physician's first responsibility to the care of his or her patient. But banks don't accept payment in oaths, as was made plain by an analyst from Nutmeg Securities, Ira Zuckerman, who reminded his prospective investors last November that the attractiveness of managed-care companies as investments changes when health plans sign up members who will actually have to see a doctor. The rule of thumb holds that a managed-care business is in trouble if more than 65 percent of its enrollees submit a significant claim in any one-year period. Little wonder then that rehabilitation for stroke victims or occupational therapy for spinal-cord injuries no longer make the list of benefits. Managed-care companies actually seek to *hide* their competencies; no HMO wishes to advertise its successes with cystic fibrosis or multiple sclerosis, or, say, the skill of its subspecialists who treat AIDS. Were a company to become known for treating complicated or expensive diseases, it would run the real risk of attracting the attention of the very sick. The blurring of priorities becomes embarrassingly obvious in the newspaper ads that promote the virtues of the country's prepaid health plans. As, for instance, last December in the Minneapolis *Star Tribune:*

> We offer an extensive and unique program of reporting quality, accessibility and satisfaction data to consumers at the clinic and physician level—through the internet and other mechanisms.
> We developed a doctor-led organization, called the Institute for Clinical Systems Integration, that develops nationally recognized medical best practices using the best medical minds in our community.
> We have received numerous national awards for our community health improvement initiatives.
> We created the nation's first comprehensive program to encourage reading and brain stimulation for infants and young children.

In less than five years, managed care has managed to eliminate from the public-policy debate any and all words that describe suffering and disease, and together with the good news about "reporting quality," and "satisfaction data," the industry defends itself against past, present, and future criticism by explaining the symptoms that afflict the country's health-care system with at least five warm and welcome fairy tales that the public apparently still chooses to believe:

All doctors are rich and omnipotent   The stereotyped image of the aloof and wealthy physician driving a Mercedes or wandering over a golf course allows the proponents of managed care to imply, usually with a good deal of success, that any doctor who speaks ill of corporatized medicine is, by definition, a greedy and callous fellow who thinks only about his fees.

As a percentage of all medical costs, the money allotted to physicians' services has remained constant over the last thirty years. Between 1993 and 1995, what the American Medical Association calls "median physician net income (after expenses, before taxes)" declined, in real terms, by 1.4 percent. Surgeons and radiologists, among them the most highly paid practitioners in any of the medical professions, earned, on average in 1995, roughly $250,000. The sums dwindle into pittances when compared with the earnings of the executives of publicly traded managed-care companies, which, on average in 1996, approached the handsome sum of $10 million. What inflates the price of medicine in the United States is the cost of corporate vice presidents, not the cost of doctors.

Which possibly explains why the number of practicing physicians in the United States has increased by no more than 20 percent in the last six years, while since 1983 the number of health-care managers has increased by 683 percent. The comparative percentages speak to the loss of authority on the part of doctors who no longer have much to say about the schedules they keep, the fees they charge, the treatments and protocols they prescribe. As often as not, they possess as little power of decision as the custodians of a hospital's linen supply.

The operation is unnecessary The rich doctor requires the unnecessary operation (as well as the superfluous test, the costly prescription, the frivolous C-section or coronary bypass) not for any sound medical reason but in order to become even more rich. Thus the nation's hospitals and operating rooms supposedly overflow with patients who have no cause for serious complaint, healthy, happy people, who, were it not for the avarice of their physicians, would be baking pies or running relay races.

Once again, actual practice contradicts the heartwarming cant. The numbers of C-sections performed in the country have more to do with the availability of fetal-monitoring equipment and the fear of malpractice suits than with the will to profit on the part of the attending obstetrician. Recent reviews of coronary-bypass operations have shown that the number of inappropriate procedures varies from 0 percent to 2.4 percent, while the number deemed "equivocal" never has exceeded 7 percent. The number of inappropriate coronary angiographies in a 1994 study conducted in New York State was 5 percent. In 1992, a Medicare pre-authorization program was discontinued when, following a review of Medicare requests for coronary-bypass procedures in the state of Texas, a negligible number were found to be inappropriate.

Health-care executives like to say that doctors get away with performing needless operations because their monopoly of the standard surgical repertoire excuses them from having to explain or justify their actions. The canard ignores the fierce but societally beneficial struggle between different medical specialties, a struggle that constantly forces the argument about what is necessary and what is not. Internists develop drugs to reduce the need for the cardiovascular surgeons' bypass procedure; neonatalists use chemicals to get premature infants off respirators quicker and keep them out of the hands of pulmonologists; infectious-disease specialists develop oral regimens and home antibiotic therapies as alternatives to orthopedic surgery or in-hospital IV medications.

The doctor is a mechanical device The systems planners at the Pentagon construed the Vietnam War as a manufacturing problem—victory a product, death a means of production, soldiers listed in the inventories like truck tires or boxes of ammunition. A similar habit of mind inclines our health-care managers to classify doctors as interchangeable pieces of hospital equipment. As with light bulbs and bottles of saline solution, so also with heart specialists and neurosurgeons. Every doctor serves as well as every other doctor. The proposition is patently false, but it allows the HMOs to limit their patients' choice of physician. Like nineteenth-century coal miners obliged to buy their necessities from a company store, subscribers to late-twentieth-century health plans must go to the doctors named on a company list. A number of HMOs improve the policy with a further refinement of cost-saving simplification. Not content with the assignment of absolute equality to doctors in all degrees of specialty, they suggest that the only physician whom any patient ever needs to see is the primary-care physician—i.e., the doctor who knows a little of this and a little of that, who is so well rounded that he points in no direction at all, a compliant soul content to follow a memo or a guideline because he isn't sure when an MRI is really appropriate or whether, in the attempt to rule out Lyme disease, it is best to do the expensive Western Blot test or the cheaper ELISA essay.

The patient loves going to the hospital   As corollary to the story of the rich doctor, the health-care companies tell the story of the patient as spendthrift fool, who, if left to his or her own devices, will bankrupt the country with an "infinite demand" for heart transplants, kidney dialysis, and liposuction. But as with the health-care industry's other probings of imaginary symptoms, the diagnosis has been proven false. Most people check into hospitals only when they have no choice in the matter, and the nonexistent phenomenon of infinite demand doesn't lead to the unproven result of infinite cost. New medical treatments and surgical procedures, no matter how expensive when first introduced, retain their original costly forms for astonishingly short periods. Less expensive and less complicated therapies invariably replace the early experiments.

The evolving art of kidney dialysis offers the textbook case in point. Long before the advent of managed care, kidney specialists looking for an alternative to hemodialysis—with its inconvenience, risks of infection, clotting, and blood loss, as well as its complicated machinery—pursued the development of the less demanding peritoneal dialysis. So also with balloon angioplasty, which today has become the preferred alternative to the expensive coronary bypass. So also with every other specialty that anybody but an insurance agent cares to name.

An axiom of economics holds that nothing can be rationed that is itself not scarce, and, absent evidence of infinite demand and infinite cost, you can't ration health care when there are more than enough doctors, hospitals, and high-tech equipment distributed through the country to do everything and anything that needs to be done. American health care is an unsaturated demand market, and in such markets "rationing" is simply a code word for not spending the money to take care of the poor, the uninsured, the underinsured, and the high-risk patient.

Sickness is the patient's fault, and death is a preventable disease   Because we live in a society that equates youth and wellness with intelligence and superior moral character, the health-care industry can pretend that it really isn't supposed to do anything at all. If the patient hadn't been so careless—if he or she had given up smoking and drinking, read the complete works of Andrew Weil, cut down on the day's fat intake, checked the blood pressure, ridden the stationary bicycle, ingested the correct amounts of garlic and zinc, gotten in touch with the inner child—then the patient wouldn't be making so many awful noises, wouldn't be conspiring to harm the "medical-loss ratio," wouldn't be bothering doctors (busy and important people, albeit overpaid) with the miserable proofs of their weakness and stupidity.

No health plan advertises the fact that a good many patients admitted to the hospital with a diagnosis of a myocardial infarct have few or none of the so-called risk factors for a heart attack: they are not smokers; they are not overweight; they are not hypertensive; they exercised; they have normal cholesterol. No plan sends out notices or memos that one in twenty-five births will have a congenital defect, or that a third of patients with diabetes run the risk of going blind.

In truth, it is a dangerous world out there. Slip through the ice, get hit on the freeway, wake up with blood in your urine, have trouble breathing, stumble about after a splitting headache, lose the ability to feel, have trouble remembering things, experience ringing in your ears, find mucus in your stools, start gasping at night, and garlic pills will be of little help. But wellness is the panacea of the 1990s, and the health plans promote the wonders of aerobic exercise and fat-free diets in order to obscure the real purpose of medicine, which is the treatment of illness and the relief of suffering. To the extent that the plans can shift the burden of health care to the private sectors of personal hygiene and morality, they excuse themselves from the tedious and increasingly expensive chores of providing a public service or addressing the common good.

⋖◉⋗

For the last twenty years the theory and practice of managed care has enjoyed the protection of the political and financial interests—insurance companies, the pharmaceutical industry, large business corporations, suppliers of hospital equipment, members of Congress—eager to keep the Ponzi scheme profitably in place. Assured of the approval of the best people that money can buy, the HMOs have gone calmly about the business of eliminating one treatment after another and adding one doctor after the next to their rosters. For the time being they probably can count on their formularies of false diagnosis to preserve the illusions of compassion and competence. But every month another 315,000 Americans reach the age of fifty, a figure that will rise over the next fifteen years. Of the money spent on medical care during the course of an average American's lifetime, the bulk of it is spent during the last two or three years of that life, and by the year 2010, people over the age of sixty-five will constitute the most rapidly multiplying sector of the population. They will want, expect, and need medical care, but who will pay the bill? The government has been steadily depleting the funds intended to meet the future costs of Social Security and Medicare, and the working children of what promises to be the most long-lived generation in the country's history can't be counted on to come up with either the money or the will to support a pyramid scheme.

Because Americans as they grow older tend to become more political, the demographics also imply the likelihood of active protests on the part of large numbers of people (surprisingly vigorous, remarkably well informed) bent on redressing what they will come to perceive, not without reason, as a balance of wrongs. The reaction already has begun. A few months ago the Massachusetts physicians published their manifesto, and the American College of Rheumatology recently recommended that chronic arthritis patients should be seen at least once by a rheumatologist both for confirmation of the diagnosis and the development of an adequate treatment plan. The American College of Cardiology has compiled its own guidelines for heart disease and posted them on the Internet in the hope that Americans might learn from a computer what they never will learn from a doctor sworn to silence by an HMO.

All the symptoms of protest confirm the same diagnosis—a health-care industry sickened with the virus of "medical-loss ratio" and unlikely to recover until cured of its addiction to the profit motive. A physician is not by nature a commodities broker, a clinic is not a meat-packing plant, and unless the health-care industry quits caring for money instead of people, its chronic pathology almost certainly will be referred to the consulting rooms of government. Not that the politicians will want to take the case, but let enough people make strong enough complaint, and the therapeutics committees in the country's legislatures might be forced to write a new and not so mean-spirited set of guidelines.

Notes

1. Alan Enthoven, who served as a systems analyst under Defense Secretary Robert McNamara during the Vietnam War, devised the theory of managed competition and still serves as its principal apologist, both in his capacity as chairman of California's Managed Health Care Improvement Task Force and as a professor of health-care economics at Stanford University.

2. The wealthier American zip codes continue to support a troupe of expensive physicians whose skills (at unclogging beefeater hearts or smoothing the wrinkles in a woman's neck) are so renowned, or whose clients are so prosperous, that they do not accept any form of insurance. Such practices are, in effect, boutiques, and the practitioner is able to lavish time and attention on his patients, who may in turn congratulate themselves on the quality of the care they have received.

3. Last fall, Oxford Health Plans, Inc., a "model" HMO that aggressively marketed its friendliness toward consumers, reported losses of $125 million, citing higher medical costs than expected. Not surprisingly, the stock price of Oxford lost 80 percent of its value over the span of four months. Shortly thereafter, investors accused Oxford executives of withholding information about the company's balance sheet while they sold large blocks of shares. The Securities and Exchange Commission and the New York Attorney General's Office are investigating the complaint.

POSTSCRIPT

Will Managed Care Improve Health Care in the United States?

Should managed care scare the typical health care consumer? Will our access to necessary care be denied in favor of the bottom line? Many experts think that is the case since managed care plans reward physicians for providing less care. In some plans, gag orders have been imposed on member doctors. The doctors are forbidden, or "gagged," from disclosing expensive treatment options not covered by the plan. As more and more workers are enrolled in managed care programs by their employers, can we assume that companies can make better health care choices than their employees would individually? On the other hand, can we as a nation cope with rising health costs, especially as our population ages?

An overview of managed care is provided in "The Rise and Fall of Managed Care: History of the Mass Medical Movement," *Choice* (February 2003); "Managed Care or Managed Inequality? A Call for Critiques of Market-Based Medicine," *Medical Anthropology Quarterly* (December 2002); "Managed-Care Plan Performance Since 1980: A Literature Analysis," *Journal of the American Medical Association* (May 18, 1994); and "Managed Care: Do Health-Care Firms Sacrifice Quality to Cut Costs?" *CQ Researcher* (April 12, 1996).

Although there are dissatisfied consumers, several articles assert that the quality of care through managed care is comparable with fee-for-service care. These include "The Fortune 500 Model for Health Care: Is Now the Time to Change?" *Journal of Health Politics, Policy and Law* (February 2002); "Controlling Health Care Expenditures," *The New England Journal of Medicine* (February 15, 2002); "Managed Care Means Shared Responsibilities," *St. Louis Post-Dispatch* (January 29, 1996); and "Learning to Accentuate the Positive in Managed Care," *The New England Journal of Medicine* (February 13, 1997).

Many articles, books, and reports, however, counter that patients suffer under managed care. These include "Unhealthy Partnership: How Managed Care Wrecks Mental Health for Kids," *The American Prospect* (January 1, 2001); "Bedside Mania: Medicine Turned Upside Down," *The American Prospect* (March/April 1997); "The Sick Business: Why For-Profit Medicine Couldn't Care Less," *The New Republic* (December 29, 1997); "Why HMOs Are the Opposite of Free Markets," *Human Events* (January 30, 1998); "Should We Accept Mediocrity?" *The New England Journal of Medicine* (April 9, 1998); and "Health Care Update," *American Enterprise* (March/April 1998).

If managed care is not the solution for reforming medical services in the United States, are there alternatives? The Canadian system has often been considered the solution to rising health care costs in the United States. The Canadian medicare program, however, has been under attack for not providing necessary services for its patients, especially in regard to making referrals to specialists. For information on the Canadian system, read "Bitter Medicine: Canada Is Taking an Ax to Its Popular Health Care System," *In These Times* (January 20, 1997).

ISSUE 2

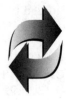

Should Health Care for the Elderly Be Rationed?

YES: Alan Williams, from "The Rationing Debate: Rationing Health Care by Age: The Case For," *British Medical Journal* (March 15, 1997)

NO: Patricia Lanoie Blanchette, from "Age-Based Rationing of Healthcare," *Generations* (Winter 1996–1997)

ISSUE SUMMARY

YES: Professor Alan Williams contends that rationing health care in old age has some merit. He asserts that the treatment of young people should be a priority.

NO: Patricia Lanoie Blanchette, a physician and a professor of medicine and public health, argues that health care should not be rationed by age and that age bias should be recognized and confronted.

In 1980, 11 percent of the U.S. population was over age 65, but they utilized about 29 percent ($219 billion) of the total American health care expenditures. By the beginning of the new millennium, the percentage of the population over 65 had risen to 12 percent, which consumed 31 percent of total health care expenditures, or $450 billion. It has been projected that by the year 2040, people over 65 will represent 21 percent of the population and consume 45 percent of all health care expenditures.

Medical expenses at the end of life appear to be extremely high in relation to other health care costs. Studies have shown that nearly one-third of annual Medicare costs are for the 5–6 percent of beneficiaries who die that year. Expenses for dying patients increase significantly as death nears, and payments for health care during the last weeks of life make up 40 percent of the medical costs for the entire last year of life. Some studies have shown that up to 50 percent of the medical costs incurred during a person's entire life are spent during their last year!

Many surveys have indicated that most Americans do not want to be kept alive if their illness is incurable and irreversible, for both economic and humanitarian reasons. Many experts believe that if physicians stopped using high technology at the end of life to prevent death, then we would save billions of dollars, which could be used to insure the uninsured and provide basic health care to millions.

In England the emphasis of health care is on improving the quality of life through primary care medicine, well-subsidized home care, and institutional programs for the elderly and those with incurable illnesses, rather than through life-extending acute care medicine. The British seem to value basic medical care for all rather than expensive technology for the few who might benefit from it. As a result, the British spend a much smaller proportion of their gross national product (6.2 percent) on health services than do Americans (10.8 percent) for a nearly identical health status and life expectancy.

In the following selection, Alan Williams argues that prioritizing health care in favor of the young will disadvantage the elderly, but depriving the young seems far worse.

In the second selection, Patricia Lanoie Blanchette maintains that health care must be appropriate, not rationed. She stresses that covert rationing of medical care based on age is a serious concern and must be addressed.

Alan Williams 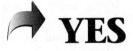 **YES**

The Rationing Debate:
Rationing Health Care by Age:
The Case For

$\mathbf{A}$s we grow older our recuperative powers diminish. Thus we accumulate a distressing collection of chronic incurable conditions. Some of these are no more than a minor nuisance, and we adapt as best we can; and when adaptation is not possible we learn to tolerate them. Some are more serious, involving severe disability and persistent pain, and may eventually become life threatening.

We are also at risk of various acute conditions (like influenza or pneumonia) which are more serious threats to the health of elderly people than to younger people. We also have more difficulty recovering from what younger people would regard as minor injuries (such as falls). When you add to all this the increased likelihood that illness (and other disruptions of our normal lifestyle) will leave us rather confused and in need of more rehabilitative and social support than a young person it is hardly surprising that NHS [National Health Service] expenditure per person rises sharply after about age 65.

The Vain Pursuit of Immortality

People are also living longer, and people aged over 65 now form a much bigger proportion of the population than they used to. From the viewpoint of NHS expenditure this would not matter if the extra years of life were predominantly healthy years but it would if the extra years were ones of disability, pain, and increasing dependence on others.

The evidence on this is ambiguous. Many people remain fit and independent well into their 80s. Others enter their 60s already afflicted with the aftermath of stroke, heart disease, arthritis, or bronchitis. It is not clear whether things are getting worse at each year of age, or whether expectations are rising and people are now more likely to report disabilities once shrugged off as the inevitable consequence of getting old. That many of these conditions are incurable does not mean they are untreatable. Much can be done to reduce their adverse consequences, including many remedial activities which lie outside the NHS (such as home adaptations, domestic support, and special accommodation).

It is important to get away from the notion of "cure" as the criterion of benefit and adopt instead measures of effectiveness that turn on the impact of treatments on people's health related quality of life. Such an approach concentrates on the features that people themselves value, such as mobility, self care, being able to pursue usual activities (whatever they are), and being free of pain and discomfort and anxiety and depression.

Improving the quality of life of elderly people in these ways may not be very costly, but these unglamorous down to earth activities tend to lose out to high tech interventions which gain their emotional hold by claiming that life threatening conditions should always take priority. This vain pursuit of immortality is dangerous for elderly people: taken to its logical conclusion it implies that no one should be allowed to die until everything possible has been done. That means not simply that we shall all die in hospital but that we shall die in intensive care.

Reasonable Limits

This attempt to wring the last drop of medical benefit out of the system, no matter what the human and material costs, is not the hallmark of a humane society. In each of our lives there has to come a time when we accept the inevitability of death, and when we also accept that a reasonable limit has to be set on the demands we can properly make on our fellow citizens in order to keep us going a bit longer.

It would be better for that limit to be set, with fairly general consent, before we as individuals get into that potentially harrowing situation. When the time comes we shall probably each want an exception made in our case, because few of us are strong willed enough to act cheerfully in the general public interest when our own welfare is at stake. But if a limit is to be set, on what principles should it be determined? And what is their justification? And what role does age have?

In arguing for this article's proposition I have sought to make two contextual points clear: firstly, that ability to benefit should be measured in rather broader terms than cure or survival, and, secondly, that although chronological age is the best single predictor of increasing health problems, it is only a predictor, not a mechanistic determinant.

But age as an indicator of declining recuperative powers, of future health problems, of increasing need for health care, and of declining capacity to benefit from health care (because of shorter life expectancy) is only half the story. It addresses the issue of whether age is a good indicator of the extent to which people could benefit from health care but not in itself of whether they should be offered it. This more crucial step depends on what the objectives of the NHS are to be.

The NHS's Objectives

If we start with the proposition that the objective should be to improve as much as possible the health of the nation as a whole then the people who should get priority are those who will benefit most from the resources available. In some cases the old will benefit most, in others the young. But for treatments which yield benefits that last for the rest of a person's life (or for a long time) the young will generally benefit more, because the rest of a young person's life is usually longer than the rest of an old person's life. And even among old people themselves the life expectancy of a 70 year old is usually greater than that of an 80 year old. Where a treatment offers only modest benefits a person may have to live a long time to make treatment worth while—that is, to make the benefit to that person larger than the sacrifices of rival candidates who failed to get treated. So improving the health of the nation as a whole is likely, in some circumstances, to discriminate indirectly against older people.

Is this morally defensible? Well, if we behaved otherwise we would by implication be asserting that in order to provide small benefits for the elderly, young people should sacrifice large benefits. What makes old people more deserving of health benefits than young people? One argument might be that all their lives they have been paying their taxes to finance the health care system (among other things), and just when they need health care most the government lets them down. But the government—that is, their fellow citizens—did not promise to do everything possible no matter what the costs.

The NHS is part of a social insurance system, not a savings club for each individual's health care expenditures. It is the lucky ones who do not get their money's worth out of the system, and the unlucky ones who need heavy NHS expenditures all their lives. The NHS is there to meet certain contingencies but not others. And many of the treatments which the NHS now offers to old people in certain contingencies were not even invented when they started contributing 40 or 50 years ago. So to argue, from a historical viewpoint, about an entitlement to get your money's worth seems inappropriate to any insurance scheme, and in particular to a social insurance scheme such as the NHS.

A different line of argument might be that as the number of years left becomes smaller and smaller, each is more precious. The implication of this argument is that elderly people value their small improvements more highly than young people do their much larger improvements. This raises a fundamental problem about whose values should count in a social insurance setting. Suppose that it were true that older people would spend relatively more on health care to get health improvements rather than other things, whereas younger people would spend relatively more on (say) education for their children and rather less on health benefits for themselves. Rational self interest drives individual citizens operating in private markets precisely in that direction.

But did we not take the NHS out of that context precisely because as citizens (rather than as consumers of health care) we were pursuing a rather different ideal—namely, that health care should be provided according to people's needs, not according to what they were each willing and able to pay. A person's needs (constituting claims on social resources) have to be arbitrated by a third party, whose unenviable task it is to weigh different needs (and different people's needs) one against another. This is precisely what priority setting in health care is all about. So the values of the citizenry as a whole must override the values of a particular interest group within it.

A Fair Innings

So I can find no compelling argument to justify the view that the young should sacrifice large benefits so that the old can enjoy small ones. But I can find an argument which goes in the opposite direction. It is that one of the objectives of the health care system should be to reduce inequalities in people's lifetime experience of health. The popular folklore is rich in phrases indicating that we all have some vague notion of a "fair innings" in health terms. Put at its crudest, it reflects the biblical idea that the years of our life are three score and ten. Anyone who achieves or exceeds this is reckoned to have had a fair innings, whereas anyone who dies at an earlier age "was cut off in their prime" or "died tragically young." As has been observed, while it is always a misfortune to die if you wish to go on living, it is both a misfortune and a tragedy to die young. Why?

From my perspective (approaching the age of 70) I see clearly why it is a tragedy, because someone who dies young has been denied the opportunities that we older people have already had. If reducing inequalities in lifetime health is a worthy social objective, it will lead us to be willing to do more to enable young people to survive than we are willing to do to enable old people to survive.

But I do not think that the notion of a "fair innings" should be restricted to matters of survival and life expectancy. Quality of life considerations concerning health may be just as important. Someone who has suffered a lifetime of pain and disability cannot be said to have had a fair innings even if she did live to be 80, and I would therefore extend the concept to embrace something more than just years of life. My preferred concept would be the number of quality adjusted life years a person had enjoyed. On the whole people's earlier years are healthy years, and their later years less healthy years, so this does not affect the general tenor of my argument. What it implies is that we need to consider, alongside age itself, the quality of a person's lifetime experience of health. The worse it has been, the more consideration they deserve, age for age.

Age Matters

So my overall conclusion is that age matters in two respects. Firstly, it affects people's capacity to benefit, and therefore places them at a general disadvantage if the objective is to maximise the benefits of health care. Secondly, the older you are the more likely you will have achieved what your fellow citizens would judge to have been a fair innings, and this will place old people at a disadvantage if the objective is to minimise the differences in lifetime experience of health. I would be the first to admit that I personally have had a fair innings and that it would not be equitable to deny a younger person large benefits in order to provide small ones for me. Indeed, I would go further: it would be equitable to provide small benefits for a young person even if by so doing I were denied large benefits, provided that the young person in question had a low probability of ever achieving a fair innings. Note that this argument does not mean that benefits to young people take absolute priority over benefits to old people. It simply means that we give rather more weight to them than to us.

Surveys of public opinion commonly find that most people, if pushed into a tight situation, would give priority to the young over the old when distributing a given amount of health care benefit. There is also little doubt that health care professionals share this general attitude. It does not, of course, stop them from being kind, considerate, and caring when old people need health care, but it manifests itself at the level of clinical policymaking, when different needs have to be prioritised. For the professionals what may be in their minds may be mostly old people's impaired capacity to benefit from health care. But I strongly suspect that some variant of the fair innings argument also underlies such views, and this is especially likely to be the case among the general public. When the views of older respondents in such surveys have been reported separately, they too give priority to the young over themselves.

So I am encouraged to hope that, in the interests of fairness between the generations, the members of my generation will exercise restraint in the demands we make on the health care system. We should not object to age being one of the criteria (though not the sole criterion) used in the prioritisation of health care, even though it will disadvantage us. The alternative is too outrageous to contemplate—namely, that we expect the young to make large sacrifices so that we can enjoy small benefits. That would not be fair.

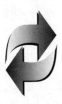

NO ⤶

Patricia Lanoie Blanchette

Age-Based Rationing of Healthcare

Given the temporal relationship between the increasing numbers of older people and the nation's focus on the costs of healthcare, it might seem evident that aging is the major determinant of increasing costs. The image of demented oldsters avariciously consuming the legacy of our children springs to mind, and indeed, an incomplete and biased recitation of healthcare statistics would appear to support this conclusion, leading to serious proposals to ration healthcare for older people (Callahan, 1987). A careful examination of the facts begins with an acknowledgement of the potential for bias, the willingness to question what appears obvious, and a search beyond those data that are assembled to support a predetermined conclusion. Decisions about healthcare must be guided by objective information and by the ethical and moral principles that can enlighten decisions about limits on the public money allocated for people of all ages.

In considering the costs of healthcare, it is easy to be drawn into a debate that labels this an intergenerational contest, pitting the costs of providing increasingly sophisticated care to increasingly younger, potentially chronically impaired neonates, for example, against the costs of caring for the nation's elders. In such a debate, it might be argued that although the potential life expectancy of babies in general is much longer than that of elders, this is often not true when individual lives are compared. It is also possible to make the argument that elders may have contributed to the public good for many years and are now more deserving of care. However, basing decisions on whether an individual is deserving of care presupposes a wisdom that we have not yet attained and is to be strenuously avoided.

Another issue that might be raised in such a debate is that in a country concerned with overpopulation, we may question the use of public monies or health insurance for infertility treatment. However, our culture is one that cherishes children and families, and the social benefits of establishing families with children may return the output in full measure. We are most likely to accept the costs of raising a child and seldom stop to total up the costs of the years of dependency. We are less likely to appreciate the personal fulfillment, redefinition of productivity, and intergenerational significance in old age. The importance of completing psychological development and establishing roots for successive generations by the presence of elders as well as children is undervalued.

However, in considering the allocation of resources it is futile and intellectually inadequate to pursue the avenues of intergenerational conflict. People's lives are priceless at any age. A fully developed society must be guided by principles equally valid across an age spectrum. A consideration of the allocation of resources requires that we examine the quality of the data, guard against the old-age prejudice that exists in our culture, and be primarily guided by the ethical bases for limiting care at any age.

Population Aging and Costs

Is there a primary cause-and-effect relationship between the rapid aging of the population and healthcare costs? People over age 65 today constitute something over 12 percent of the U.S. population and account for one-third of the nation's annual federal healthcare expenditures, or $300 billion of an estimated $900 billion in 1993 (National Academy on Aging, 1994). By 2020, when baby boomers will be in their mid to late 70s, the population over 65 is estimated to be 20 percent of the total population, with the actual number of people over 65 doubling from today.

However, when examined closely, less than 10 percent of the increased costs of healthcare can be accounted for by population aging (National Academy on Aging, 1994; Newhouse, 1996). Further, while it would appear that 12 percent of the population is using one-third of all public resources, state and local governments spend ten times the amount on education and children's programs than is spent on programs benefitting elders, including Medicaid (Gist, 1992).

Futility and the Costs of Caring for the Dying

It has become a widespread belief that a majority of healthcare resources are spent on high-technology care for elderly people in their last year of life. However, the facts show that medical costs in the last year of life for people aged 80 and older are less than for younger people. In 1989, 2,150,466 persons died in the United States. Of these, 29 percent were younger than 65, 22 percent were aged 65–74, 28 percent were aged 75–84, and 21 percent were aged 85 and older. In one study of 500 persons who died, people over 80 had only half the hospital costs of those at younger ages, and costs for those age 65 to 79 were only slightly higher than for those under age 65 (Scitovsky, 1988). The beliefs about the costs of caring for the dying come from a series of papers showing that about 30 percent of Medicare costs are spent on about 6 percent of people who die (Lubitz and Prikoda, 1994; Lubitz and Riles, 1993). However, only 6 percent of those who died had costs of over $15,000, and in all age groups, a high proportion of costs are incurred for a small number of beneficiaries who are either sick enough to be at risk of dying or chronically ill. This is not an exclusive old-age phenomenon (Cohen, 1994).

There is also the argument that precious healthcare resources are squandered on demented elders who would be better off dead and that caring for older people is generally not only expensive, but futile.

Although the exact prevalence of dementia is still to be determined, it probably is present in 10 percent of people over age 65. It increases in prevalence with age, usually doubling in prevalence with each decade over 65, so that by age over 85, estimates of the proportion with dementia range between 30 and 50 percent. Conversely, then, from 50 to 70 percent of people over age 85 are not demented. Even in those who have dementia, with forgetfulness and disorientation as prominent features, the quality of life can be quite acceptable with proper assistance. Those whose lives are more burdensome than pleasurable would be best served by providing care according to their self-determined wishes and advanced directives than by an external application of rationing standards. Although advanced directives, such as living wills, have been developed to further autonomy and privacy, early studies of costs are beginning to show some savings, without the need to impose rationing (Goldstein, 1994).

If the cost of care is spread over an entire age spectrum, it still might seem obvious that there would be poorer outcomes of treatment in people of advanced age. But again, we see the value of hard data. In numerous studies of outcomes from surgical procedures and renal dialysis, counter to intuition, chronological age drops out as an independent predictor of results of treatment. Outcomes are more closely tied to the presence of several diseases or conditions and functional status (Cassel, 1991). Past studies on the results of cancer treatment showing poorer outcomes in older patients have now been shown to be flawed by a systematic undertreatment of elders. One study of the impact of eliminating aggressive, life-prolonging treatments for patients beyond certain ages revealed that if the age limit for treatment were set at 80, the overall costs would be reduced 14 percent; if set at 90 years, the charges would be reduced only 0.4 percent. The study points out the wide range in fitness among individuals of the same age, with some at 80 years comparing favorably to others at 65, and some at 65 more like others at 95 (Goldstein, 1994). Although age may be a marker for comorbidity and poorer functional status, the results of these studies underline the need to assess individuals one-by-one for appropriateness of treatment, and they caution against an across-the-board age exclusion.

Overt Rationing

Despite the lack of data to support age-based rationing of care, it is common to hear or read comments about holding down healthcare costs by overtly withholding high-tech, high-cost services for older people. As noted above, there are no data to support chronological age as an independent criterion for the effectiveness of treatment. There is also the concern that a limitation of high-tech care will lead to a limitation on other types of care—the "slippery slope" phenomenon. In 1994, the British newspapers spotlighted the story of a 73-year-old man refused physiotherapy for arthritis. Subsequently, the Royal College of Physicians published its study of equity care for the elderly. They declared that "there is no biological rationale for separating older people from the rest of the human race: they should get the same quality of care as anyone else." In both the United States in the 1960s and in Great Britain until the 1980s there is a history of people over age 45 being excluded from renal dialysis (Moss, 1994). Subsequently, this age was gradually increased. In the early days of renal dialysis, in both places, with few resources to offer, an age bias was overt. It was assumed that older people would have a reduced life expectancy and derive less overall benefit from treatment. Subsequent information has shown that as a group, older people do have a shorter life expectancy in treatment, but, after careful study, the Institute of Medicine Committee for the Study of the Medicare ERSD (End-Stage Renal Disease) Program (Levinsky and Rettig, 1991) has specifically rejected age as a criterion for patient acceptance to dialysis, noting that comorbidities and functional status are the primary predictors of benefits from treatment, not age. Data influencing the decision include, as predicted, the finding that one-year and five-year survival of people on dialysis decreases with age. However, this decrease is to be expected because, of course, older people on or off dialysis have a shorter life expectancy than do younger people. In addition, the likelihood that other major medical events will occur is greater in the elderly, leading to a greater prevalence of older people voluntarily choosing to go off dialysis and dying from withdrawal of dialysis. However, whereas older people's life expectancy may be less, studies have shown that older people may value their continued lives on dialysis more than younger people do, with a higher well-being index, more positive feelings, and a greater life satisfaction in general, including being more satisfied with their marriages, family life, savings and investments, and standard of living (Office of Technology Assessment, 1987).

Covert Rationing

As carefully as we must defend against unwarranted, overt age-based rationing, we must be evermore vigilant against covert rationing. Consider the following actual case:

A 75-year-old married man in overall good health except for mild emphysema chooses to be admitted to a long-term-care facility with his wife, who has severe, crippling arthritis and frail health. They have been married for over fifty years, and he would rather be admitted to a nursing home to be with her than remain at home alone. In addition, the nursing facility is run by a religious organization and offers the further opportunity to study and to live his faith and culture. While at the facility, he chances upon the occurrence of a friend receiving cardiopulmonary resuscitation. He is frightened by the event, and in counseling him staff take the opportunity to discuss advance directives. After careful consideration, with lots of questions asked and answered, he decides that his life is of high quality, and that he wishes to receive medical intensive care if he should ever need it, but without chest compressions. Some time later, he suffers a relatively uncomplicated inferior myocardial infarction and is transferred to the hospital. He is expected to recover fully, but, because of the emphysema and some respiratory fatigue, it is decided to "rest him" for a short while with elective pulmonary intubation (insertion of a breathing tube). He fully agrees to this plan with the stipulation that if weaning cannot be accomplished easily within a few days, he not be allowed to remain on the ventilator indefinitely. According to hospital policy, the intensive care unit medical director, who does not know the patient, becomes the attending physician of record. The next day, the patient is visited by his primary physician who finds him without the ventilator, cyanotic (bluish because of lack of oxygen), and near death, having been discharged from the intensive care unit.

The following explanation is offered to the primary physician by the unit resident trainee who was on duty the previous night. It was he who decided, without consultation, to extubate the patient. "Our society cannot afford to keep these elderly nursing home residents alive indefinitely. Besides, he's a 'no code' patient [meaning a notation of 'do not resuscitate' was on his chart]; what's he doing in an ICU?" The patient died shortly thereafter, leaving a grieving wife who fully expected to have him back with her within a few weeks and a stunned family and primary physician who were not consulted in the ICU decision.

While there are many aspects to criticize about this case, among them poor supervision of the unit trainee and the lack of consultation with the family and primary physician, the main factor at work was age discrimination. In-depth discussion with this misinformed and dangerously unsupervised trainee revealed a person who was both lacking in judgment and profoundly influenced by the comments he had heard and read about the cost and futility of healthcare for the elderly.

Covert actions to withdraw care are dangerous, must be anticipated, and must result in policies to prevent such situations as the above. Even more dangerous are the more concealed, less dramatic, case-by-case decisions in which healthcare providers choose to limit the treatment options they offer older people, strictly because of age, that erode options presented to older people. These providers may be well-intentioned, erroneously believing that the treatments will fail to have an acceptable outcome, or they may be responding to an excessive concern for costs. There is a growing concern that the pressure to tightly control costs in managed-care settings in particular will result in limits being placed on the marketing of these plans to older people or will stay the hand of care once these individuals are enrolled. We must guard against both systematized and individual discrimination.

The Answer: Appropriate Care

The concerns regarding costs and rationing are usually phrased in the context of the allocation of limited resources among individuals within a group. In cultures where personal autonomy and rights of the individual are priorities, the discussion of allocation of resources according to age is unsettling. In other cultures, utilitarianism, in which the interests of the individual are secondary to the interests of the group, predominates, and different ethical decisions are made. Despite the current substantial percentage of the national resources allocated to healthcare, some would question whether we are near the actual limits of the resources. They raise the "guns versus butter" argument, noting ". . . the cost of stealth bombers," for example, as compared to health-related expenditures. But given that the amount of resources available for healthcare does have some reasonable limit, and assuming that we are at or near maximum, the argument about allocation rages. The issue at hand is how to control costs within an acceptable ethical and cultural framework.

There is every reason to believe that good care, self-determination, and autonomy can prevail at the same time that costs are reduced. This desirable combination can be achieved by focusing on providing the most appropriate care. Appropriate care requires the following: careful and comprehensive assessment; prevention as well as intervention; clinicians enlightened with evidence-based, unbiased data; and liberation from financial or other incentives to provide excessive care. A major concern at present is the lack of integration of geriatric principles and knowledge into the usual healthcare of many elders, and the limited geriatrics training received by many primary and specialist providers. Promoting quality care and self-determination and autonomy while containing costs also requires a systematic way to encourage patients to understand and to choose the extent of care they desire.

Healthcare should be appropriate, not rationed. Appropriate care requires that (1) decisions to accept or reject care be truly informed with good data, (2) the tendency to an age bias be recognized and confronted, and (3) advance directives and health proxies or surrogate decision-makers be explained and recommended for adults of all ages. While there does not appear to be any move to institute overt rationing by age in the United States, the possibility of covert rationing is of serious concern. Health policy must be enlightened so that the possibility of overt or covert rationing to people of all ages who may need appropriate high-cost care will be acknowledged and rejected.

This work was supported in part by a Geriatric Education Center grant from the U.S. Public Health Service, Department of Health and Human Services, Health Resources and Services Administration, Bureau of Health Professions.

References

Callahan, D. 1987. *Setting Limits: Medical Goals in an Aging Society.* New York: Simon and Schuster.

Cassel, C.K., et al. 1991. "Ethical Issues." In R. A. Rettig and N. Levinsky, eds., *Kidney Failure and the Federal Government.* Washington, D.C.: National Academy Press.

Cohen, G.D. 1994. "Health Care at an Advanced Age: Myths and Misconceptions." *Annals of Internal Medicine* 121:146–47.

Gist, J. 1992. "Entitlements and the Federal Budget Deficit: Setting the Record Straight." Washington, D.C.: AARP Public Policy Institute.

Goldstein, M. K. 1994. *Reduction in Health Care Costs in the Last-Year-of-Life: Impact of Three Alternative Policies.* Master's thesis, Department of Health, Research and Policy, Stanford University.

Levinsky, N., and Rettig, R. A. 1991. "The Medicare End-Stage Renal Disease Program: A Report from the Institute of Medicine." *New England Journal of Medicine* 324:1143.

Lubitz, J., and Prikoda, R. 1994. "The Use and Costs of Medicare Services in the Last Two Years of Life." *Health Care Financing Review* 5:117–31.

Lubitz, J., and Riles, G. 1993. "Trends in Medicare Payments in the Last Year of Life." *New England Journal of Medicine* 328:1092–96.

Moss, A. H. 1994. "Dialysis Decisions and the Elderly." *Clinics in Geriatric Medicine* (August): 56–9.

Newhouse, J. P. 1996. "An Iconoclastic View of Healthcare Cost Containment." *Generations* 10(2):61–3.

National Academy on Aging. 1994. *Old Age in the 21st Century: A Report to the Assistant Secretary for Aging.* U.S. Department of Health and Human Services. Syracuse, N.Y.: The Maxwell School, Syracuse University.

Office of Technology Assessment. 1987. "Dialysis for Chronic Renal Failure." In *Life-Sustaining Technologies and the Elderly.* OTA-BA-306. Washington, D.C.: Government Printing Office.

Scitovsky, A. A. 1988. "Medical Care in the Last Twelve Months of Life: The Relation Between Age, Functional Status, and Medical Care Expenditures." *Milbank Memorial Fund Quarterly: Health and Society* 66: 40–60.

POSTSCRIPT

Should Health Care for the Elderly Be Rationed?

In October 1986 Dr. Thomas Starzl of Pittsburgh, Pennsylvania, transplanted a liver into a 76-year-old woman at a cost of over $200,000. Soon after that, Congress ordered organ transplantation to be covered under Medicare, which ensured that more older persons would receive this benefit. At the same time these events were taking place, a government campaign to contain medical costs was under way, with health care for the elderly targeted.

Not everyone agrees with this means of cost cutting. In "Public Attitudes About the Use of Chronological Age as a Criterion for Allocating Health Care Resources," *The Gerontologist* (February 1993), the authors report that the majority of older people surveyed accept the withholding of life-prolonging medical care from the hopelessly ill but that few would deny treatment on the basis of age alone. Two publications that express opposition to age-based health care rationing are "Rationing by Any Other Name," *The New England Journal of Medicine* (June 5, 1997) and "Fighting for Health Care," *Newsweek* (March 30, 1998).

Currently, about 40 million Americans have no medical insurance and are at risk of being denied basic health care services. At the same time, the federal government pays most of the health care costs of the elderly. While it may not meet the needs of all older people, the amount of medical aid that goes to the elderly is greater than any other demographic group, and the elderly have the highest disposable income.

Most Americans have access to the best and most expensive medical care in the world. As these costs rise, some difficult decisions may have to be made regarding the allocation of these resources. As the population ages and more health care dollars are spent on care during the last years of life, medical services for the elderly or the dying may become a natural target for reduction in order to balance the health care budget. Additional readings on this subject include "Managed Care Organizations and the Rationing Problem," *The Hastings Center Report* (January/February 2003); "Medicine, Public Health, and the Ethics of Rationing," *Perspectives in Biology and Medicine* (Winter 2002); "Rationing: Don't Give Up; It's Not Only Necessary, but Possible, if the Public Can Be Educated," *The Hastings Center Report* (March–April 2002); "Health Care Rationing Affecting Older Persons: Rejected in Principle but Implemented in Fact," *Journal of Aging & Social Policy* (Summer 2002); and "What Do We Owe the Elderly: Allocating Social and Health Care Resources," *Hastings Center Report* (March/April 1994). Articles dealing with age bias include "Recognizing Bedside Rationing:

Clear Cases and Tough Calls," *Annals of Internal Medicine* (January 1, 1997); "Measuring the Burden of Disease: Healthy Life-Years," *American Journal of Public Health* (February 1998); "Rationing Health Care," *British Medical Journal* (February 28, 1998); and "Truth or Consequences," *The New England Journal of Medicine* (March 26, 1998).

ISSUE 3

Does Employer-Based Health Insurance Provide Adequate Coverage for Most Americans?

YES: William S. Custer, Charles N. Kahn III, and Thomas F. Wildsmith IV, from "Why We Should Keep the Employment-Based Health Insurance System," *Health Affairs* (November/December 1999)

NO: Uwe E. Reinhardt, from "Employer-Based Health Insurance: A Balance Sheet," *Health Affairs* (November/December 1999)

ISSUE SUMMARY

YES: Insurance and policy analysts William S. Custer, Charles N. Kahn III, and Thomas F. Wildsmith IV assert that the employment-based health care system in the United States offers a solid, proven foundation on which to base any reform, and that attempts to break the link between employment and health insurance coverage may greatly increase the number of uninsured Americans.

NO: Economist Uwe E. Reinhardt counters that, overall, the benefits of an employer-based health insurance system are outweighed by the problems, and that a new system could ultimately replace the current system.

Recently, South Africa has legislated universal access to medical services, leaving the United States as the only industrialized nation that does not guarantee its citizens access to health care. In the United States, voluntary private health insurance, mostly offered through one's employer, has traditionally been seen as the answer for covering health costs. In all other developed countries, private insurance was replaced in favor of government-supported, universally accessed medical care.

The American health care system is the most expensive and among the least equitable in the world. No other country spends as much—14 percent of

the gross national product—on health care, including some of the most techno-
logically advanced care possible. Yet approximately 40 million Americans, that
is, one in six, have no medical insurance. Many are workers whose employers
chose not to supply health insurance to their employees. Others are unemployed or part-time workers and ineligible for insurance. Still others are unin-
surable because of current or prior health problems such as cancer, heart
disease, or AIDS. Among those with medical insurance, there are some who have
policies that do not pay for expensive items such as prescription drugs, mental
health or dental care, or home care. A recent study found that 40 percent of
bankruptcies were related to illness and medical bills, and that most of the people who declared bankruptcy had some form of health insurance.

Public programs do provide some care for specific population groups.
Medicare (for the elderly and those with end-stage kidney disease) and Medicaid (for the very poor) were enacted in the 1960s. Because these programs grew
so rapidly, legislators have recently tried to curb their costs. The same is true for
private, employer-based coverage. Insurance companies assert that for private
insurers in the United States to remain competitive they have to increase premiums or reduce or minimize benefits and coverage for known disabilities and illnesses. This is the difference that other countries have addressed that we have
not. The bottom line for private insurers is to minimize coverage for those who
have the greatest need.

Until the mid-1990s most American health insurance plans used the "fee
for service" model. Doctors and hospitals billed patients or their insurance
companies at the going rate, and the insurance covered all or most of the costs.
Because of this system's escalating and uncontrolled costs, some form of managed care has largely replaced it. Managed care comes in many varieties, but the
common features are limits on hospital stays, restricted referrals to specialists,
limited choice of providers, and other cost controls. Employers who offer
health insurance now typically provide a choice of a few managed care plans.
These plans pass on a portion of the health care costs to employees through co-
pays for services, higher deductibles, and utilization limits.

Although there have been many attempts to reform health care nationwide, none have succeeded in making the system more equitable. Congress rejected the 1994 Clinton administration's health care reform plan as too
sweeping and bureaucratic. The Bush administration does not appear to have a
significant cost-cutting or burden-shifting plan in the offing. But disenchant-
ment with many aspects of managed care has led to reconsideration of some of
the fundamental premises of the American system, among them the reliance on
employer-based insurance.

The following two selections address whether health insurance should be
based on employment. William S. Custer, Charles N. Kahn III, and Thomas F.
Wildsmith IV emphasize the strengths of workplace-based insurance and private market solutions to the problem of the uninsured. Uwe E. Reinhardt disagrees and maintains that employment-based health insurance is afflicted with
a variety of inequities and imbalances.

**William S. Custer,
Charles N. Kahn III, and
Thomas F. Wildsmith IV**

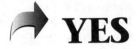 **YES**

Why We Should Keep
the Employment-Based
Health Insurance System

Today 168 million nonelderly Americans—old and young, wealthy and poor, healthy and sick—enjoy the security of private health insurance; the vast majority are covered through employer-sponsored health plans. Yet despite the many advantages of this system, it has come under increasing criticism.

While some see the employment-based system as limiting consumer choice, others argue that inequities within it are contributing to the growing number of uninsured Americans, estimated to rise from forty-three million to fifty-three million in the coming decade, even under favorable economic conditions.[1] But although some wish to address this problem through a health care program run by the federal government, others maintain that a health care financing structure based on individual choice would both expand private coverage and improve accountability, efficiency, and quality through a system that functions more like a "pure" free market.

This Commentary explores the benefits of the employment-based system and explains why it provides the best foundation for expanding coverage to more Americans. We note that given Americans' preference for private, voluntary health coverage, neither a government-run system nor a government-mandated individual system is a desirable option.[2]

Americans generally prefer to allocate resources using private markets, in large part because decision making is decentralized. This is especially beneficial in health care, where decisions often involve personal trade-offs. Moreover, when competition in the private market works well, it rewards innovation and punishes both low-quality and high-cost providers. Under perfect conditions, market-based systems allocate scarce resources across competing demands for those resources, thereby balancing the cost of production with consumers' preferences.

Real-world markets, however, are not always perfect, and some characteristics of our health care system limit the market's ability to allocate resources efficiently or equitably. Nevertheless, employer-sponsored health plans' ability to pool risks and influence both the quality and the cost of care offers significant administrative efficiencies and results in coverage that costs less than the equivalent individual coverage does. This, combined with the fact that the public benefits when each individual consumes health care services, makes the employment-based system important to national health care policy.

Tax Preference for the Employer-Based System

In 1997, 61 percent of Americans (64 percent of those under age sixty-five) were covered through an employment-based plan, as either employees or dependents. Among the nonelderly, more than 90 percent of those who have private insurance received it from an employment-based plan.[3]

The favorable tax treatment of health insurance as an employee benefit has encouraged the proliferation of employer-sponsored health plans. Since 1954 employers' contributions for employee health insurance have been excluded from income for the purpose of determining payroll taxes and federal and state income taxes. This exclusion is essentially a subsidy for the purchase of health insurance for those who receive coverage through the workplace.

Most employers that offer health coverage contribute to its cost; in larger firms this contribution typically represents about 75 percent of the cost of individual coverage and about 65 percent of the cost of family coverage.[4] This means that there is little benefit from not participating in a health plan, even for those who perceive their health risk as low. Participation rates are consequently very high, and persons generally considered to be good health risks remain in the employer's risk pool, which effectively reduces the premium and makes employment-based health insurance more cost-effective than the alternatives.[5] . . .

Employment-based insurance spreads risk more broadly and therefore more efficiently than individual health insurance, and, consequently, is less affected by adverse selection. The problems created for the individual health insurance market by consumers' particular health care needs, which shape the purchasing decision, are well documented.[6] In contrast, employer-sponsored health plans are offered to employees and their dependents as part of a compensation package—and a person's self-assessment of risk is only one of many factors leading to acceptance or rejection of a job offer.[7]

The tax subsidy promotes participation in health plans by those who otherwise would experience large net losses from participation. Some evidence exists that without tax subsidies, low-risk persons might leave pools at a higher rate than high-risk persons do because the cost of coverage would exceed its value.[8] If enough employees chose not to participate, employers might simply terminate their health plans, especially if those who dropped out tended to be better risks.[9]

If the tax subsidy were removed with no other changes in the tax code, twenty million adults would no longer have employment-based health insurance.[10] About 3.5 million more adults would purchase individual health insurance policies. But those in poor health—according to self-reported measures of health status—would be hit hard: The number of employer-insured adults with at least one family member in poor health would fall from 47 percent to 31 percent, a drop of sixteen percentage points.

Even more telling, the percentage of good risks with private coverage outside the employment-based system would increase by three percentage points, while the percentage of poor risks with other private coverage would fall slightly. Even the percentage of employer-insured adults with healthy families would fall twelve percentage points if the exclusion were repealed. These results further support the notion that the tax subsidy reinforces the risk pooling inherent in employment-based health insurance, thereby increasing the number of Americans with coverage.

In short, an inherent economic dynamic favors employment-based group coverage over individual coverage. Employers' decisions to offer health insurance depend on the demand for coverage by the workforce they wish to attract and retain. Although good risks have a lower demand for health insurance than poorer risks have, the tax preference for employer-sponsored coverage in effect lowers its price. This induces more good risks to demand insurance; as the demand rises, more employers offer coverage. And when coverage is offered as a part of compensation, the vast majority of employees participate, thereby reducing the effects of adverse selection. Thus, the group purchase of health insurance through the workplace makes that coverage affordable to poorer risks—the more vulnerable members of society. Individual purchase of insurance would not achieve this societal good.

Finally, some economists have argued that the tax preference provides an incentive for the purchase of too much insurance, resulting in a distorted market for health services, inefficient allocation of scarce resources, and increased health care cost inflation.[11] This argument ignores the social benefit provided by a person's access to health care services. Clearly, the current public policy debate centers on increasing health insurance coverage, not limiting it. . . .

The Employer-Based System: Basis for Reform

The employment-based health insurance system is not a historical accident. Its characteristics flow directly from our society's desire to maximize access to health care, our commitment to voluntary private markets, and the market advantages of employer-sponsored health insurance.

The inherent structural advantages of the employment-based private health insurance market, coupled with complementary tax and public policies, have allowed employers to help control health care costs, improve quality, and maximize health benefits for a wide range of Americans from diverse economic and social backgrounds. The success of these efforts, during the past decade in particular, shows that the employer-based system harnesses the unique risk factors and other attributes of the health insurance market, for the benefit of the public. These advantages simply are impossible to replicate in any alternative based on a voluntary system.

Voluntary markets will continue for the foreseeable future, markets in which each purchaser must compare the value of the coverage received with the cost of the premiums and decide whether or not coverage makes sense. With a voluntary market, any implicit subsidy that requires some people to pay more for health insurance so that others can pay less is, in effect, a "tax" that can be avoided simply by not buying health insurance.

Continued reliance on the employment-based health insurance system, with its ability to attract a broad range of individuals, in conjunction with targeted subsidies for specific population segments who are not eligible for, or cannot afford, employer coverage, would seem to be the best strategy for increasing access in a voluntary market. Access to affordable coverage needs to be extended to far more Americans, but such efforts should supplement and strengthen the current employment-based system, not replace it.

~◆~

Our society continues to face important challenges in moving toward a more efficient, cost-effective, and universal health care system. Perhaps the most difficult challenge is to maintain the balance between private and public coverage to maximize access to health care services, control costs, and reward innovation. As long as we continue to rely on the voluntary purchase of health insurance, the natural tendency of consumers to make financial decisions that are in their own economic best interest will limit the size of the implicit subsidies that can be generated, particularly in the individual market, without greatly reducing the number of persons who choose to purchase coverage. The employment-based health care system offers a solid, proven foundation upon which to build any reform, and it should be preserved. On the other hand, reforms based on attempts to break the link between employment and health insurance coverage are unlikely to be successful and have the potential to greatly increase the number of Americans who lack health insurance.

Notes

1. W. Custer, *Health Insurance Coverage and the Uninsured* (Washington: Health Insurance Association of America, January 1999).
2. An exhaustive literature exists on the disadvantages of a government system and the antipathy of Americans to such a system. See, for example, R. Blendon et al., "Voters and Health Care in the 1998 Election," *Journal of the American Medical Association* (14 July 1999): 189–194; M. Walker and M. Zelder, *Waiting Your Turn: Hospital Waiting Lists in Canada (9th Edition)*, Critical Issues Bulletin (Vancouver, B.C.: Fraser Institute, September 1999); S. Hall, "For British Health System, Bleak Prognosis," *New York Times*, 30 January 1997, A1; K. Donelan et al., "The Cost of Health System Change: Public Discontent in Five Nations." *Health Affairs* (May/June 1999): 206–216; T. Jost, "German Health Care Reform: The Next Steps," *Journal of Health Politics, Policy and Law* (August 1998): 697–711; and C. Dargie, S. Dawson, and P. Garside, *Policy Futures for UK Health: Pathfinder* (Draft) (London: Nuffield Trust for Research and Policy Studies in Health Services, September 1999).
3. Custer, *Health Insurance Coverage and the Uninsured.*
4. *National Survey of Employer-Sponsored Health Plans, 1997* (New York: William M. Mercer, 1998).

5. A. Monheit et al., "How Are Net Health Insurance Benefits Distributed in the Employment-Related Insurance Market?" *Inquiry* (Winter 1995/96): 372–391.

6. A consumer's choice of health insurance coverage in an individual market is determined by a self-assessment of his or her own risk and income. Those with the greatest demand for health insurance are thus most likely to use health care services. Premiums in the individual market therefore are higher, to cover the costs of the greater risks. *Providing Universal Access in a Voluntary Private-Sector Market,* Public Policy Monograph (Washington: American Academy of Actuaries, February 1996); L. Nichols, "Regulating Non-Group Health Insurance Markets: What Have We Learned So Far?" (Paper presented at the Robert Wood Johnson Foundation/Alpha Center meeting, The Evolution of the Individual Insurance Market: Now and in the Future, Washington, D.C., 20 January 1999); S. Zuckerman and S. Rajan, "An Alternative Approach to Measuring the Effects of Insurance Market Reforms," *Inquiry* (Spring 1999): 44–56; L.J. Blumberg and L.M. Nichols, "First, Do No Harm: Developing Health Insurance Market Reform Packages," *Health Affairs* (Fall 1996): 35–53; and L. Blumberg and L. Nichols, *Health Insurance Market Reforms: What They Can and Cannot Do* (Washington: Urban Institute, 1995).

7. Although employment itself may act as a health screen, given employment-based coverage's favorable selection, just under half of Americans with employment-based coverage are dependents of workers. P. Fronstin, *Features Of Employment-Based Health Insurance,* EBRI Issue Brief no. 201 (Washington: Employee Benefit Research Institute, 1998).

8. Monheit et al., "How Are Net Health Insurance Benefits Distributed?"

9. *Tax Reform and the Impact on Employee Benefits,* Public Policy Monograph (Washington: American Academy of Actuaries, Spring 1997).

10. This estimate is based on variations in state marginal income tax rates. See W. Custer and P. Ketsche, "The Tax Preference for Employment-Based Health Insurance Coverage," Working Paper (Center for Risk Management and Insurance Research, Georgia State University, April 1999).

11. M. Feldstein, "The Welfare Loss of Excess Health Insurance," *Journal of Political Economy* (March/April 1973): 251–280; M. Feldstein and B. Freidman, "Tax Subsidies, the Rational Demand for Insurance, and the Health Care Crisis," *Journal of Public Economics* (April 1977):155–178; and M. Pauly, "Taxation, Health Insurance, and Market Failure in the Medical Economy," *Journal of Economic Literature* 24, no. 2 (1986): 629–675.

NO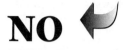

Uwe E. Reinhardt

Employer-Based Health Insurance: A Balance Sheet

As the United States faces the dynamic global economy of the next millennium, many policy analysts and even some members of Congress have begun to wonder whether employment-based health insurance can remain a cornerstone of the U.S. health care system.

The employer-based system traces its origins to World War II, when Congress illogically allowed employers to use fringe benefits as a means of evading the wage caps that it had imposed at the time. The system thrived in the postwar years, when the U.S. economy ruled the world and American workers enjoyed virtually tenured jobs. Its growth has been further abetted by a tax preference that allows employers to treat the group-insurance premiums paid on behalf of employees as tax-deductible expenses without requiring employees to pay income taxes on this part of their compensation. In effect, this tax preference allows employed Americans to purchase health insurance out of pretax income, a privilege not extended to self-employed or unemployed Americans.

Although the employer-based insurance system covers about two-thirds of the U.S. population, it accounts for less than one-third of total national health spending. This is because public insurance programs have become the catch basins for relatively high cost Americans—the elderly, the poor, and the disabled. Government's relative importance as a payer for health care is likely to grow in the next century, as the population ages.

Doubts about the employer-based health insurance system's future have grown during the 1990s, because the system actually shrank as the economy and total employment expanded apace. About 18 percent of working adults are not now offered any health insurance by their employer.[1] The more nonelderly Americans are eclipsed and left uninsured by the employer-based system, the more compelling is the search for a robust alternative to that system. . . .

The System's Debits

"Unsurance" Unquestionably the worst shortcoming of the employer-based system is that the health insurance protection of entire families, including children, is tied to a particular job and lost with that job. By international standards, privately insured Americans cannot really be considered "insured." They are "temporarily insured," or "unsured" for short.

In virtually all other industrialized nations, young people know that, come what may, they will have permanent, fully portable health insurance. The United States has never been able to afford its citizens that luxury. Would any private health insurer today be able to offer a young American a life-cycle health insurance contract, akin to the whole-life insurance policies that are available to young Americans? The job-based system has been a major roadblock to the development of fully portable, life-cycle health insurance contracts.

Job lock   Because the employer-based system ties health insurance to a particular job, it can induce employees to remain indentured in a detested job simply because it is the sole source of affordable health coverage. As Jonathan Gruber and Maria Hanratty have shown empirically, relative to the U.S. health system, the fully portable health insurance provided by the Canadian provinces actually facilitates greater labor mobility.[2] Fully portable health insurance, of course, is not contingent on government provision. Within a proper statutory framework, it should be possible to develop fully portable private health insurance that is detached from the workplace.[3]

Inequity   The tax preference enjoyed by the employer-based system is inequitable for two reasons. First, it has never been fully extended to self-employed and unemployed Americans, which is unfair on its face. Second, even among employed Americans with employer coverage, those with high incomes benefit proportionately more from the tax preference than do low-income employees in lower marginal tax brackets.

This inequity is most glaring in connection with the flexible spending accounts available only through the employer-based system. At the beginning of the year employed Americans may deposit into these accounts, out of pretax income, specified amounts to cover out-of-pocket health spending. With this set-aside, well-to-do families can purchase a dollar's worth of, say, orthodontic work or plastic surgery at an after-tax cost of only about fifty cents, whereas low-income families would pay eighty-five cents or more after taxes for the same work. Furthermore, the law includes the inflationary provision that unspent year-end balances in the accounts accrue to the employer. One suspects that Congress enacted this inequitable, inflationary provision at the behest of private employers, which found the arrangement helpful in their quest to make their workers accept more overt cost sharing for their health care.

Lack of choice   Whatever benefits employees derive from the current paternalistic system, one price they pay is limits on their choices in the health insurance market. As Stan Jones, Lynn Etheredge, and Larry Lewin reported in 1996, close to half of American employees are offered only one health plan by their employers.[4] They are in what one may call a private single-payer system. Another quarter or so of employees are offered a choice of only two health plans. A more recent Kaiser/Commonwealth national survey of health insurance corroborates these estimates.[5] This lack of choice makes a mockery of the idea of "managed competition."

Lack of privacy   In many instances, the employer-based system gives private employers access to their employees' medical records.[6] It is one thing to know that a private insurance carrier has information on the most intimate details of one's life. It is quite another to think that the personnel department of one's employer can get access to that information as well. Whatever one may think about health systems abroad, patients in those countries do not worry about this invasion of privacy.

Administrative complexity   The defenders of employer-based health insurance tend to view it as more "efficient" than alternative arrangements. That proposition is incredible, given the current system's administrative complexity. [As a result] of a multiyear study by McKinsey and Company of the American and German health systems, the latter of which is based on private, not-for-profit sickness funds that operate within a tight statutory framework,[7] [t]he McKinsey research team concluded that the U.S. system is more productively efficient than Germany's system is. It based that conclusion on the finding that in 1990 Germans actually spent $390 more per capita on strictly medical inputs (hospital days, physician visits, drugs, and the like) than did Americans. [H]owever, the U.S. system burned up more than the entire savings from its allegedly superior clinical productivity on higher administrative expenses ($360 per capita) and on higher outlays on the catch-all category "other" ($259). Because Medicare and Medicaid are known to spend relatively little on administration, the higher U.S. figure must reflect mainly private insurance. Given that the U.S. system outranks no other system in the industrialized world in either measured health status indicators or patient satisfaction, it can fairly be asked: In what sense is employer-based health insurance "efficient"?

Lack of transparency   Standard economic theory and empirical research have convinced economists that the premiums paid by employers on behalf of employees are merely part of the total price of labor and, over the longer run, are shifted back to employees collectively through commensurate reductions in take-home pay. Unfortunately, it is not known precisely how employers do this. That may be why employees typically assume that their employer fully absorbs the part of the premium that is not explicitly deducted from their paycheck. Unaware of how much their health insurance actually costs them in terms of forgone take-home pay, employed Americans have never showed nearly enough self-interest in health care cost containment. This may explain why over the long run the employer-based system has so frequently acted as the inflationary locomotive in American health care. . . .

Although different evaluators may come up with different debits, credits, and account balances for the employer-based health insurance system, I conclude from the exercise that the debits outweigh the credits. This conclusion does not call for the outright abolition of the current system, but it does suggest the need for a parallel system that would be detached from the workplace and that might, over time, absorb the bulk of the current system. With a proper regulatory framework, such a parallel system need not be public; it could rely on private insurance as well.

Notes

1. Kaiser/Commonwealth 1997 National Survey of Health Insurance, "Working Families at Risk: Coverage, Access, Costs, and Worries" (8 December 1997), 40.
2. J. Gruber and M. Hanratty, "The Labor Market Effects of Introducing National Health Insurance," *Journal of Business and Economic Statistics* (April 1995): 163–174.
3. M.V. Pauly et al., "A Plan for 'Responsible National Health Insurance'," *Health Affairs* (Spring 1991): 5–25; and U.E. Reinhardt, "An 'All-American' Health Reform Proposal," *Journal of American Health Policy* (May/June 1993):11–17.
4. L. Etheredge, S.B. Jones, and L. Lewin, "What Is Driving Health System Change?" *Health Affairs* (Winter 1996): 94.
5. Kaiser/Commonwealth 1997 National Survey of Health Insurance.
6. E.E. Schultz, "Medical Data Gathered by Firms Can Prove Less Than Confidential," *Wall Street Journal,* 18 May 1994, A1, A5.
7. McKinsey Global Institute, *Health Care Productivity* (Los Angeles: McKinsey and Company, October 1996).

POSTSCRIPT

Does Employer-Based Health Insurance Provide Adequate Coverage for Most Americans?

Managed care began replacing fee-for-service in the early 1990s. Costs were reduced by capping payments to health care providers and by limiting patients' access to expensive tests and medical specialists. Annual growth in national health spending between 1993 and 2000 fell to 5.7 percent, down from the peak 9.7 percent growth seen between 1988 and 1993. Unfortunately, cost reductions came at a price. Employers, health providers, and consumers rebelled against the HMOs' excessive cost-saving measures. By 1997 this caused medical inflation to grow once again.

Employers have fought back, implementing higher payroll deductions, co-payments, and deductibles for physician and hospital visits. Companies are also moving employees into "consumer-driven" health plans with a health care spending account that is funded by the employer. The goal is to turn employees into more careful shoppers when it comes to health care. It is also an attempt to reduce the expense caused by going to specialists, having numerous tests performed, and going through costly procedures. For further reading on this subject, see "Private Medical Insurance in Need of Radical Surgery," *Personnel Today* (January 28, 2003); "Mental Health Cuts Could Bring Quick Savings, Long-Term Regrets," *Business Insurance* (January 20, 2003); "Health Insurance Declining Among Workers," *Case Management Advisor* (January 2003); and "The Improbable Future of Employment-Based Insurance," *The Hastings Center Report* (May 2000).

For other views on employer-based health insurance, see "The Tough Decisions That No One Wants to Make: Workplace Health and Benefits," *Medical Benefits* (March 30, 2003) and "Employers Have New Weapon to Fight Health Care Cost Increases," *The Kiplinger Letter* (April 17, 2003). In "How Large Employers Are Shaping the Health Care Marketplace (Second of Two Parts)," *The New England Journal of Medicine* (April 9, 1998) and "Who Really Pays for Employment-Based Health Insurance?" *The Hastings Center Report* (May 2000), the authors discuss the influence of employers on health care services. They assert that employers have largely succeeded in their first cost-cutting strategy—channeling employees into managed care plans. However, the success of their second strategy—bringing employers together in large regional plans and contracting directly with health care providers—is still in doubt. See also "Health Care for All: A Conservative Case," *Commonweal* (February 22, 2002) and "The Breaking Point: Worker Health Costs Will Rise a Staggering 24% This Year: Companies Can No Longer Afford to Pick Up the Bill," *Fortune* (March 3, 2003).

ISSUE 4

Is the Pharmaceutical Industry Responsible for the High Cost of Prescription Drugs?

YES: Christopher F. Koller, from "Prescription for Trouble: Why Drug Prices Keep Exploding," *Commonweal* (June 15, 2001)

NO: Ronald Bailey, from "Goddamn the Pusher Man," *Reason* (April 2001)

ISSUE SUMMARY

YES: Christopher F. Koller, CEO of Neighborhood Health Plan of Rhode Island, a health plan serving Medicaid enrollees based in Providence, asserts that the pharmaceutical industry has achieved its rapid growth by political protection and by exploiting the vulnerabilities of patients.

NO: Ronald Bailey, science correspondent for *Reason* magazine, states that spending on prescriptions is rising rapidly because Americans are buying more drugs. Bailey maintains that the drug companies have actually enriched the quality of our lives.

Prescription drug spending continues to grow at a faster pace than any other component of health care in the United States, and this trend is expected to continue for at least the next several years. The nation's prescription drug bill has been rising 14 to 18 percent a year and is expected to exceed $160 billion in 2003. About 50 percent of Americans have no prescription drug coverage, and government programs such as Medicare lack a pharmacy benefit. Unfortunately, some people solve the problem of high drug costs by cutting back on buying food or paying for utilities. Others simply go without some or all of their medications. A survey conducted recently by AARP (the American Association of Retired Persons) found that one in five older Americans did not fill one or more prescriptions for financial reasons.

There are two primary reasons that drug spending has increased: higher use and a higher average cost per prescription. Research indicates that each year drug spending will account for 18 percent to 25 percent of overall health care spending. Prescription drug costs have increased from less than 10 percent of total health care costs to over 15 percent and could approach 20 percent of total health care costs in the future. There are several key drivers of these cost increases, including the significant increase in the elderly population. People tend to use more drugs as they grow older to treat chronic conditions and, on average, tend to use drugs that cost more. Also, interestingly, the thresholds for determining diabetes and high cholesterol were recently lowered. As a result, more than 38 million additional people fell under the guidelines for prescription drug treatment. While this should have a positive impact on patients' health in the long-term, the short-term impact on drug spending is significant.

Costs for prescription drugs continue to escalate to allow pharmaceutical companies to recoup costs for advertising, research, and development. Drug companies have invested heavily in advertising directly to consumers the latest heartburn, allergy, arthritis, and pain medications, to name a few. This has led to a nation of consumers who enter their doctors' offices with a particular brand-name drug in mind that they believe will cure their ailment.

At an estimated annual cost of $2.5 billion, pharmaceutical advertising on television and in the popular press has made drug companies and their brands household names. Analysis from the managed care industry has shown that from 1999 to 2000, prescriptions written for the 50 most heavily advertised drugs rose nearly 25 percent, compared to 4.3 percent for all other drugs combined. Drug manufacturing, a $122 billion industry, is becoming more dependent on advertising to sell their products.

In addition to advertising expenditures, the drug companies assert that they must heavily spend on research and development to bring new, better drugs to market. More new drugs are being released, with additional drugs in clinical trials. In 2000 the Food and Drug Administration (FDA) approved 27 new drugs plus many improved or enhanced versions of existing drugs. Currently, more than 1,000 drugs are in the pipeline. The pharmaceutical companies contend that it costs an average of $800 million to bring a new drug to market. Critics state that much of the research and development needed to bring a drug to market is supported by taxpayers via support by the federal government. Also, a study by the National Institute for Health Care Management Foundation found, that two-thirds of the prescription drugs approved by the FDA between 1998 and 2000 were modified or enhanced versions of existing drugs. Only 15 percent of the approved drugs were both new and improved over existing medications.

While it is clear that drug prices have risen dramatically, there are some positive effects to this trend to consider. Many key drugs will lose their patent protection in the next couple of years, providing an opportunity to switch to generics. While the initial cost of the generic alternatives for some of these drugs may be expensive, it does provide for a more competitive environment. In addition, some of the drugs being introduced will significantly improve the health of patients.

In the following selections, Christopher F. Koller maintains that drug companies' policies have inflated the cost of prescription drugs, putting many medications out of reach for vulnerable Americans, particularly the elderly. Ronald Bailey argues that the pharmaceutical industry has a sound track record of raising the quality of life.

Christopher F. Koller 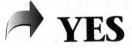 **YES**

Prescription for Trouble:
Why Drug Prices Keep Exploding

Consider Walter. At seventy, he has a history of high blood pressure, heart trouble, high cholesterol, stomach pains, and seasonal allergies. He used to smoke but gave it up a while back. He is only moderately overweight. For his various ailments, Walter has a variety of prescriptions from his doctor. His real problem, however—as for 26 percent of his fellow Americans, particularly the elderly, those most in need of medications—is that Walter has no insurance coverage for his medications. Medicare does not provide it.

Drug coverage makes a real difference in people's lives, for two reasons. Those who have it use prescriptions at a 50-percent higher rate than those without it, presumably to their benefit; and people without it spend on average $220 *more* per year for the few drugs they do get. Combine these facts and you have a recipe for not only moral but political outrage. Hence the increased attention being paid to a drug benefit for those on Medicare.

Yet there is something else at work here. Only eleven years ago, the percentage of Americans with no drug coverage was almost twice as high (48 percent) as it is today. By most measures of equity, then, things have gotten better: more people have coverage, and—for advocates of smaller government, something even more positive—this improvement has come about through private health insurance.

So why has drug coverage become a national issue? In 1999, $100 billion was spent on prescription drugs in the United States—8.3 percent of the total health-care ticket. By 2010, that figure is expected to rise to $366 billion (14 percent of total expenses). This works out to a predicted average annual growth rate of 11.3 percent for the next nine years—more than twice the growth rate of the country's economy as a whole. (Last year alone, spending for prescription drugs rose a stunning 18.8 percent.) The real problem we are facing, therefore, is providing not simply prescription-drug coverage but the total bill for such expenses. And this reality is finally registering with American consumers, previously shielded from the real costs of such services. Naturally, the first to feel it are uninsured, high utilizers—namely, the elderly.

Every drama needs its shadowy character, and in this story the pharmaceutical industry is ripe for the role. Under increasing scrutiny, "big pharma" is reaping what it has sown. Through the 1990s, it grew at an average of 12.5 percent per year—two and one-half times the rate of the economy as a whole—and posted profits between 15 and 20 percent, making it one of the most profitable businesses around. The industry achieved this growth by delivering new hope to people, by securing political protection for itself, and by exploiting the vulnerabilities of both patients and an insurance-based payment system that inured customers to price sensitivity.

How much can Americans afford to pay for their medications? Who benefits from the growth of the prescription-drug industry? Might consumers trade slower pharmaceutical innovation for lower costs and broader coverage? To explore these issues, let's return to Walter, our chronically unwell subject.

✦

The accompanying table illustrates the range Walter might pay for his drug regime, depending on the drugs prescribed and his insurance coverage. The table also serves to illustrate the difficulties associated with resource allocation in health care, particularly how to balance social benefit and individual need.

The table is based on generally accessible and accurate (but hardly definitive) information on drug pricing estimates, as they relate to the theoretical treatment of Walter's particular symptoms. Depending on insurance coverage, Walter could end up paying as little as nothing, or as much as $911 for his ninety-day course of drugs. The "system costs" (that is, the revenues to the drug

Table 1

		Approximate Costs for 90-Day Supply				
		Private Insurance		**Medicaid**		**Medicare**
Symptoms/ Condition	*Medicine*	*Patient*	*Company*	*Patient*	*State*	*(all paid by patient)*
Stomach Pains/	Prilosec	$10	$273	0	$201	$336
Heartburn	Ranitidine	$5	$119	0	$92	$141
Hypertension	Accupril	$10	$94	0	$67	$112
	Atenolol	$5	$6	0	$2	$4
High Cholesterol	Lescol	$10	$137	0	$99	$183
Allergic Rhinitis	Claritin	$10	$232	0	$168	$280
(runny nose)	Semprex	$10	$66	0	$46	$78
Maximum paid		$40	$736	0	$535	$911
Minimum paid		$30	$328	0	$239	$406

Source: Author's research of average wholesale price (AWP) and standard industry discounts and copayments.

companies) could range from $239 to $911, based on what is prescribed and who pays. A look at the table also indicates that there are few other markets for goods and services where product pricing varies so significantly, and largely to the benefit of the seller. Nonuniversal, third-party coverage compounds this issue by exposing some people to full costs while insulating other consumers from any sort of price sensitivity.

There are six elements at play in the pharmaceutical industry which contribute not only to its growth but also to the pressures it puts on the financing and delivery of health care in general.

- **Product Development** The key to growth in the pharmaceutical industry is the introduction of new products. Drug companies are masters at creating such innovations. They spent $25 billion in 1999—a whopping 25 percent of sales—on research and development. Their production pipeline is full of future products targeted for widespread chronic conditions like Walter's—heart disease, depression, and arthritis—where utilization will be high and sustained. It is estimated that 46 percent of the rate of increase in prescription-drug spending each year comes from the introduction of new products. Companies search for blockbuster drugs that will deliver new benefits to patients and that will sustain their research and development programs. Of the $21 billion increase in spending for prescription drugs from 1999 to 2000, one-half was due to increased sales of just twenty-three individual drugs.

- **Marketing** Once a drug is developed, it is marketed intensively to differentiate it from its competition. In 1999, pharmaceutical companies spent more than $10 billion on marketing activities. Over 80 percent of this outlay was directed at physicians, trying to get them to recognize when to prescribe, and then to recommend a particular brand of drug. Company "detailers" (sales people) aggressively court doctors with information and entertainment. And marketing works. Between 1993 and 1998, sales of the ten most heavily marketed drugs contributed to more than one-fifth of the total increase in drug expenditures.

  Yet the benefits of these blockbuster drugs are often overstated. Four out of five of Walter's conditions can be treated with much cheaper regimens of generally similar efficacy. There is, however, little incentive in the health system for doctors not to prescribe the latest thing, once it is proven safe and effective. Furthermore, today's fastest-growing marketing effort is direct-to-consumer advertising—getting *patients* to ask a physician for Claritin for a runny nose because they saw Joan Lunden recommend it on television. First permitted on television four years ago, consumer advertising was a $2.5 billion ticket in the year 2000. Such advertising campaigns offer only partial information about the products to the consumer, yet he or she can exert effective pressure on a physician to write a particular prescription.

- **Differential Pricing and Cost Responsibility** In a typical market, price is based on the consumer's perceived value of a particular good or service. But in pharmaceuticals, the consumer is not the only purchaser.

His or her insurance plan also plays a part, and this has had the unintended consequence of contributing significantly to price insensitivity for pharmaceuticals—all the while enhancing the industry's profits. As Walter's table indicates, third-party insurance coverage has created significant opportunities for differential pricing by the industry, again resulting in increased revenues. By law, Medicaid gets the lowest price, but uninsured individual consumers may end up paying a retail price typically almost twice that of Medicaid.

If the market can't arrive at a fair or consistent price, is there some other workable mechanism? Efforts at price controls, common in Canada and Europe, are anathema in the United States. Every other major developed country employs some form of aggressive price and utilization control in its pharmaceutical program—whether as the provider of national health insurance or as a matter of industrial policy. (These include individual or product-group price controls, profit caps, monitoring the prescribing patterns of doctors, establishing national formularies, and patient cost sharing.) The results are significant: per capita spending for prescription drugs in other major developed countries is 70 percent of the U.S. total—and growing at a slower rate. No wonder stories abound about Americans making shopping trips to Canada to purchase cheaper medicines. The U.S. pharmaceutical industry maintains that price controls in other countries force U.S. consumers to shoulder a disproportionate share of future product and development costs. But the industry is silent when it comes to whether Americans pay a greater share of its profits. The global reach of the industry may present an occasion for a global trade and industry policy.

- **Patent Protections** After a blockbuster drug is invented, marketed, and priced, a company works hard to protect its privileged position. Patent law exists to encourage innovation by preserving exclusivity and its benefits to the innovator for some time. The profits which accrue to the pharmaceutical industry, however, are truly extraordinary. Through diligent legislative activity, the industry has been able to more than double the potential effective patent life of a new drug, from 8.1 years in 1984 to 18.4 years in 2000. While not all drugs enjoy 18 years of exclusivity, the benefits of even six months of additional protection are considerable for a manufacturer, for once generic competition arrives on the market, prices can drop from 75 to 90 percent.

- **Political Spending** The pharmaceutical industry spent some $74 million for lobbying activities in 1998. The result? In addition to the patent protections noted above, federal tax credits for research resulted in the industry's massive profits being taxed at only 15 percent, almost half of the average corporate tax rate. In the recent presidential election, the industry contributed more than $6 million to the Bush campaign, and coughed up another $1.7 million for Bush's inaugural. Perhaps it is no surprise that an industry executive was named director of the Office of Management and Budget, or that three industry representatives served on the Department of Health and Human Services transition team—important positions from which to preserve current advantages and ensure that, for instance, a Medicare prescription-drug benefit proposal would steer away from governmental price controls.

- **The Technological Imperative** The last piece at work is probably the most difficult to harness: our collective desire for science to make our lives easier and to save us from our fears. The most important things Walter can do to help himself are to eat correctly, stay away from cigarettes, and get plenty of exercise and sleep. But these habits are hard to build and maintain. Virtue often loses to the quick fix promised by a pill, especially when it is cleverly marketed and the user does not directly pay for its full cost. Ultimately, of course, even good habits are no match for disease, let alone death. On the other hand, the benefits of medication, while not permanent, are incontestable. Still, we are guilty of a collective deceit when we let our faith in technology supplant a healthy respect for our bodies, both their strengths and their limitations. This deceit cannot be treated with a pill, and its results may be just as corrosive to the human spirit as any disease.

❧

None of this helps Walter directly when he is trying to figure out how to pay for Lescol so he can lower his cholesterol and reduce the risk of a heart attack. And though it may make sense for him to pay a share of his costs, few of us would be comfortable with the idea that access to an effective drug should be rationed based on the ability to pay, let alone proof of a person's exercise habits. How, then, do we get ourselves out of this mess?

The focus on prescription-drug coverage for the elderly is the best place to begin thinking about costs and coverage, for clearly the needs are real and, finally, it is federal policy that shapes the market for health care.

Currently, the only prescription-drug coverage options available for the elderly are retiree coverage for the lucky few; small state-based, sliding-scale programs; and Medicaid (for the impoverished). If actuarial estimates are correct, however, simply adding a full benefit for the elderly could raise program costs by 25 percent, an untenable prospect. How then do we close this gap between the real and growing needs of an aging population, and our ability to pay for those needs? Prescription drugs for the elderly thus become a more focused version of the larger dilemma raised by advocates of universal health insurance.

Current proposals break down less over the size of federal participation than over how allocation decisions get made; that is, the extent to which one believes the private market can and should work. The Bush administration's original "Immediate Helping Hand Program" called for an annual block grant of $12 billion to the states. This would provide for means-tested subsidies to the needy elderly for purchasing necessary drugs—augmenting what some states already have in place. After a period of denial over the need for any federal role, the pharmaceutical industry has embraced this approach as the least intrusive of potential evils. It is easily administrable and is philosophically compatible with a limited and preferably state-based governmental role. It also lets the private sector take care of health, starts to create a lower tier of care and financing for the elderly, and does nothing to address the fact that prescription-drug costs are driving the system as a whole.

For their part, advocates of a broader Medicare prescription-drug coverage have a hard time making the numbers work. Means testing for any Medicare benefit would reduce the cost burden, but is politically difficult, given Medicare is a universal entitlement. Some proposals call for a separate, privately administered prescription insurance program. Medicare enrollees could use a voucher to buy into different types of coverage in a newly created "market" of privately administered, government-certified drug benefit programs. These policy administrators would hammer out their best deals for enrollees with the manufacturers. But advocates for these private-sector purchasing techniques conveniently overlook the fact that it is the private health-insurance sector that has produced the 15–20 percent per year growth rates that now threaten the whole system.

Installing greater patient cost-sharing mechanisms to foster price sensitivity is one potential means of lowering medical expenditures. But such a program would have to be carefully administered, lest people forgo needed drugs because of the expense. Finally, reducing costs by limiting the extent of the benefit becomes dicey. Just imagine the reaction when the first elderly patient with the need for an excluded medicine shows up on the nightly news.

Reform of the present system, therefore, will require money and real political will. Still, almost anything would represent an improvement over what is currently in place for the elderly. Medicare prescription drug plans should follow some of the time-tested patterns already established by Medicare.

- First, coverage rules should apply to all. A safety-net type of program would represent a break from Medicare's commitment to equitable treatment. Medicare, along with Social Security, is the strongest example of social solidarity we have in the United States. It must be preserved.

- Second, we must get as comprehensive a benefit plan as we can afford. Half a loaf is better than none, but we have to make sure everyone gets it. Let those who can afford it buy a bigger loaf.

- Third, program operations must address the factors that have landed us in this fix. Federal purchasing or price controls for prescriptions should be instituted, as is already done for hospitals and physicians under the Medicare program. Admittedly, such price setting is ugly and inelegant, but it has worked for thirty-five years. For all their antimarket appearances, Medicare's physician and hospital fees are the standard reference metrics used throughout the private health-care industry. In addition, let Medicare recipients buy those drugs not covered under Medicare for the same price Medicaid pays. The industry will howl in protest, but it will adjust.

- Fourth, a Medicare prescription drug program should install effective and means-tested patient cost sharing at the point of consumption. This will encourage more price sensitivity. Patients need a limited incentive to weigh the costs and benefits of various treatments. For example, in Germany the first $20 of the cost of any prescription is covered by public insurance, but all costs above that are privately financed.
- Finally, we should acknowledge that pharmacy costs—the fastest-rising element in health care—are emblematic of our infatuation with the technological fix and unlimited choices. Proposals for prescription-drug coverage—and any other health-care coverage—must address a fundamental tectonic force at work: the proliferation of products and technologies that push costs upward. Particularly at a time when health-care utilization is likely to increase as the population ages and diagnostic technologies, often gene-based, improve, we should recognize that the industry has no need for the protections it has been afforded legislatively in the form of excessive patent protection and tax credits. Furthermore, no credible argument has been made that direct-to-consumer advertising for drugs does anything more than increase costs and create unrealistic and partially informed demands on physicians by patients.

In the end, health care is a supply-driven business: The more options our friend Walter has, the more he will use. The unchallenged assumption is that the more we use, the better off we are. That assumption must be questioned. But the prescription drug industry has embraced that paradigm and profited immensely from it. At the same time, the commercial insurance sector has failed to control prescription costs, assuming, as we all have, that the benefits provided are worth the expense. How much different would our lives be, however, if lower industry profits and fewer legislative protections meant less capital for research and slower product development cycles? Can the American public learn to love last year's antihistamine if it means that Walter can get most of his medication paid for?

NO ←

Ronald Bailey

Goddamn the Pusher Man

Drug companies saved my marriage.

Get that smirk off your face, for this is not a tale of Viagra. Two years ago, I asked Pamela to marry me. She said yes, making me a happy man—arguably the happiest man on Earth. But that tender moment was only possible because of what I am more than willing to call a miracle drug. You see, Pamela owns two cats, and she had made it clear that if I was going to live with her, I was going to have to live with her two cats as well. "I gave up my cats for my first husband, and I'm not going to do it for a second one," she declared.

The problem is that I am allergic to cats. The solution is the new antihistamine Zyrtec, developed by Pfizer in 1995. I take one pill a day and the felines can rub their fluffy tails across my nose without provoking so much as a sniffle. (Zyrtec doesn't cause drowsiness, either.) So now we are living happily ever after in wedded bliss. A month's supply costs $66.25 at my local pharmacy, but what price love?

Yet the development of products such as Zyrtec—not to mention Viagra and birth-control pills—has not bought pharmaceutical companies a lot of love. Quite the opposite. When Al Gore listed "Big Drug Companies" along with "Big Oil, Big Tobacco, and Big Polluters" as foes of the American people in his acceptance speech at [the 2000] Democratic National Convention, he wasn't going out on a limb. He was tapping into widespread bad feelings toward pill makers. John Le Carré, the best-selling British writer famous for his Cold War spy novels, casts pharmaceutical companies as the new global villains in his 2000 novel *The Constant Gardener.* Communist dictators are out as bad guys and drug company CEOs are in.

The pill-pushing industry is now one of the top targets of politicians and much of the public for ire, wrath, and (possibly) regulation. The most frequent complaint is that prescription drugs cost too much, that their costs are spiraling out of control. There's no question that Americans are spending more on prescription drugs than they used to. In 1997, our total spending on drugs increased by 14.2 percent from the previous year; in 1998, it went up 15.7 percent; and in 1999, it rose again by 18.8 percent. During that same time span, the overall inflation rate never rose above 3 percent per annum.

So the drug companies must be gouging patients and health care providers, right? No. Many critics have made the mistake of confusing more spending with higher prices. In other words, prices aren't going up—we're buying more. Spending on prescription drugs is rising rapidly because Americans like me are buying more pills; our medicine cabinets are bulging with new treatments for whatever ails us.

Between 1993 and 1999, overall inflation rose 19 percent while drug prices increased 18.1 percent. In some years inflation outstripped drug price increases, while in others drug prices rose faster than inflation. For example, in 1996 inflation was 3.3 percent and drug prices increased only 1.6 percent; in 1998, inflation rose 1.6 percent and drug prices went up 3.2 percent. The vast majority of the spending increase on drugs—some 78 percent—has occurred because doctors and patients are taking advantage of the more and better drugs that are now available.

During the 1990s, the pharmaceutical industry developed nearly 400 new drugs, many of which act as substitutes for older, more expensive medical treatments. When other industries develop new products that people want—personal computers, say, or cell phones—we typically laud them for their innovation and willingly plunk down our money.

So why are pharmaceutical companies in the doghouse, especially since they are making products that save and enrich our lives? The answer includes political opportunism, large doses of ignorance regarding the drug industry's economics, and an entitlement mindset among many consumers. Those are potent sentiments that, in today's policy climate, are particularly troubling. If enacted, the most common proposed solutions to the prescription drug "problem" would actually undermine an industry that has greatly enriched our quality of life.

Cost Analysis

Just how much are Americans spending on prescription medicines, and what are they getting in return? According to the Bureau of Labor Statistics, the average consumer spends just over 1 percent of her annual income on pharmaceuticals, about the same amount that gets spent on tobacco and alcohol. The elderly, who are by far the largest consumers of medicine, spend roughly 3 percent of their annual income on drugs, about the same amount they spend on entertainment. Households with seniors 65 to 74 years old spend $1,587 on entertainment and $698 on drugs, while those over 74 years old spend $875 on entertainment and $719 on drugs. (The average income for 65–74-year-olds is $28,928; for those over 74 it is $23,937.)

As mentioned before, Americans are indeed spending more on prescription medicines in absolute terms. Average expenditures per household were $301 in 1993 and $370 in 1999. But spending totals aren't the end of the analysis. A more important question is whether we are getting value for our money. According to Columbia University economist Frank Lichtenberg, the answer is absolutely yes. Between 1960 and 1997, life expectancy at birth for Americans rose from 69.7 years to 76.5 years. "Increased drug approvals and health expenditure per person jointly explain just about 100 percent of the observed long-run longevity increase," writes Lichtenberg in a working paper done last year for the National Bureau of Economic Research. Lichtenberg found that for an expenditure of $11,000 on general medical care, there is a gain of one life-year on average. (A life-year in this context is simply an extra year of life that a patient gains by being treated.) However, spending just $1,345 on pharmaceutical research and development gets the same result. Economists have calculated that, on average, people value an extra year of life at about $150,000. (That figure is based on people's willingness to engage in risky jobs.) Assuming an average value of $150,000 per life-year, the benefits from medical care expenditures outweigh the costs by a factor of more than 13; the benefits of drug R&D are more than 100 times greater than its costs. As important, drugs can also reduce health care costs. In "Do (More and Better) Drugs Keep People Out of the Hospital?"—a 1996 study published in the *American Economic Review*—Lichtenberg found that "a $1 increase in pharmaceutical expenditure is associated with a $3.65 reduction in hospital-care expenditure."

The story of stomach-acid-blocking drugs such as Tagamet and Zantac illustrates how drugs save money by keeping patients out of the hospital. In 1977, the year in which such drugs were introduced, surgeons performed some 97,000 operations for peptic ulcers. In 1993, despite population growth, that number had shrunk to 19,000. The shift from surgery to highly effective pills—a change that has made life better for tens of thousands of people with stomach problems—is the sort of quiet development that escapes much attention. The Boston Consulting Group's health care practice reported that it saves patients and insurers at least $224 million in annual medical costs.

Other examples abound. In 1991, for instance, the benefits that drugs offered became painfully apparent when New Hampshire, in a cost-saving measure, adopted spending caps on the number of reimbursable medications that Medicaid patients could receive. The result was that nursing home admissions doubled among chronically ill elderly patients and raised government costs for institutional care by $311,000, which was 20 times more than was "saved" by imposing spending caps on drugs. As John Calfee, a drug policy analyst at the market-oriented American Enterprise Institute [AEI], has noted, drugs that break apart blood clots cut hospitalization and rehabilitation costs for stroke victims by about four times the cost of the drug. In his recent monograph *Prices, Markets and the Pharmaceutical Revolution,* Calfee also reports that schizophrenia drugs costing $4,500 per year save more than $70,000 in annual institutional treatment costs.

A yearlong study of 1,100 patients done by Humana Hospitals found that using drugs to treat congestive heart failure increased pharmacy costs 60 percent, but cut hospital costs by 78 percent, for an overall savings of $9.3 million. Better still, the death rate dropped from an expected 25 percent to 10 percent. In Virginia, an asthma study found that new asthma drugs cut emergency room visits by 42 percent. And, relevant to my cat situation, a study by the consulting firm William M. Mercer concluded that every $1 spent on non-sedating antihistamines yielded a $3.07 return to employers, due to increased productivity and reduced accident costs.

"The ability of pharmaceuticals to reduce the total expenditures for health care, as well as business costs, is important but secondary," concludes Calfee. Modern drug therapy means "patients and consumers . . . are gaining . . . better health, longer life, reduced pain and discomfort, and other blessings."

Obscene Profits

OK, grant some critics of the industry. Drugs dramatically cut some medical costs, they say, but the drug makers are reaping huge—obscene, really—profits. In fact, drug company profits as conventionally calculated do run to as much as 20 percent, while 5 percent profit margins are typical of many other American industries. That 20 percent figure, however, is deceptive, since the standard accounting procedures used to calculate drug company profits write off R&D [research and development] costs as "current expenses." No other industry has nearly as high R&D expenses, so when other industries write off their R&D it doesn't have as much effect on their rate of return calculations. If pharmaceutical R&D were depreciated over time, then annual profits for the industry drop to around 9 percent.

That's still almost double the average rate of return. What explains it? Drug discovery and development is a notoriously risky business. "Some 5,000 to 10,000 molecules are screened and only one will make it to being a drug," explains Kees Been, vice president for business and marketing at Biogen Inc., a leading biotech pharmaceutical company based in Cambridge, Massachusetts. "From discovery to launch takes 12 to 16 years. Only 30 percent of all products ever invented returned more than what was invested in them," adds Been. That means that 70 percent of the drugs currently available for treating and curing people are in fact economic losers for the companies that developed them.

A 1999 study by Duke University economists Henry Grabowski and John Vernon for the Tufts University Center for the Study of Drug Development analyzed the sales of a cohort of drugs introduced between 1988 and 1992. The study found that the top 10 percent of new drugs accounted for more than half the total sales revenues of drugs. "The returns to R&D projects in pharmaceuticals have similar properties to that of venture capital investments," conclude Grabowski and Vernon. In other words, drug companies, like venture capital firms, throw money at a lot of different high-risk projects knowing that virtually none will pan out, but that a few may score real jackpots.

These jackpots cover the losses on the other projects and, perhaps more important, pay for future bets. In this way, revenues from such blockbuster drugs as Prozac for depression, Celebrex for arthritis pain, Viagra for erectile dysfunction, and Lipitor for controlling cholesterol levels do more than cover the costs of the majority of drugs that do not make a profit; they also fuel further research.

Investment in R&D for any given drug is not trivial. Typically, it costs between $300 million and $500 million to bring a single drug from being a gleam in a lab jockey's eye to delivery to the marketplace. Yet one argument that critics often make is that drug companies sell their pills for dozens, if not hundreds, of times more than it costs to make them. The liberal policy magazine *American*

Prospect made just this case in its September 11, 2000, issue, in an article titled, "The Price Isn't Right." The piece cites an analysis that claims Bristol-Myers Squibb can manufacture a patient's 18-month supply of the popular cancer drug Taxol for just $500, but charges over 20 times more than the manufacturing costs.

This kind of "analysis" is just willfully stupid. For many products whose value is essentially embodied in intellectual property—drug makers get a 20-year patent on new drugs—copies can be manufactured very cheaply once the product has been developed. Hence, it may cost hundreds of millions of dollars to create the first copy of a computer program, but the second copy is little more than the cost of the CD onto which it can be downloaded. The same holds true for most pharmaceuticals. Manufacturing that first pill takes millions in conducting research and clinical trials, in processing regulatory filings and building a factory, in establishing distribution channels and generating advertising. The second pill may indeed take only pennies to make physically, but virtually all the money to create it has already been spent by the time that second pill goes into a pharmacist's bin.

"A pill is very small, so people have the intuition that it shouldn't have a high price," says Alison Keith, who recently stepped down as head of economic and science policy analysis at pharmaceutical giant Pfizer. "But a better way to think about our medications is that they are small tablets wrapped in huge envelopes of information."

Double Billing?

A related charge regarding pharmaceutical costs is the idea that patients are actually paying for drugs twice—the first time as taxpayers through government-funded scientific research and again as patients, when they go to their local drugstore to pick up their prescriptions. "Research funded by the public sector—not the private sector—is chiefly responsible for a majority of the medically significant advances that have led to new treatments of disease," argues *The American Prospect.*

Is that true? The annual budget of the National Institutes of Health [NIH], the major government grant-giving institution for medical research, was $17.8 billion in 2000 and is expected to rise to $20.5 billion this year. Meanwhile, the pharmaceutical companies' R&D budgets totaled $26.4 billion last year—almost 50 percent more than the 2000 NIH budget. (Industry R&D expenditures equal more than 20 percent of what pharmaceutical companies make in total sales, making the industry the most research-intensive business in the world.) What roles do government and private-sector research actually play in the drug discovery and development process?

"Government-supported research gets you to the 20-yard line," explains Duke's Grabowski. "Biotech companies get you to the 50-yard line and [the big pharmaceutical companies] take you the rest of the way to the goal line. By and large, government labs don't do any drug development. The real originator of 90 percent of prescription drugs is private industry. It has never been demonstrated that government labs can take the initiative all the way" to drug-store shelves.

George Whitesides, a distinguished professor of biochemistry at Harvard University, similarly appreciates the role of often-government-funded research labs at universities in the early stages of drug development. But he stresses that "pure" research rarely translates into usable products. "The U.S. is the only country in the world that has a system for transmitting science efficiently into new technologies," he argues. That system includes research universities that produce a lot of basic science and get a lot of government money. In turn, startup companies take that lab science and develop it further. "Startups take 50 percent of the risk out of a product by taking it up to clinical trials," explains Whitesides. "Industry has an acute sense of what the problems are that need addressing." Without private industry to mine the insights of university researchers, taxpayers would have paid for a lot of top-notch scientific papers, but few if any medicines.

Frank Lichtenberg, the Columbia economist, has a slightly different take on the question of whether patients are paying twice for drugs. He cites the example of Xalatan, a glaucoma drug developed by Pharmacia & Upjohn. Last April, *The New York Times* ran a news story suggesting that although some of the original research on Xalatan was backed by a $4 million NIH grant in 1982, the "taxpayers have reaped no financial reward on their investment." Not so fast, says Lichtenberg. In 1999, Xalatan represented 7 percent of sales for Pharmacia & Upjohn, so Lichtenberg reasonably assumes that 7 percent of the company's $344 million in corporate income tax payments that year can be attributed to Xalatan. Thus Pharmacia & Upjohn paid about $24 million in income taxes on its 1999 sales of Xalatan. Just counting that one year of increased taxes as if it were the only return ever for a 17-year-old investment, Lichtenberg calculates that this yields a very respectable 11 percent return on the taxpayers' money. In fact, future sales are very likely to be higher, "so the return on the taxpayers' investment is likely to be considerably greater."

Placebo Effect

"Big drug companies are putting more money into advertising and promotion than they are into research and development," said Al Gore on the campaign trail, neatly summarizing another popular complaint against the pharmaceutical industry. This widespread assertion, however, is just plain wrong. In 1999, for instance, the pharmaceutical industry spent $13.9 billion on advertising and promotion. (Half the promotion costs, incidentally, were for drug samples that doctors give to patients for free.) R&D expenditures for 1999 were more than $24 billion.

There are, to be sure, more drug ads around these days. In 1997, the Food and Drug Administration, concerned about a couple of First Amendment lawsuits against its regulations, relaxed its restrictions on advertising prescription drugs. Since then, there has been an explosion of direct-to-consumer television and print ads for prescription drugs. In 1999, pharmaceutical companies spent $1.8 billion appealing directly to consumers. Industry critics charge that advertising directly to consumers causes patients to demand drugs they don't need. As Gore put it, drug makers were nefariously "spending hundreds of millions of dollars on television and on magazine advertising to persuade people to buy newer and more expensive medications when less expensive versions work just as well."

Such charges raise several issues. First, do less-expensive medicines work just as well as those "newer and more expensive ones"? In a study of the benefits and costs of newer drugs, Lichtenberg shows that older drugs are, in general, not as good as newer drugs. Using data from the 1996 Medical Expenditure Panel Survey, an in-depth national survey of the health care expenditures of more than 22,000 people, Lichtenberg developed an econometric model to compare the costs and benefits of using older and newer drugs to treat similar medical conditions. He concluded that "the replacement of older by newer drugs results in reductions in mortality, morbidity, and total medical expenditure." Lichtenberg also found that *"denying people access to branded drugs* [as opposed to cheaper generic drugs] *would increase total treatment costs, not reduce them, and would lead to worse outcomes"* (emphasis in original). Newer is clearly better.

What about the claim that advertising simply tricks consumers into demanding more expensive drugs? Obviously, advertising can generate interest in a product—that, after all, is the whole point. But the idea that advertising can simply create a demand for a worthless product is no less convincing when it comes to medical care than it is for other goods and services. If anything, it is less so in this case, since the advertiser needs to convince two buyers—the patient and her doctor—to make a sale.

More to the point, such criticisms ignore basic realities of the health care market. "There are substantial societal benefits to health from consumer advertising," says Alison Keith from Pfizer. "Patients have a lot of information about themselves that otherwise would not go into the medical system." A survey in 1999 by *Prevention* magazine estimated that direct-to-consumer advertising encouraged nearly 25 million patients to talk with their doctors about illnesses or medical conditions that they had never discussed before. In my case, a television ad for Zyrtec showing people being pursued by herds of allergen-generating cats alerted me to its marriage-saving possibilities. As important, by providing information outside of the traditional doctor-patient relationship, direct-to-consumer advertising can also give patients some protection against incompetent or indifferent physicians who have failed to keep up with new developments.

"The industry . . . also downplays the fact that many 'new' drugs aren't medical breakthroughs," complains *The American Prospect,* jabbing away at the pharmaceutical industry, looking to win its argument on points if not by knockout. "About half of industry research is aimed at developing me-too drugs," that treat problems already addressed by existing medications, it adds. The implication is that companies are simply trying to take market share away from each other without providing any "real" benefits to patients.

Such a scenario ignores the simple fact that companies are likely to be researching similar drugs to begin with and that one firm has to be first to market.

But so-called me-too drugs actually benefit patients, not simply by offering different treatments for similar conditions—Tagamet and Zantac, for instance, have different active ingredients—but by driving down prices in a given treatment category. "The period of one-brand dominance for an innovating drug within a breakthrough therapeutic category has unmistakably shortened," writes AEI's Calfee. This faster competition leads to price cuts among competing medicines. Hence, when new anti-depressant medications were introduced in the mid-1990s, they cost only 53 percent as much as Prozac did when it first hit shelves in 1988 and had the field more or less to itself. Similarly, new cholesterol-lowering drugs that came to market in the mid-1990s cost 60 percent less than pioneering effort Mevacor did when it first showed up in 1987.

First, Do No Harm

The Hippocratic Oath famously insists that doctors do nothing to worsen a patient's condition: First, do no harm. Unfortunately, when it comes to most policy recommendations regarding prescription drugs, the potential for harm, usually in the form of price controls and universal, mandatory coverage, lurks everywhere.

Central to virtually all "reform" agendas is reining in those drug company profits. Will that contain health care costs? "Suppose we seize all pharmaceutical profit," suggested Sidney Taurel, CEO of Eli Lilly & Co., in a speech last October [2000]. "Drugs are just 8 percent of total health care. To simplify the arithmetic, let's stretch and say [profits are] 20 percent of sales. Twenty percent of 8 percent equals just 1.6 percent of total health care costs. Does that sound like a solution to you?" Despite its political appeal, it's not much of one. In fact, that sort of thing would almost certainly retard the development of new drugs by destroying the incentive for research. (It's not called the profit *motive* for nothing.)

Given their relatively small cost as a percentage of health care dollars and overall household consumption, why have drugs raised the ire of politicians and populists so forcefully? The short answer is third-party payments. "Most of the drugs are not being paid for by users. Third parties are paying but not getting the benefits, so they are very concerned about costs," explains AEI's Calfee. As doctors prescribe more drugs to cure and ameliorate the ills that afflict their patients, this means that health insurance and managed-care providers are spending more on drugs. Insurers, in turn, pass along the additional spending to their customers, companies who provide job-based medical coverage, whose bottom lines are squeezed by the additional spending.

In many cases, spending on drugs does lower health care costs, but often enough the new drugs do cost more than earlier, less effective therapies, so third-party payers are shelling out more money while patients are getting greater benefits. From a strictly actuarial point of view, it's cheaper for patients to drop dead of heart attacks than for the government or insurers to pay for years of cholesterol-lowering life-extending drugs. Employers who don't want to pay the rising costs for employee health insurance, and politically potent seniors who have been schooled by Medicare to think that all health care is a right, complain to legislators that drug costs are out of control. Such complaints focus on increased spending on drugs, while ignoring the costs saved through pharmaceutical treatments and the suffering and disability that afflicted patients before pharmaceutical companies developed the new drugs.

The policy initiatives that respond to such complaints are fraught with problems. Those that simply award consumers more money specifically earmarked for drugs amount to little more than corporate welfare, by giving pharmaceutical companies a new revenue stream. More typically, though, policies that address prescription drugs end in some sort of price control scheme that, by undercutting the possible return to investment in the pharmaceutical industry, will over time harm patients by reducing the supply of new drugs. Trying to devise some sort of drug benefit for seniors—a major goal of the Bush administration—is treacherous policy territory, since misguided or ham-handed regulation can have serious consequences, especially with respect to not-yet-invented drugs. During the debate over the Clinton health plan, notes AEI's Calfee, just the threat of price controls spooked pharmaceutical R&D. "Growth in research spending dropped off dramatically from 10 percent annually to about 2 percent per year," according to Calfee.

Yet the perception that drug prices—and drug company profits—are too high is likely to drive policy. Last year, Congress passed legislation allowing the reimportation of drugs manufactured in America from Canada, where drug prices are significantly lower due to price controls, which are in place in some form in virtually all developed nations outside the U.S. The law drew part of its moral authority from the fact that American drug companies routinely sell their drugs abroad at lower prices than they do in the U.S. Why shouldn't Americans get as good a deal? asked lawmakers.

Essentially, companies are selling their products abroad at prices well below their long-run development costs, but above their current manufacturing costs. While the drug companies can make some money this way, it's not enough to generate the profits necessary to fund their enormous R&D costs. Indeed, it is because of our relatively unregulated market that the U.S. provides the rest of the world with new drugs. Over the past two decades, companies in the U.S. have produced nearly 50 percent of the world's leading pharmaceuticals. Today, U.S. drug companies make all 10 of the world's best-selling drugs. Due to other countries' price controls, pharmaceutical research and development has increasingly been centered in the United States.

With regard to Congress' reimportation scheme, former Secretary of Health and Human Services [HHS] Donna Shalala refused to certify the program on the grounds that she "could not demonstrate that it is safe and cost effective." However, if Tommy Thompson, the new HHS secretary, approves the program, it will be Canadians and not Americans who will be in for a rude price shock. "The drug companies will not sell to Canada at the current rate," says Calfee. "They will raise their prices to Canada in order to not undercut their markets in the U.S." As evidence, he cites a 1999 General Accounting Office report which found that a "law requiring drug companies to grant Medicaid the best price offered to managed care firms effectively raised the managed care prices rather than lowered Medicaid prices." Instead of lowering prices, reimportation and matching-discount requirements eliminate any incentive to give discounts at all.

We are entering a golden age of pharmaceutical research. With the completion of the Human Genome Project, "all pharmaceutical targets until the end of time are now known," said Biogen's Kees Been, at a presentation in December at the Massachusetts Institute of Technology. At the same meeting, Sean Lance, CEO of Chiron, a biopharmaceutical company located near San Francisco, predicted, "We are going to win over HIV, malaria, and tuberculosis because of biotech."

Such certitude—bordering on arrogance—would be irredeemably smug, if not for the pharmaceutical industry's track record in raising the quality of life. "In the 1950s and '60s, doctors performed millions of tonsillectomies and put grommets in the ears of children to prevent earaches. Now we know that they don't work," said Lance. "In 10 years' time, we're going to look back and laugh at what we're thinking are complicated issues and technologies today."

If we want the pharmaceutical and biotech companies to find and market new life-saving, life-enhancing drugs to cure and treat heart disease, cancer, dementia, diabetes, AIDS, and other illnesses, then Congress and President Bush would be wise to let the sort of relatively unfettered market competition that has worked well in the past continue into the future. "There is no substitute for the profit motive for inducing and guiding research," says Calfee. In a recent article in *Science,* Jurgen Drews, chairman of International Biomedicine Management Partners and former head of global research at Hoffman-La Roche, concludes that "free markets will be capable of generating the technical and institutional instruments that are needed to apply scientific advances to the solution of societal problems." True enough. But only if we let them.

POSTSCRIPT

Is the Pharmaceutical Industry Responsible for the High Cost of Prescription Drugs?

There appears to be a drug war in America. Rapidly escalating prescription costs are affecting the most vulnerable among us—the elderly. The lack of a pharmacy benefit in Medicare coverage plus the rising costs of many medications causes too many seniors to make tough choices between prescription drugs and other necessities, such as food. Some states, including Maine, Florida, and Michigan, have taken on the drug companies to lower the cost of prescription medications. The pharmaceutical industry has vowed to fight the states on every front. More states are ready to address the problem of rising drug prices under the Medicaid program, and a battle may be looming. See the "War on Drug Prices: States Are Taking Up the Fight to Reduce Prescription Drug Costs," *State Legislatures* (March 2002); "Needed: Rx for Drug Costs," *The Nation* (July 16, 2001); and "Drug Makers See Branded Generics Eating Into Profits," *The Wall Street Journal* (April 17, 2003).

Some American consumers are also fighting back. They are traveling to Mexico and Canada in search of lower prices. Others are asking for generic versions of their medications and also requesting double-dosage pills and splitting them. Often the larger dose pills have a lower unit cost. Still others are shopping online, by mail, or through prescription drug groups. While all of these techniques may save money, critics of the pharmaceutical industry assert that drug companies' rising profits, monopolies on patented drugs, high advertising costs, and political contributions all play a role in creating high prescription costs. See "Undue Influence: Regulation of the Pharmaceutical Industry," *The American Prospect* (August 13, 2001); "Stripping Away Big Pharma's Fig Leaf," *Multinational Monitor* (June 2002); and "Teaching Clinic Lowers Pharmacy Costs: How to Achieve More Cost-Effective Prescribing of Prescription Drugs," *Physician Executive* (January–February 2003).

While new prescription drugs may save lives, it can also be argued that the pharmaceutical industry, via advertising to consumers and physicians, has increased the demand for their products. Television advertisements for heartburn medicine imply that overeating is not a problem if one takes the right pill. Shifting to a healthier lifestyle may help many Americans avoid and reduce their need for costly prescription medications. See "Seven Ways to Save Money on Prescription Drugs," *Harvard Heart Letter* (January 2003).

On the Internet . . .

ACLU In Brief: Workplace Drug Testing

This American Civil Liberties Union site offers information on workplace drug testing and its legal ramifications. Click on the links for the article entitled "Privacy in America: Workplace Drug Testing" and the Legislative Briefing Kit on Drug Testing.

http://www.aclu.org/WorkplaceRights/
WorkplaceRights.cfm?ID=9074&c=178

Euthanasia World Directory

This site is about euthanasia and contains a newsletter and a main page featuring Dr. Jack Kevorkian. There is also a discussion on the book *Final Exit* and numerous citations about different laws regarding assisted suicide.

http://www.finalexit.org

Center for Science in the Public Interest

The Center for Science in the Public Interest is a nonprofit education and advocacy organization that focuses on improving the safety and nutritional quality of our food supply.

http://www.cspinet.org

National Institutes of Health Guide: NIH Policy on Reporting Race and Ethnicity Data: Subjects

This site offers information on the National Institutes of Health's policy on the use of subjects in medical research.

http://grants1.nih.gov/grants/guide/notice-files/
NOT-OD-01-053.html

National Bioethics Advisory Commission: Publications

The full text of the National Bioethics Advisory Commission report *Cloning Human Beings* is available on this site.

http://www.bioethics.gov/reports/

PART 2

Health and Society

*P*ublic policy and medical ethics have not always kept pace with rapidly growing technology and scientific advances. This part discusses some of the major controversies concerning the role of society in health concerns. Should companies automatically test prospective and current employees for drug use? This issue has raised concerns over individual privacy and the overall benefit to employers. Do doctors have a moral obligation to use whatever technology is available to prolong life? This topic has caused agony for the families of terminally ill patients and the families of babies born with severe birth defects. Two other issues concern whether or not the government should regulate the sale, advertisement, and distribution of junk food and what role race should play in the treatment and study of disease. Also discussed in this part is whether human cloning would be of more harm or help to society.

- Is Drug Testing Vital to the Workplace?

- Should Doctors Ever Help Terminally Ill Patients to Commit Suicide?

- Should the Government Regulate the Sale, Advertisement, and Distribution of Junk Food?

- Should Race Play a Role in the Treatment and Study of Disease?

- Should Human Cloning Ever Be Permitted?

ISSUE 5

Is Drug Testing Vital to the Workplace?

YES: William F. Current, from "Cut Costs and Increase Safety With Pre-Employment Drug Testing," *Occupational Hazards* (July 2002)

NO: Jacob Sullum, from "Urine—Or You're Out," *Reason* (November 2002)

ISSUE SUMMARY

YES: William F. Current, president of WFC & Associates, a national consulting firm specializing in drug-free workplace policies, states that pre-employment drug testing is accepted by employees, hassle free, and beneficial to employers.

NO: Jacob Sullum, senior editor of *Reason* magazine, argues that employment-based drug testing is insulting to employees and mostly irrelevant to future job performance.

Drug abuse in the workplace is reported to cost American businesses as much as $60 billion to $100 billion each year and impacts the safety of the work environment. A typical "casual" substance user in the workforce is over twice as likely to take time off, twice as likely to be absent eight or more days each year, three times more likely to be tardy, and three times more likely to have an accident or injure another person. Overall, these workers are less productive on the job. In addition to these measurable costs, there are indirect losses related to impaired judgment, theft, turnover, recruitment and training costs, reduced quality of services and goods, and low morale. It appears that worksite substance abuse seriously affects a company's profits and reduces the company's ability to successfully compete in global markets.

Drug testing has a lot of support from both employers and employees who are concerned about a safe environment on the job. The Institute for a Drug-Free Workplace commissioned a national study that found that close to 100 percent of workers polled believed that drug testing was necessary and should be conducted under certain circumstances. Most employees supported drug testing for transportation workers, including airline pilots and those in safety-sensitive jobs. Both employees and employers believe that workplace drug testing programs are also an effective way to reduce substance abuse.

However, while most employees accept drug testing, and most firms believe that drug testing saves them a significant amount of money, a 1999 report from the American Civil Liberties Union (ACLU) argues that it is an invasion of privacy and a bad investment for employers. The report indicates that the billions of dollars in lost productivity each year is based on a flawed study that compared the annual incomes of households containing marijuana users to households containing nonusers. Absenteeism is the one measure in which drug users and nonusers differ on a consistent basis, according to studies. However, since most studies lump together workers of all ages, this finding may be related to the fact that drug users tend to be young men who are more likely to have high absentee rates regardless of whether or not they use drugs.

While the cost savings of drug testing are difficult to verify, the cost of drug testing is clearer. In 1990 a study of drug testing at government agencies noted that it cost nearly $80,000 for every positive test. Since, according to the ACLU, most drug users are not abusers, the money needed to identify an employee whose substance abuse is actually affecting his or her work could be 10 times as high. The ACLU also asserts that mandatory drug testing makes it harder to attract qualified job seekers, undermines morale, and may force recreational drug users into treatment. In 1998 a study of high-tech companies found that worksite drug testing was actually related to reduced productivity.

In the following selections, William F. Current maintains that establishing and maintaining a drug testing program shows a positive return on investment. Jacob Sullum counters that testing for drugs at the workplace is generally unrelated to job performance and is an invasion of privacy.

William F. Current 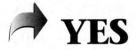 **YES**

Cut Costs and Increase Safety With Pre-Employment Drug Testing

$\mathbf{M}$aintaining a drug-free workplace is an important component of a safe working environment. In this year of major cost-cutting and shrinking budgets for occupational health and safety programs, however, how do you justify drug-screening initiatives? Most significantly, can you show a positive return-on-investment for establishing or continuing a comprehensive drug-testing program?

The good news is yes, you can. The following should help make the case for drug screening.

Pre-Employment Drug Screening: Is It Effective?

Pre-employment testing continues to be, by far, the most common type of drug testing. Pre-employment testing is required as part of several federal government drug-testing programs and regulations, including the Department of Transportation (DOT). It is also required by almost every state that offers workers' compensation premium discounts to employers who conduct drug testing in accordance with specific state guidelines.

Pre-employment testing is virtually hassle-free. Employers are free to conduct pre-employment drug testing just about whenever and of whomever they choose. It's outside the dictates of collective-bargaining agreements per the National Labor Relations Board. Individual state laws that regulate employment drug testing typically allow employers wide latitude when it comes to screening applicants.

A good deal of research supplies evidence for the value of pre-employment drug testing from a pure business standpoint. Drug users are far more costly to employ than nonsubstance-abusing workers. As employers avoid hiring drug users, they save thousands of dollars each year through reduced accidents, absenteeism, theft, violence and health care costs.

American Management Report

According to the American Management Association (AMA), the percentage of the nation's largest companies that conduct drug testing increased from 21.5 percent in 1987 to nearly 88 percent in 1997, the final year the association conducted its annual survey on corporate drug testing practices.

AMA found that nearly 68 percent of firms that drug test screen all applicants, while others only screen applicants for certain positions. The AMA survey also found that between 4 percent and 5 percent of applicants test positive for illicit drugs, which is in line with other national reports, including DOT drug-testing figures. Further, AMA reports that the vast majority of employers do not hire an applicant who tests positive (95 percent), thus avoiding the associated costs of employing a substance abuser.

The Cost of Hiring Drug Users

There are numerous studies on the effectiveness of drug testing and pre-employment testing in particular. One of the most compelling of these surveys was conducted by the U.S. Postal Service (USPS).

In September 1987, the Postal Service initiated a major pre-employment drug testing study sponsored by the federal government. The purpose of the study was to determine the relationship, if any, between drug use and job performance. USPS tested 5,465 applicants between September 1987 and May 1988. Of the 4,375 applicants who were hired, 395 tested positive (63 percent for marijuana, 24 percent for cocaine and 11 percent for all other drugs combined). No one in the Postal Service was aware of the test results except those conducting the study.

After 1.3, 2.4 and 3.3 years, the Postal Service noted remarkable differences between the "test-positive" group and those who tested negative:

- **Involuntary turnover.** At the 1.3-year mark, 15 percent of the test-positive group had been terminated. That represented a 47 percent higher rate than the test-negative group. At 2.4 years, the rate was 69.4 percent higher. At 3.3 years, the rate was 77.4 percent higher.
- **Absenteeism.** After 1.3 years, the test-positive group was 59.4 percent more likely to be heavy users of leave. Those who tested positive for cocaine were four times more likely to be heavy leave users. Those who tested positive for marijuana were 1.5 times more likely to be heavy leave users. After 2.4 years, the positive testers were absent almost 10 percent of the total work hours scheduled. At 3.3 years, they were absent 11 percent of the scheduled work hours.
- **EAP.** After three years of employment, 14 percent of the test-positive group had been referred to the company's employee assistance program (EAP), compared to 7 percent of the test-negative group. If the EAP identified an alcohol problem, the referral rate was 3.5 times higher. If a problem with illicit drugs was identified, the referral rate jumped to 5.7

times higher. Interestingly, the referrals rate between the two groups for emotional, marital or stress-related problems was virtually the same.

- **Disciplinary actions.** The test-positive group had a tendency to face disciplinary action more often than the test-negative group. At the 3.3-year mark, 37 percent of the test-positive group had been disciplined, compared to 19 percent of the test-negative group.

The findings of the Postal Service study show a direct tie to the cost of doing business. USPS projected it would have saved approximately $52 million by 1989 if it had not hired the known drug users in 1987. By 1991, the estimated savings increased to $105 million.

The Liquid I.Q. Test

A strong vote in favor of pre-employment drug testing is found in a study conducted by the federal government of its annual U.S. Household Survey on Drug Abuse. The survey identified regular drug users as employed or unemployed. The employed drug users were asked a series of questions specific to their employment (e.g., Does your employer drug test? How many employers have you had in the past year?).

When the regular drug users employed full-time were asked if they were more likely or less likely to work for a company that conducted drug testing, the answer was beyond what most experts would have predicted. Thirty percent admitted that they were less likely to work for a company that conducted pre-employment screening.

For years, some employers have joked that a pre-employment drug screen is nothing more than a "liquid I.Q." test—a "whiz quiz" for stupid people. The truth is not that simple. Many people who use drugs have a very serious problem with addiction. Although drug users may know that an employer will conduct a pre-employment drug screen, they can't even abstain from drug use for two or three days to increase their chances of obtaining employment.

Undoubtedly, companies that do not conduct pre-employment testing hire more drug users than those that do. That is among the reasons why there has been such an increase in all types of drug testing among smaller companies. For many years, because these smaller firms did not drug test and the larger companies did, the small employers discovered that they had a disproportionate percentage of drug users among their employees. Consequently, these smaller firms were experiencing more of the problems commonly associated with drug abuse in the workplace.

A 220-employee company, Warner Plumbing of Washington, D.C., came to this conclusion and initiated a drug-testing program that included pre-employment, pre-transfer and post-accident screening. The company estimates that it saved approximately $385,000 in one year just from lowering workers' compensation and insurance premiums. Workers' compensation claims fell from an annual average of 111 to 35.

It may be that pre-employment drug testing is some kind of an intelligence test, but it's not the drug-abusing applicant whose intelligence is being tested, it's the employer's. With the most recent reports indicating noteworthy increases in substance abuse in America since Sept. 11, the need for drug testing, and pre-employment screening in particular, may be at one of its highest levels in more than a decade.

While it is a smart business practice to cut costs, it is also a smart business practice to make your organization's workplace as safe as possible. Drug testing can assist you with both.

Jacob Sullum

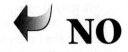 **NO**

Urine—Or You're Out

"I ain't gonna pee-pee in no cup, unless Nancy Reagan's gonna drink it up."

—from the 1987 song "I Ain't Gonna Piss in No Jar," by Mojo Nixon

In 1989 the U.S. Supreme Court upheld a drug test requirement for people seeking Customs Service positions that involved carrying a gun, handling classified material, or participating in drug interdiction. Justice Antonin Scalia dissented, calling the testing program an "immolation of privacy and human dignity in symbolic opposition to drug use." Scalia noted that the Customs Service policy required people to perform "an excretory function traditionally shielded by great privacy" while a monitor stood by, listening for "the normal sounds," after which "the excretion so produced [would] be turned over to the Government for chemical analysis." He deemed this "a type of search particularly destructive of privacy and offensive to personal dignity."

Six years later, Scalia considered a case involving much the same procedure, this time imposed on randomly selected athletes at a public high school. Writing for the majority, he said "the privacy interests compromised by the process of obtaining the urine sample are in our view negligible."

Last March [2002] the Supreme Court heard a challenge to a broader testing program at another public high school, covering students involved in any sort of competitive extracurricular activity, including chess, debate, band, choir, and cooking. "If your argument is good for this case," Justice David Souter told the school district's lawyer, "then your argument is a fortiori good for testing everyone in school." Scalia, who three months later would join the majority opinion upholding the drug test policy, did not seem troubled by that suggestion. "You're dealing with minors," he noted.

That factor helps explain Scalia's apparent equanimity at the prospect of subjecting every high school student to a ritual he had thought too degrading for customs agents. But his nonchalance also reflects the establishment of drug testing as an enduring fact of American life. What was once the "immolation of privacy and human dignity" is now business as usual.

While the government has led the way, the normalization of drug testing has occurred mainly in the private sector, where there are no constitutional barriers to the practice. Today about half of all U.S. employers require applicants, workers, or both to demonstrate the purity of their bodily fluids by peeing into a cup on demand. For defenders of liberty, this situation arouses mixed feelings.

On the one hand, freedom of contract means that businesses should be allowed to set whatever conditions they like for employment. People who don't want to let Home Depot or Wal-Mart sample their urine can take their labor elsewhere. The fact that drug testing is widespread suggests either that applicants and employees do not mind it much or that it enhances profits enough to justify the extra cost of finding and keeping workers, along with the direct expense of conducting the tests.

On the other hand, the profit motive is clearly not the only factor driving the use of drug testing. Through mandates and exhortation, the government has conscripted and enlisted employers to enforce the drug laws, just as it has compelled them to enforce the immigration laws. In 1989 William Bennett, then director of the Office of National Drug Control Policy, cited drug testing by employers as an important element of the government's crackdown on recreational users. "Because anyone using drugs stands a very good chance of being discovered, with disqualification from employment as a possible consequence," he said, "many will decide that the price of using drugs is just too high." The Institute for a Drug-Free Workplace, a coalition that includes companies that supply drug testing services as well as their customers, echoes this line. "Employers and employees have a large stake and legitimate role to play in the 'war on drugs,'" the institute argues. "A high level of user accountability . . . is the key to winning the 'war on drugs.'"

Why Test?

Federal policies requiring or encouraging drug testing by private employers include transportation regulations, conditions attached to government contracts, and propaganda aimed at convincing companies that good corporate citizens need to take an interest in their workers' urine. From the government's perspective, it does not matter whether this urological fixation is good for a company's bottom line. And given the meagerness of the evidence that drug testing makes economic sense, it probably would be much less popular with employers if it were purely a business practice rather than a weapon of prohibition. If it weren't for the war on drugs, it seems likely that employers would treat marijuana and other currently illegal intoxicants the way they treat alcohol, which they view as a problem only when it interferes with work.

Civilian drug testing got a big boost in 1986, when President Reagan issued an executive order declaring that "drugs will not be tolerated in the Federal workplace." The order asserted that "the use of illegal drugs, on or off duty," undermines productivity, health, safety, public confidence, and national security. In addition to drug testing based on "reasonable suspicion" and following accidents, Reagan authorized testing applicants for government jobs and federal employees in "sensitive positions." Significantly, the order was based on the premise that "the Federal government, as the largest employer in the Nation, can and should show the way towards achieving drug-free workplaces." Two years later, Congress approved the Drug-Free Workplace Act of 1988, which demanded that all federal grant recipients and many contractors "maintain a drug-free workplace." Although the law did not explicitly require drug testing, in practice this was the surest way to demonstrate compliance.

Private employers, especially big companies with high profiles and lucrative government contracts (or hopes of getting them), soon followed the government's lead. In its surveys of large employers, the American Management Association found that the share with drug testing programs increased from 21 percent in 1987 to 81 percent in 1996. A 1988 survey by the Bureau of Labor Statistics estimated that drug testing was required by 16 percent of work sites nationwide. Four years later, according to a survey by the statistician Tyler Hartwell and his colleagues, the share had increased to nearly half. In the 1997 National Household Survey on Drug Abuse (the source of the most recent nationwide data), 49 percent of respondents said their employers required some kind of drug testing.

As many as 50 million drug tests are performed each year in this country, generating revenue in the neighborhood of $1.5 billion. That's in addition to the money earned by specialists, such as consultants and medical review officers, who provide related services. Drug testing mainly affects pot smokers, because marijuana is much more popular than other illegal drugs and has the longest detection window. Traces of marijuana can be detected in urine for three or more days after a single dose, so someone who smoked a joint on Friday night could test positive on Monday morning. Daily marijuana smokers can test positive for weeks after their last puff. Because traces linger long after the drug's effects have worn off, a positive result does not indicate intoxication or impairment. (See [box].)

The relevance of such test results to job performance is by no means clear. But in the late 1980s and early '90s, government propaganda and alarmist press coverage combined to persuade employers that they could no longer rely on traditional methods for distinguishing between good and bad workers. "When employers read in *Time* and *Newsweek* and *U.S. News & World Report* that there was an epidemic of drug abuse in America, they got scared like everyone else," says Lewis Maltby, president of the National Workrights Institute and a leading critic of drug testing. "They didn't want some pot-head in their company causing a catastrophe and killing someone. Drug testing was the only answer that anyone presented to them, so they took it." Because drug testing was seen as an emergency measure, its costs and benefits were never carefully evaluated. "Most firms are understandably rigorous about making major investment decisions," Maltby says, "but drug testing was treated as an exception."

My interviews with officials of companies that do drug testing—all members of the Institute for a Drug-Free Workplace—tended to confirm this assessment. They all seemed to feel that drug testing was worthwhile, but they offered little evidence to back up that impression.

Link Staffing Services, a Houston-based temp agency, has been testing applicants since the late 1980s. "In the industry that we are in," says Amy Maxwell,

Link's marketing manager, "a lot of times we get people with undesirable traits, and drug testing can screen them out real quick." In addition to conducting interviews and looking at references, the company does background checks, gives applicants a variety of aptitude tests, and administers the Link Occupational Pre-employment Evaluation, a screening program that "helps identify an applicant's tendency towards characteristics such as absenteeism, theft and dishonesty, low productivity, poor attitude, hostility, and drug use or violence." Although the drug testing requirement may help impress Link's customers, it seems unlikely that urinalysis adds something useful to the information from these other screening tools. Asked if drug testing has affected accident rates or some other performance indicator, Maxwell says, "We probably don't track that, because we have other things that [applicants] have to pass."

TESTING LIMITS:
ALTERNATIVES TO DRUG SCREENING

In the 1980s, when everyone was talking about the dangers posed by addicts in the workplace, Lewis Maltby was executive vice president and general counsel of Drexelbrook Engineering, a Pennsylvania company that designs and manufactures control systems for toxic chemicals. "This company makes a product that, if it doesn't work properly, could cause a Bhopal [1984 tragedy in India in which toxic chemicals burst from a tank at a Union Carbide plant and injured thousands] in the United States," says Maltby, now president of the National Workrights Institute. "Almost every job in the company is safety-sensitive."

Not surprisingly, Drexelbrook considered drug testing. Maltby, long active with the American Civil Liberties Union, was leery of the idea, but he could not deny that the company needed to make sure that its products were assembled properly. Ultimately, he says, "we decided that drug testing was a red herring. The real issue was building an organization that inherently produces quality and reliability."

That meant paying careful attention to every step of the process, including recruitment, hiring, training, supervision, and quality assurance. "We had a very systematic, company-wide program to make sure that everything we did was right," Maltby says. "If we had drug testing, it just would have been a distraction from the real business of safety."

Maltby's experience at Drexelbrook convinced him that drug testing was not the right answer even for employers with serious safety concerns. As an alternative, he has tried to promote impairment testing. Unlike urinalysis, which detects traces of drugs long after their effects have worn off, impairment testing is aimed at assessing an employee's current fitness for duty. The idea is to identify employees who are not up to snuff, whether the cause is illegal drugs, alcohol, medication, illness, personal troubles, or inadequate sleep.

Several different systems are currently available, including an electronic shape recognition test and a device that measures the eye's response to light. But Maltby was able to identify only 18 employers that have ever used such systems, and he suspects the total is not more than 25.

One reason impairment testing has never caught on is its lack of a track record, which poses something of a Catch-22. Although it seems to address safety concerns more directly than urinalysis does, employers are not inclined to adopt a new technology without solid evidence that it works—unless, like drug testing, it has the government's stamp of approval. That factor is especially important for federally regulated industries such as aviation and trucking, where employers who adopted impairment testing would still have to do drug tests.

Impairment testing also could raise new problems for employers, workers, and unions. "The information that impairment testing provides is the information that employers most need, but employers wouldn't know what to do with it," Maltby argues. "Running any kind of a business, you know 5 percent of your employees are showing up not really on the ball every day: sick kids, colds, divorces, death in the family, drugs, alcohol, hangovers. Figuring out what to do about 5 percent of your employees being unfit to work every day is a monumental challenge."

Michael Walsh, a Maryland-based drug testing consultant, calls impairment testing "sort of a holy grail." It's a sound idea in theory, he says, but "I haven't seen a good one that is usable. . . . I have never seen any data that would convince a general audience of scientists that this is the way to go." But then, the same could be said of drug testing.

Eastman Kodak, which makes photographic supplies and equipment, tests all applicants in the U.S. but tests employees (except for those covered by Department of Transportation regulations) only when there's cause for suspicion of drug-related impairment. Wayne Lednar, Eastman Kodak's corporate medical director, says safety was the company's main concern when it started doing drug testing in the 1980s. "Our safety performance has substantially improved in the last 10 years on a worldwide basis, not just in the United States," Lednar says. "That improvement, however, is not one [for which] the drug testing approach in the U.S. can be the major explanation. A very large worldwide corporation initiative driven by line management is really what I think has made the difference in terms of our safety performance."

David Spratt, vice president for medical services at Crown Cork & Seal, a Philadelphia-based packaging manufacturer, says that when the company started doing drug testing in the early 1990s, "there was a concern that employees who used drugs were more likely to have problems in the workplace, be either the perpetrators or the victims of more accidents or more likely to be less productive." But like Eastman Kodak, Crown Cork & Seal does not randomly test employees; once they're hired, workers can use drugs without getting into trouble, as long as they do their jobs well. "What drives our concern is work performance," Spratt says. "If there is such a thing [as] 'recreational use,' we would probably not find that out."

Asked if the company has any evidence that drug testing has been effective, Spratt says: "That's not typically the way these things start out. They typically start out with, 'We gotta do drug testing, because the guy up the street is doing drug testing, and the people who walk in and see his sign will come down and sign up with us for a job.' We're going to get the skewed. . . . They will be a different group who may be less than desirable."

Margot Brown, senior director of communications and public affairs at Motorola, which makes semiconductors, cell phones, and two-way radios, says that when the company started doing drug testing in 1988, "They were trying to control the quality of their products and the safety of their work force." Asked whether the goals were accomplished, she says: "Our productivity per employee did go up substantially. . . . Who knows if that was coincidental or not? Those were good years for Motorola."

Phantom Figures

As those remarks suggest, drug testing became broadly accepted without any firm evidence that it does what it's supposed to do: improve safety, reduce costs, and boost productivity. "Despite beliefs to the contrary," concluded a comprehensive 1994 review of the scientific literature by the National Academy of Sciences, "the preventive effects of drug-testing programs have never been adequately demonstrated." While allowing for the possibility that drug testing could make sense for a particular employer, the academy's panel of experts cautioned that little was known about the impact of drug use on work performance. "The data obtained in worker population studies," it said, "do not provide clear evidence of the deleterious effects of drugs other than alcohol on safety and other job performance indicators."

It is clear from the concessions occasionally made by supporters of drug testing that their case remains shaky. "Only limited information is available about the actual effects of illicit drug use in the workplace," admits the Drug Free America Foundation on its Web site. "We do not have reliable data on the relative cost-effectiveness of various types of interventions within specific industries, much less across industries. Indeed, only a relatively few studies have attempted true cost/benefit evaluations of actual interventions, and these studies reflect that we are in only the very early stages of learning how to apply econometrics to these evaluations."

Lacking solid data, advocates of drug testing tend to rely on weak studies and bogus numbers. The Office of National Drug Control Policy, for example, claims a 1995 study by Houston's Drug-Free Business Initiative "demonstrated that workplace drug testing reduces injuries and worker's compensation claims." Yet the study's authors noted that the "findings concerning organizational performance indicators are based on numbers of cases too small to be statistically meaningful. While they are informative and provide basis for speculation, they are not in any way definitive or conclusive, and should be regarded as hypotheses for future research."

Sometimes the "studies" cited by promoters of drug testing do not even exist. Quest Diagnostics, a leading drug testing company, asserts on its Web site that "substance abusers" are "3.6 times more likely to be involved in on-the-job accidents" and "5 times more likely to file a worker's compensation claim." As

Queens College sociologist Lynn Zimmer has shown, the original source of these numbers, sometimes identified as "the Firestone Study," was a 1972 speech to Firestone Tire executives in which an advocate of employee assistance programs compared workers with "medical-behavioral problems" to other employees. He focused on alcoholism, mentioning illegal drugs only in passing, and he cited no research to support his seemingly precise figures. Another number from the Firestone speech appears on the Web site of Roche Diagnostics, which claims "substance abusers utilize their medical benefits 300 percent more often than do their non-using co-workers."

Roche also tells employers that "the federal government estimates" that "the percentage of your workforce that has a substance abuse problem" is "about 17 percent." This claim appears to be a distortion of survey data collected by the National Institute of Mental Health (NIMH). As summarized by the American Psychiatric Association, the data indicate that "nearly 17 percent of the U.S. population 18 years old and over will fulfill criteria for alcohol or drug abuse in their lifetimes." By contrast, Roche is telling employers that 17 percent of the population meets the criteria *at any given time.* Furthermore, the vast majority of the drug abusers identified by the NIMH were alcoholics, so the number does not bolster the case for urinalysis aimed at catching illegal drug users.

According to a study published last February [2002] in the *Archives of General Psychiatry,* less than 8 percent of the adult population meets the criteria for "any substance use disorder" in a given year, and 86 percent of those cases involve alcohol. The study, based on data from the National Comorbidity Survey, found that 2.4 percent of respondents had a "substance use disorder" involving a drug other than alcohol in the previous year. So Roche's figure—which is also cited by other companies that profit from drug testing, such as RapidCup and eVeriTest—appears to be off by a factor of at least two and perhaps seven, depending upon whether "substance abuse problem" is understood to include alcohol.

Drinking Problems

This ambiguity seems to be deliberate. To magnify the size of the problem facing employers, the government and the drug testing industry routinely conflate illegal drugs with alcohol. But it's clear that employers are not expected to treat drinkers the way they treat illegal drug users. Although drinking is generally not allowed on company time, few employers do random tests to enforce that policy. In 1995, according to survey data collected by Tyler Hartwell and his colleagues, less than 14 percent of work sites randomly tested employees for alcohol. And while 22 percent tested applicants for alcohol, such tests do not indicate whether someone had a drink, say, the night before. In any case, it's a rare employer who refuses to hire drinkers.

When it comes to illegal drugs, by contrast, the rule is zero tolerance: Any use, light or heavy, on duty or off, renders an applicant or worker unfit for employment. "With alcohol, the question has always been not 'Do you consume?' but 'How much?'" notes Ted Shults, chairman of the American Association of

Medical Review Officers, which trains and certifies physicians who specialize in drug testing. "With the illegal drugs, it's always, 'Did you use it?'"

The double standard is especially striking because irresponsible drinking is by far the biggest drug problem affecting the workplace. "Alcohol is the most widely abused drug among working adults," the U.S. Department of Labor notes. It cites an estimate from the Substance Abuse and Mental Health Services Administration that alcohol accounts for 86 percent of the costs imposed on businesses by drug abuse.

In part, the inconsistency reflects the belief that illegal drug users are more likely than drinkers to become addicted and to be intoxicated on the job. There is no evidence to support either assumption. The vast majority of pot smokers, like the vast majority of drinkers, are occasional or moderate users. About 12 percent of the people who use marijuana in a given year, and about 3 percent of those who have ever tried it, report smoking it on 300 or more days in the previous year. A 1994 study based on data from the National Comorbidity Survey estimated that 9 percent of marijuana users have ever met the American Psychiatric Association's criteria for "substance dependence." The comparable figure for alcohol was 15 percent.

According to the testing industry, however, any use of an illegal drug inevitably leads to abuse. "Can employees who use drugs be good workers?" Roche asks in one of its promotional documents. Its answer: "Perhaps, for a while. Then, with extended use and abuse of drugs and alcohol, their performance begins to deteriorate. They lose their edge. They're late for work more often or they miss work all together. . . . Suddenly, one person's drug problem becomes everyone's problem." This equation of use with abuse is a staple of prohibitionist propaganda. "It is simply not true," says the Drug-Free America Foundation, "that a drug user or alcohol abuser leaves his habit at the factory gate or the office door." The message is that a weekend pot smoker should be as big a worry as an employee who comes to work drunk everyday.

Employers respond to the distinctions drawn by the government. Under the Americans With Disabilities Act, for example, alcoholics cannot be penalized or fired without evidence that their drinking is hurting their job performance. With illegal drugs, however, any evidence of use is sufficient grounds for disciplinary action or dismissal.

A Crude Tool

A more obvious reason government policy shapes employers' practices is that many do not want to hire people who break the law. A positive urinalysis "proves someone has engaged in illegal behavior," observes drug testing consultant Michael Walsh, who headed the task force that developed the federal government's drug testing guidelines. "All companies have rules, and this is a way of screening out people who are not going to play by the rules." He concedes that "you are going to rule out some people who would have made really good employees, and you are going to let in some people who make lousy employees." Still, he says, "in a broad way, it's a fairly decent screening device."

Perhaps the strongest evidence in support of drug testing as a screening device comes from research involving postal workers conducted in the late 1980s. A study reported in *The Journal of the American Medical Association* in 1990 found that postal workers who tested positive for marijuana when they were hired were more prone to accidents, injuries, absences, disciplinary action, and turnover. The differences in these rates were relatively small, however, ranging from 55 percent to 85 percent. By contrast, previous estimates had ranged from 200 percent for accidents to 1,500 percent for sick leave. "The findings of this study suggest that many of the claims cited to justify pre-employment drug screening have been exaggerated," the researchers concluded.

Even these comparatively modest results may be misleading. The study's methodology was criticized on several grounds, including an accident measure that gave extra weight to mishaps that occurred soon after hiring. A larger study of postal workers, reported the same year in the *Journal of Applied Psychology,* confirmed the finding regarding absenteeism but found no association between a positive pre-employment drug test and accidents or injuries. On the other hand, workers who had tested positive were more likely to be fired, although their overall turnover rate was not significantly higher.

It's hard to know what to make of such findings. As the National Academy of Sciences noted, "drug use may be just one among many characteristics of a more deviant lifestyle, and associations between use and degraded performance may be due not to drug-related impairment but to general deviance or other factors." On average, people who use illegal drugs may be less risk-averse or less respectful of authority, for example, although any such tendencies could simply be artifacts of the drug laws.

In any case, pre-employment tests, the most common kind, do not catch most drug users. Since people looking for a job know they may have to undergo a drug test, and since the tests themselves are announced in advance, drug users can simply abstain until after they've passed. For light users of marijuana, the drug whose traces linger the longest, a week or two of abstinence is probably enough. Pot smokers short on time can use a variety of methods to avoid testing positive, such as diluting their urine by drinking a lot of water, substituting someone else's urine, or adulterating their sample with masking agents. "Employers are very concerned that there's always a way to cheat on a drug test," says Bill Current, a Florida-based drug testing consultant. "The various validity testing methods that are available are always one step behind the efforts of the drug test cheaters."

Generally speaking, then, drug users applying for jobs can avoid detection without much difficulty. "The reality is that a pre-employment drug test is an intelligence test," says Walsh. The people who test positive are "either addicted to drugs, and can't stay away for two or three days, or just plain stupid. . . . Employers don't want either of those." Alternatively, applicants who fail a drug screen may be especially reckless or lazy. In short, it's not safe to draw conclusions about drug users in general from the sample identified by pre-employment tests. By the same token, however, such tests may indirectly measure characteristics of concern to employers.

The upshot of all this is something that neither supporters nor opponents of drug testing like to admit: Even if drug use itself has little or no impact on job performance—perhaps because it generally occurs outside the workplace—pre-employment testing still might help improve the quality of new hires. If so, however, it's a crude tool. As an index of undesirable traits, testing positive on a drug test could be likened to having a tattoo. Refusing to hire people with tattoos might, on balance, give a company better employees, but not because tattoos make people less productive or more prone to accidents.

How Much?

Maltby, president of the National Workrights Institute, argues that such benefits are too speculative to justify drug testing, and he believes employers are starting to realize that. "Times are tougher than they were 15 years ago," he says. "Money is tighter, and employers are scrutinizing all of their expenditures to see if they are really necessary. Initially, in the late '80s or early '90s, employers looked at drug testing and said, 'Why not?' Now employers look at drug testing like everything else and say, 'Where's the payoff?' And if nobody sees a payoff, programs get cut—or, more often, cut back."

One example is Motorola, which has seen its profits slide recently and plans to eliminate a third of its work force by the end of the year. When Motorola started doing drug testing, the company's communications director says, "The cost wasn't really a factor because we really felt like it was something we should attend to at the time." But Motorola recently scaled back its urinalysis program, which for a decade included random testing of employees; now it tests only applicants.

Motorola's decision may be part of a trend. The share of companies reporting drug testing programs in the American Management Association's surveys of large employers dropped from a peak of 81 percent in 1996 to 67 percent last year. Some of that drop may reflect a new questionnaire the organization started using in 1997. The new survey is less focused on testing, which could have changed the mix of companies that chose to participate. But the downward trend continued after 1997.

Once drug testing became common, it acquired a certain inertia: Employers who didn't do it worried that they might be at a disadvantage in attracting qualified workers or maintaining a positive public image. Employers who did it worried that stopping would hurt their recruitment or reputations. Yet without abandoning drug testing completely, a company can save money by giving up random tests. Even if it keeps random tests, it can save money by testing less frequently—the sort of change that would not be widely noticed.

Still, one reason drug testing endures is that it does not cost very much, especially from the perspective of a large employer. Eastman Kodak, which has more than 100,000 employees worldwide, pays just $12 to $15 per test. Even considering additional expenses (such as the medical review officer's time), and even with thousands of applicants a year, the total cost is a drop in the bucket. Drug tests cost Cork Crown & Seal, which has nearly 40,000 employees worldwide, $25 to $30 per applicant, for a total of less than $100,000 a year. Motorola, which will have about 100,000 employees after this year's cutbacks, spent something like $1 million a year when it was doing random testing of employees—still not a significant concern to a corporation with billions of dollars in revenue (at least, not until profits took a dive).

Small companies, which have always been less inclined to do drug testing, have to pay more per test and are less able to afford it. They also have lower profiles. "If G.M. were to be on the front page of *The Wall Street Journal,* announcing that they dropped their drug testing program, I wouldn't want to own their stock," Maltby says. He recalls a conversation in which the president of a *Fortune* 500 company told him that a few million dollars a year was a small price to pay for the reassurance that drug testing gives stockholders.

The direct costs of drug testing are not the whole story, however. Wayne Sanders, CEO of the paper products giant Kimberly-Clark, has to keep shareholders in mind, but he also worries about the message that drug testing sends to employees. In 1986, when Sanders was the company's head of human resources, managers pressured him to start doing drug testing, arguing that otherwise Kimberly-Clark would get all the addicts rejected by other employers. According to *The Dallas Morning News,* Sanders, "who wasn't about to pee in a bottle," thought the notion was "utter bunk." He successfully argued that "the idea of urine testing was demeaning and completely alien in a culture based on trust and respect."

There is some evidence that the atmosphere created by drug testing can put employers at a disadvantage. A 1998 *Working USA* study of 63 high-tech companies found that pre-employment and random drug testing were both associated with *lower* productivity. The researchers, economists at LeMoyne College in Syracuse, speculated that drug testing programs may create a "negative work environment" that repels qualified applicants and damages employee morale.

The Familiarity Factor

Yet survey data suggest that most Americans have gotten used to the idea that their urine may be part of the price they pay to get or keep a job. In the National Household Survey on Drug Abuse, the share of employees who said they would be less likely to work for a business that tested applicants fell from 8 percent in 1994 to 5 percent in 1997. Random testing of employees was somewhat less popular, with 8 percent saying it would be a negative factor in 1997, compared to 14 percent in 1994. Even among current users of illegal drugs, only 22 percent said pre-employment testing would make a job less appealing in 1997 (down from 30 percent in 1994), while 29 percent said random testing would (down from 40 percent in 1994)—which suggests how ineffective testing is at identifying drug users.

For those who object to drug testing, the natural tendency is to give in and take the test, on the assumption that a few protests are not likely to change a well-established business practice. But in jobs that require a high level of training or experience, even one person's objection can make a difference. An executive with a global management consulting company says he discussed his use of psychedelics with senior management early on "because I didn't want any negative repercussions later." When the company considered starting a drug testing program, he recalls, "I said, 'I'm not going to subject myself to mandatory testing because I don't have a problem. You know I don't have a problem, so testing me is not going to fly. And I think testing a bunch of people you pay upper five figures to mid to upper six figures is silly.' . . . The idea was dropped. I like to think I had some impact on that."

A former librarian who works in sales for a publisher of reference works says he was offered an appealing job with another publisher but balked at taking a drug test, although he has not used illegal drugs in years. He told the company, "I want to take this job, but I can't take a drug test. I think it's invasive. I think it's insulting." The employer dropped the requirement, telling him he could instead sign a statement saying that he doesn't use illegal drugs. Although he ended up not taking the job, he sees the experience as evidence that applicants can have more impact than they might think. "Every single person I've talked with [about drug testing], they don't like it, but they concede," he says. "Even when they say, 'I don't have anything to hide,' they say, 'I really don't like this, but I want the job.'"

Since it sharply reduces the cost that has to be weighed against the uncertain benefits of drug testing, this willingness to go along may be the most important reason, aside from the drug laws, that the practice endures. When push comes to shove, even those who recognize the political roots of drug testing are not inclined to take a stand. A strategic marketer in her 20s who used a variety of drugs in college and still smokes pot occasionally says her attitude toward drug testing has changed. "I think maybe three years ago I would have said, 'Fuck the man. No way am I taking a drug test. I'm standing up for my principles,'" she says. "But now I have to pay my rent, and I have to figure out what's important to me in life: Do I want a really nice apartment, or do I want to hold onto my principles?"

POSTSCRIPT

Is Drug Testing Vital to the Workplace?

Many companies conduct employee drug testing with the belief that the company will save money. These companies also believe that testing is perceived as a means of fighting substance abuse in society. In many firms, employers and workers have committed themselves to create a drug-free work environment and to help many employees in their efforts to stop abusing substances. Drug abuse experts agree that a workplace is an excellent place to reach people and to help them change their lifestyles. Supporting that statement is the recent reductions in the number of workers who tested positive for drugs. In the late 1980s approximately 18 percent of workers tested positive for drugs. Five years later, that number dropped by 50 percent. While other factors may have been responsible, many believe that worksite drug testing played a role in reducing substance abuse.

However, while many companies continue to drug test, alternatives have been proposed. One option, known as impairment testing, is aimed at assessing an employee's current fitness for work. Unlike urinalysis, which detects traces of drugs long after their effects have worn off, the goal of impairment testing is to identify workers who are not performing well and determining the cause. While some poorly performing employees may be substance abusers, others may be suffering from personal problems, lack of sleep, or illness. While impairment testing may be a more holistic approach, the concept could raise new problems, such as what to do with the information. Knowing that employees are working poorly due to personal problems and figuring out how to help them could be a major challenge. See "Testing Limits: Alternatives to Drug Screening," *Reason* (November 2002).

For further reading on the cost factor related to drug testing, see "Money Lost to Addictions: Over $3 Billion in Losses to Ontario Companies Annually," *Northern Ontario Business* (December 2001); "Ontario to Impose 'Urinary Witch-Hunt'?" *The Lancet* (November 25, 2000); and "Pissing Contest," *Reason* (January 2000). For an overview of the issue, see "Drug Testing Is Vital in the Workplace," *USA Today Magazine* (January 1995). Articles that address the privacy issue include "Safety Trumps Privacy in Employee Drug Testing Debates," *Arkansas Business* (March 24, 2003) and "Kentucky Court Upholds Firing Based Solely on Lab Report," *Drug Detection Report* (August 12, 1999).

ISSUE 6

Should Doctors Ever Help Terminally Ill Patients to Commit Suicide?

YES: Richard T. Hull, from "The Case For Physician-Assisted Suicide," *Free Inquiry* (Spring 2003)

NO: Margaret Somerville, from "The Case Against Physician-Assisted Suicide," *Free Inquiry* (Spring 2003)

ISSUE SUMMARY

YES: Richard T. Hull, professor emeritus of philosophy at the State University of New York at Buffalo, asserts that physician-assisted suicide is the only resource terminally ill patients have with which to communicate that their end-of-life care is inadequate.

NO: Margaret Somerville, Gale Professor of Law and professor in the faculty of medicine at the McGill University Centre for Medicine, Ethics, and Law in Montreal, Canada, argues that basic reasons to oppose euthanasia include the sanctity of human life and the harms and risks to individuals and to society. Somerville contends that these reasons outweigh any possible benefits.

Should doctors ever help their patients die? Whereas doctors should provide every support possible to their dying patients, do they have the right or obligation to actually hasten the process of death even if a patient requests it? This topic has been the subject of numerous debates over the past decade.

Some of the practices that were controversial a short time ago in the care of terminally ill patients have become accepted and routine. Many doctors now believe that it is ethical to use "do-not-resuscitate" orders on dying patients, while others feel that it is also acceptable to withhold food and water from patients who are hopelessly ill and dying. The word *euthanasia,* which comes from Greek roots—the prefix *eu,* meaning good, fortunate, or easy, and the word *thanatos,* meaning death—describes a good or easy death. Withdrawing care or treatment (referred to as *passive euthanasia*) may be acceptable to many doctors, but *active euthanasia,* or playing an active role in a patient's death, may not.

One form of active euthanasia, physician-assisted suicide, has been the subject of numerous debates in recent years.

The *Journal of the American Medical Association* published a short article entitled "It's Over, Debbie" (January 8, 1988), which was written by an anonymous physician who described administering a lethal dose of morphine to a young woman with terminal cancer. The doctor stated that her suffering was extreme and that there was absolutely no hope of recovery. The morphine was requested by the patient, who said, "Let's get this over with." The patient died within minutes of receiving the drug, while the doctor looked on. This article generated a great deal of criticism because the doctor had met the patient for the first time that evening and had not consulted with colleagues or family members before making his decision. The doctor did, however, believe he was correctly responding to the patient's request.

Soon after this incident, Dr. Jack Kevorkian assisted in the suicide of an Oregon woman who suffered from Alzheimer's disease. Dr. Kevorkian supplied the woman with a device that he developed—a "suicide machine"—that allowed her to give herself a lethal dose of drugs. Intense criticism followed regarding the ability of Dr. Kevorkian to diagnose the patient's illness (which was not immediately terminal) and whether or not the patient was able to make an informed decision to end her life.

Other physicians contend that many hopelessly ill patients contemplate taking their own lives because their doctors do not help them manage their pain. Pain is one of the principal reasons the sick ask their doctors to help them to die. Many doctors believe that the best antidote to the appeal of doctor-assisted suicide would be better treatment of pain. In "The Quality of Mercy: Effective Pain Treatments Already Exist. Why Aren't Doctors Using Them?" *U.S. News and World Report* (March 17, 1997), the authors maintain that health providers are unwilling to treat pain adequately out of fear of litigation, fear their patients will become addicted, or because they lack adequate knowledge about pain management.

The debate over aided suicide has reached a new plateau. In June 1997 the Supreme Court justices unanimously rejected a plea to declare physician-assisted suicide a constitutional right. The justices did leave the way open for states to legalize the practice. Although most states make aided suicide a crime, legislators in nine states want to repeal the laws. In Oregon voters narrowly approved the legalization of assisted suicide in 1994; a bill to repeal the legislation was rejected in November 1997.

In the following selections, Richard T. Hull supports a patient's right to physician-assisted suicide, stating that it is the only way that a patient can convey the inadequacy of his or her end-of-life care. Margaret Somerville argues that physician-assisted suicide is wrong because it is never justified for one human to take another's life. She also contends that any benefits to physician-assisted suicide would be negated by the overall harm to individuals and society.

Richard T. Hull 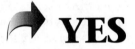 **YES**

The Case For Physician-Assisted Suicide

In early 1997, the medical community awaited the U.S. Supreme Court's decision in *Vacco v. Quill.* Ultimately the high court would overturn this suit, in which doctors and patients had sought to overturn New York's law prohibiting physician-assisted suicide. But it was fascinating to see how much attention physicians suddenly paid to the question of pain management while they were waiting.

Politicians and physicians alike felt shaken by the fact that the suit had made it as far as the Supreme Court. Medical schools scrutinized their curricula to see how, if at all, effective pain management was taught. The possibility that physician-assisted suicide would be declared as much a patient's right as the withdrawal of life-sustaining technology was a clarion call that medicine needed to "houseclean" its attitudes toward providing adequate narcotics for managing pain.

The ability to demand physician aid in dying is the only resource dying patients have with which to "send a message" (as our public rhetoric is so fond of putting it) to physicians, insurers, and politicians that end-of-life care is inadequate. Far too many patients spend their last days without adequate palliation of pain. Physicians sensitive to their cries hesitate to order adequate narcotics, for fear of scrutiny by state health departments and federal drug agents. Further, many physicians view imminent death as a sign of failure in the eyes of their colleagues, or just refuse to recognize that the seemingly endless variety of tests and procedures available to them can simply translate into a seemingly endless period of dying badly. Faced with all this, the ability to demand—and receive—physician aid in dying may be severely compromised patients' only way to tell caregivers that something inhumane stalks them: the inhumanity of neglect and despair.

Many physicians tell me that they feel it is an affront to suppose that their duty to care extends to a duty to kill or assist in suicide. If so, is it not even more an affront, as dying patients and their families tell me, to have to beg for increases in pain medication, only to be told that "We don't want to make you an addict, do we?" or that "Doctor's orders are being followed, and Doctor can't be reached to revise them." If apologists for the status quo fear that a slippery slope will lead to voluntary euthanasia, then nonvoluntary euthanasia, the proponents of change already know that we've been on a slippery slope of inadequate management of suffering for decades.

Let's examine some of the stronger arguments against physician-assisted suicide—while keeping in mind that these arguments may not be the deepest reasons some people oppose it. My lingering sense is that the unspoken problem with physician-assisted suicide is that it puts power where opponents don't want it: in the hands of patients and their loved ones. I want to see if there are ways of sorting out who holds the power to choose the time and manner of dying that make sense.

1. Many severely compromised individuals, in their depression, loneliness, loss of normal life, and despair, have asked their physicians to assist them in dying. Yet later (after physicians resisted their requests and others awakened them to alternative opportunities) they have returned to meaningful lives.

No sane advocate of physician-assisted suicide would deny the importance of meeting the demand to die with reluctance and a reflective, thorough examination of alternative options. The likelihood of profound mood swings during therapy makes it imperative to distinguish between a patient's acute anguish of loss and his or her rational dismay at the prospect of long-term descent into the tubes and machines of intensive care.

But note that, in stories like the above, it is the very possibility of legal physician-assisted suicide that empowers patients to draw attention to their suffering and command the resources they need to live on. Patients who cannot demand to die can find their complaints more easily dismissed as "the disease talking" or as weakness of character.

2. Medicine would be transformed for the worse if doctors could legally help patients end their lives. The public would become distrustful, wondering whether physicians were truly committed to saving lives, or if they would stop striving as soon as it became inconvenient.

Doubtless there are physicians who, by want of training or some psychological or moral defect, lack the compassionate sensitivity to hear a demand for aid in dying and act on it with reluctance, only after thorough investigation of the patient's situation. Such physicians should not be empowered to assist patients to die. I would propose that this power be restricted to physicians whose primary training and profession is in pain management and palliation: they are best equipped to ensure that reasonable alternatives to euthanasia and suicide are exhausted. Further, patients' appeals for assisted suicide should be scrutinized by the same institutional ethics committees that already review requests for the suspension of life-sustaining technology as a protection against patient confusion and relatives' greed.

3. Euthanasia and physician-assisted suicide are incompatible with our obligations to respect the human spirit and human life.

When I hear *all* motives for euthanasia and physician-assisted suicide swept so cavalierly into the dustbin labeled Failure to Respect Human Life, I'm prompted to say, "Really? *Always?*" Those same opponents who find physician-assisted suicide appalling will typically excuse, even acclaim, self-sacrifice on behalf of others. A soldier throws himself on a grenade to save his fellows. A pedestrian leaps into the path of a truck to save a child. Firefighters remain in a collapsing building rather than abandon trapped victims. These, too, are decisions to embrace death, yet we leave them to the conscience of the agent. Why tar all examples of euthanasia and physician-assisted suicide with a common brush? Given that we do not have the power to ameliorate every disease and never will, why withhold from individuals who clearly perceive the financial and emotional burdens their dying imposes on loved ones the power to lessen the duration and extent of those burdens, in pursuit of the values they have worked to support throughout their lives?

Consider also that some suffering cannot be relieved by any means while maintaining consciousness. There are individuals, like myself, who regard conscious life as essential to personal identity. I find it nonsensical to maintain that it is profoundly morally *preferable* to be rendered comatose by drugs while awaiting life's "natural end," than to hasten death's arrival while still consciously able to embrace and welcome one's release. If I am irreversibly comatose, "I" am dead; prolongation of "my life" at that point is ghoulish, and I should not be required to undergo such indignity.

Finally the question, "What kind of life is worth living?" is highly personal. There are good reasons patients diagnosed with a wide range of conditions might not wish to live to the natural end of their diseases. How dare politicians and moralists presume to make these final judgments if they don't have to live with the results? Of course, every demand for physician-assisted suicide must be scrutinized, and determined to be fully informed. To withhold aid in dying beyond that point is, first, barbarically cruel. Second, it only increases the risk that individuals determined to end their lives will attempt to do so by nonmedical means, possibly endangering others or further magnifying their own suffering.

4. The time-honored doctrine of double effect permits administering pain-relieving drugs that have the effect of shortening life, provided the intent of the physician is the relief of the pain and not the (foreseen) death of the patient. Isn't that sufficient?

Others may find comfort in the notion that the intention of the agent, not the consequences of his or her action, is the measure of morality. I do not. In any case, preferences among ethical theories are like preferences among religious persuasions: no such preference should be legislated for all citizens. For the thinker who focuses on consequences rather than intentions, the fact that we permit terminal care regimens to shorten life *in any context* shows that the line has already been crossed. The fact that physicians must, at the insistence of the competent patient or the incompetent patient's duly appointed surrogate, withdraw life-sustaining technology shows that physicians *can* assist patient suicides and can perform euthanasia on those fortunate enough to be dependent on machines. It becomes a matter of simple justice—equal protection before the law—to permit the same privileges to other terminal patients. That the U.S. Supreme Court has ruled against this argument did not dissuade the citizens of the State of Oregon from embracing it. States like New York that have turned back such initiatives must bear the shame of having imposed religious majorities' philosophies on all who suffer.

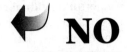
The Case Against Euthanasia and Physician-Assisted Suicide

There are two major reasons to oppose euthanasia. One is based on principle: it is wrong for one human to intentionally kill another (except in justified self-defense, or in the defense of others). The other reason is utilitarian: the harms and risks of legalizing euthanasia, to individuals in general and to society, far outweigh any benefits.

When personal and societal values were largely consistent with each other, and widely shared because they were based on a shared religion, the case against euthanasia was simple: God or the gods (and, therefore, the religion) commanded "Thou shalt not kill." In a secular society, especially one that gives priority to intense individualism, the case for euthanasia is simple: Individuals have the right to choose the manner, time, and place of their death. In contrast, in such societies the case against euthanasia is complex.

Definitions

Definitions are a source of confusion in the euthanasia debate—some of it deliberately engendered by euthanasia advocates to promote their case.[1] Euthanasia is "a deliberate act that causes death undertaken by one person with the primary intention of ending the life of another person, in order to relieve that person's suffering."[2] Euthanasia is not the justified withdrawing or withholding of treatment that results in death. And it is not the provision of pain relief, even if it could or would shorten life, provided the treatment is necessary to relieve the patient's pain or other serious symptoms of physical distress and is given with a primary intention of relieving pain and not of killing the patient.

Secular Arguments Against Euthanasia

1. *Impact on society.* To legalize euthanasia would damage important, foundational societal values and symbols that uphold respect for human life. With euthanasia, how we die cannot be just a private matter

of self-determination and personal beliefs, because euthanasia "is an act that requires two people to make it possible and a complicit society to make it acceptable."[3] The prohibition on intentional killing is the cornerstone of law and human relationships, emphasizing our basic equality.[4]

Medicine and the law are the principal institutions that maintain respect for human life in a secular, pluralistic society. Legalizing euthanasia would involve—and harm—both of them. In particular, changing the norm that we must not kill each other would seriously damage both institutions' capacity to carry the value of respect for human life.

To legalize euthanasia would be to change the way we understand ourselves, human life, and its meaning. To explain this last point requires painting a much larger picture. We create our values and find meaning in life by buying into a "shared story"—a societal-cultural paradigm. Humans have always focused that story on the two great events of each life, birth and death. Even in a secular society—indeed, more than in a religious one—that story must encompass, create space for, and protect the "human spirit." By the human spirit, I do not mean anything religious (although this concept can accommodate the religious beliefs of those who have them). Rather, I mean the intangible, invisible, immeasurable reality that we need to find meaning in life and to make life worth living—that deeply intuitive sense of relatedness or connectedness to others, the world, and the universe in which we live.

There are two views of human life and, as a consequence, death. One is that we are simply "gene machines." In the words of an Australian politician, when we are past our "best before" or "use by" date, we should be checked out as quickly, cheaply, and efficiently as possible. That view favors euthanasia. The other view sees a mystery in human death, because it sees a mystery in human life, a view that does not require any belief in the supernatural.

Euthanasia is a "gene machine" response. It converts the mystery of death to the problem of death, to which we then seek a technological solution. A lethal injection is a very efficient, fast solution to the problem of death—but it is antithetical to the mystery of death. People in postmodern societies are uncomfortable with mysteries, especially mysteries that generate intense, free-floating anxiety and fear, as death does. We seek control over the event that elicits that fear; we look for a terror-management or terror-reduction mechanism. Euthanasia is such a mechanism: While it does not allow us to avoid the cause of our fear—death—it does allow us to control its manner, time, and place—we can feel that we have death under control.

Research has shown that the marker for people wanting euthanasia is a state that psychiatrists call "hopelessness," which they differentiate from depression[5]—these people have nothing to look forward to. Hope is our sense of connection to the future; hope is the oxygen of the human spirit.[6] Hope can be elicited by a sense of connection to a very immediate future, for instance, looking forward to a visit from a loved person, seeing the sun come up, or hearing the dawn chorus. When we are dying, our horizon comes closer and closer, but it still exists until we finally cross over. People need hope if they are to experience dying as the final great act of life, as it should be. Euthanasia converts that act to an act of death.

A more pragmatic, but nevertheless very important, objection to legalizing euthanasia is that its abuse cannot be prevented, as recent reports on euthanasia in the Netherlands have documented.[7] Indeed, as a result of this evidence some former advocates now believe that euthanasia cannot be safely legalized and have recently spoken against doing so.[8]

To assess the impact that legalizing euthanasia might have, in practice, on society, we must look at it in the context in which it would operate: the combination of an aging population, scarce health-care resources, and euthanasia would be a lethal one.

2. *Impact on medicine.*[9] Advocates often argue that euthanasia should be legalized because physicians are secretly carrying it out anyway. Studies[10] purporting to establish that fact have recently been severely criticized on the grounds that the respondents replied to questions that did not distinguish between actions primarily intended to shorten life—euthanasia—and other acts or omissions in which no such intention was present—pain-relief treatment or refusals of treatment—that are not euthanasia.[11] But even if the studies were accurate, the fact that physicians are secretly carrying out euthanasia does not mean that it is right. Further, if physicians were presently ignoring the law against murder, why would they obey guidelines for voluntary euthanasia?

Euthanasia "places the very soul of medicine on trial."[12] Physicians' absolute repugnance to killing people is necessary if society's trust in them is to be maintained. This is true, in part, because physicians have opportunities to kill not open to other people, as the horrific story of Dr. Harold Shipman, the British physician–serial killer, shows.

How would legalizing euthanasia affect medical education? What impact would physician role models carrying out euthanasia have on medical students and young physicians? Would we devote time to teaching students how to administer death through lethal injection? Would they be brutalized or ethically desensitized? (Do we adequately teach pain-relief treatment at present?) It would be very difficult to communicate to future physicians a repugnance to killing in a context of legalized euthanasia.

Physicians need a clear line that powerfully manifests to them, their patients, and society that they do not inflict death; both their patients and the public need to know with absolute certainty—and to be able to trust—that this is the case. Anything that would blur the line, damage that trust, or make physicians less sensitive to their primary obligations to protect life is unacceptable. Legalizing euthanasia would do all of these things.

Conclusion

Euthanasia is a simplistic, wrong, and dangerous response to the complex reality of human death. Physician-assisted suicide and euthanasia involve taking people who are at their weakest and most vulnerable, who fear loss of control or isolation and abandonment—who are in a state of intense "pre-mortem loneliness"[13]—and placing them in a situation where they believe their only alternative is to be killed or kill themselves.

Nancy Crick, a sixty-nine-year-old Australian grandmother, recently committed suicide in the presence of over twenty people, eight of whom were members of the Australian Voluntary Euthanasia Society. She explained: "I don't want to die alone." Another option for Mrs. Crick (if she had been terminally ill—an autopsy showed Mrs. Crick's colon cancer had not recurred) should have been to die naturally with people who cared for her present and good palliative care.

Of people who requested assisted suicide under Oregon's Death with Dignity Act, which allows physicians to prescribe lethal medication, 46 percent changed their minds after significant palliative-care interventions (relief of pain and other symptoms), but only 15 percent of those who did not receive such interventions did so.[14]

How a society treats its weakest, most in need, most vulnerable members best tests its moral and ethical tone. To set a present and future moral tone that protects individuals in general and society, upholds the fundamental value of respect for life, and promotes rather than destroys our capacities and opportunities to search for meaning in life, we must reject euthanasia.

Notes

1. Margaret Somerville, "Death Talk: The Case Against Euthanasia and Physician-Assisted Suicide" (Montreal: McGill Queen's University Press, 2001), p. xiii.

2. Ibid.

3. D. Callahan, "When Self-Determination Runs Amok," *Hastings Center Report* 1992, 22(2): 52–55.

4. House of Lords. Report of the Select Committee on Medical Ethics (London: HMSO, 1994).

5. H.M. Chochinov, K.G. Wilson, M. Enns, et al. "Depression, Hopelessness, and Suicidal Ideation in the Terminally Ill," *Psychosomatics* 39 (1998):366–70, "Desire for Death in the Terminally Ill," *American Journal of Psychiatry* 152 (1995):1185–1191.

6. Margaret Somerville, *The Ethical Canary: Science, Society and the Human Spirit* (Toronto: Viking/Penguin, 2000).

7. K. Foley and H. Hendin, editors, *The Case Against Assisted Suicide: For the Right to End-of-Life Care* (Baltimore: The Johns Hopkins University Press, 2002).

8. S.B. Nuland, "The Principle of Hope," *The New Republic* OnLine 2002: May 22.

9. This section is based on Margaret Somerville, "'Death Talk': Debating Euthanasia and Physician-Assisted Suicide in Australia," *AMAJ* February 17, 2003.

10. H. Kuhse, P. Singer, P. Baume, et al. "End-of-Life Decisions in Australian Medical Practice," *Med J Aust* 166 (1997): 191–96.

11. D.W. Kissane, "Deadly Days in Darwin," K. Foley, H. Hendin, editors, *The Case Against Assisted Suicide: For the Right to End-of-Life Care,* pp. 192–209.

12. W. Gaylin, L. Kass, E.D. Pellegrino, and M. Siegler, "Doctors Must Not Kill," *JAMA* 1988; 259:2139–2140.

13. J. Katz, *The Silent World of Doctor and Patient* (New York: Free Press, 1984).

14. K. Foley and H. Hendin. "The Oregon Experiment," in K. Foley, H. Hendin, editors, *The Case Against Assisted Suicide: For the Right to End-of-Life Care,* p. 269.

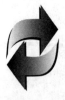

POSTSCRIPT

Should Doctors Ever Help Terminally Ill Patients to Commit Suicide?

As our population ages and the incidence of certain diseases, such as cancer and AIDS, continues to increase, it appears that the ranks of the dying and suffering will grow. In the past, there were limited means of prolonging life; however, due to advances in modern medicine and technology, the dying can be kept alive sometimes for lengthy time periods. Although some doctors are beginning to speak more often of euthanasia, the American Medical Association has unequivocally reaffirmed its opposition to the practice.

Articles that support euthanasia include "Suicide: Should the Doctor Ever Help?" *Harvard Health Letter* (August 1991); "What Quinlan Can Tell Kevorkian About the Right to Die," *The Humanist* (March/April 1997); "The Promise of a Good Death," *The Lancet* (May 16, 1998); and "The Supreme Court and Physician-Assisted Suicide: The Ultimate Right," *The New England Journal of Medicine* (January 2, 1997).

Opponents of euthanasia and physician-assisted suicide argue that all life has value and that doctors do not have the right to end it. These include "Competent Care for the Dying Instead of Physician-Assisted Suicide," *The New England Journal of Medicine* (January 2, 1997); Ezekiel Emanuel and Margaret Battin in "What Are the Potential Cost Savings From Legalizing Physician-Assisted Suicide?" *The New England Journal of Medicine* (July 16, 1998); *Death Talk: The Case Against Euthanasia and Physician-Assisted Suicide* (McGill Queen's University Press, 2001); and *The Case Against Suicide: For the Right to End of Life Care* (The Johns Hopkins University Press, 2002).

Other articles that discuss the issue include "Whose Right to Die?" *The Atlantic Monthly* (March 1997); "A National Survey of Physician-Assisted Suicide and Euthanasia in the United States," *The New England Journal of Medicine* (April 23, 1998); "Clear Thinking About Morally Complex Questions," *The World & I* (July 1998); "Was Dr. Kevorkian Right? Why Cling to a Life Without Savor? Physician-Assisted Suicide, Pro and Con," *Free Inquiry* (Spring 2003); "Quiet Killings in Medical Facilities: Detection and Prevention," *Issues in Law & Medicine* (Spring 2003); "A Dignified Exit? Discussion of Assisted Suicide Cases," *Community Care* (March 13, 2003); and "Should GPs Be Allowed to Help Patients to Die?" *GP* (March 3, 2003).

ISSUE 7

Should the Government Regulate the Sale, Advertisement, and Distribution of Junk Food?

YES: Marion Nestle and Michael F. Jacobson, from "Halting the Obesity Epidemic: A Public Health Policy Approach," *Public Health Reports* (January/February 2000)

NO: Michelle Cottle, from "Heavy Duty," *The New Republic* (May 13, 2002)

ISSUE SUMMARY

YES: Professor of nutrition, Marion Nestle, and executive director of the Center for Science in the Public Interest, Michael F. Jacobson, state that the government should be substantially involved in the regulation of nonnutritious food.

NO: Writer Michelle Cottle argues that nonnutritious food should not be regulated any more than other unhealthy products. Cottle maintains that our relationships to food are too complex for the government to oversee.

The government has taken action to help reduce the number of deaths related to smoking by passing laws that affect the sale, taxation, and advertisement of tobacco products. Should similar laws be enacted to protect the public from the consumption of nonnutritious foods? Should the sale of junk food be restricted and heavily taxed? Should the advertisement of these foods be banned, particularly on children's television?

To promote and encourage healthy dietary choices, the United States government publishes guidelines for nutritious eating, such as the Food Guide Pyramid. The government also requires that all manufactured food carry two items on food labels: nutrition facts and an ingredient list. The nutrition facts portion of the label provides quantitative information on certain nutrients in food and indicates the percentage of the recommended daily amount that is contained in the food. Despite the availability of this information, many Americans do not eat a healthy diet, and the majority of adults and an increasing number of children are overweight.

Food manufacturers, like all companies, advertise and promote their products in order to maximize sales. Many nonnutritious foods are presented to the public in a misleading way for that purpose. For instance, low-fiber, high-sugar breakfast cereals may be sprinkled with vitamins and marketed as a low-fat, nutritious breakfast. Some school districts, working with food manufacturers and producers, sell fast-food items in school cafeterias. Soft drink companies have provided monies and other support to schools that promote their products. Nonnutritious foods, including sugary breakfast cereals, fast food, and candy are heavily advertised on television shows catering to children.

Ethical and legal standards for the food industry, mandated by the government, could address some of these concerns. For instance, clearer food labels that would allow consumers to better understand what they are eating might help to reduce excessive consumption of calories, fat, and sugar. Many nonnutritious food labels seem to have incredibly small or unrealistic serving sizes. A more accurate serving size might be beneficial to consumers. A ban on the advertising of junk foods in public schools, specifically soft drinks, candy, and other items with a high sugar content, could also be enacted as well as increased taxes on these foods. Alcohol and tobacco advertisements are not allowed on children's television, so it would seem reasonable to many to ban the promotion of foods that encourage overeating and obesity. In addition, nonnutritious foods could have health warnings similar to the warnings on cigarette packs or bottles of alcoholic beverages.

However, while there are some similar health outcomes between tobacco use and junk-food consumption, nonnutritious foods are not harmful to nonusers as is environmental tobacco smoke. Tobacco contains an addictive element while a counterpart in food has not been identified. Finally, we do not have to smoke to survive, but we must eat on a regular basis. Some argue that legislating food consumption would be considerably more difficult than implementing tobacco restrictions.

Marion Nestle and Michael F. Jacobson contend that a public health approach is needed to encourage Americans to eat a healthy diet. Michelle Cottle counters that the government should not be regulating food products any more than manufacturers of other unhealthy items.

Marion Nestle and
Michael F. Jacobson

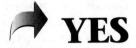 **YES**

Halting the Obesity Epidemic:
A Public Health Policy Approach

In 1974, an editorial in The Lancet *identified obesity as "the most important nutritional disease in the affluent countries of the world,"[1] yet a quarter century later, its prevalence has increased sharply among American adults, adolescents, and children.[2-4] The deleterious effects of obesity on chronic disease risk, morbidity, and mortality[5,6]; its high medical, psychological, and social costs[7,8]; its multiplicity of causes[9]; its persistence from childhood into adulthood[10]; the paucity of successful treatment options[11]; the hazards of pharmacologic treatments[12]; and the complexities of treatment guidelines[13] all argue for increased attention to the prevention of excessive weight gain starting as early in life as possible. Prevention, however, requires changes in individual behavioral patterns as well as eliminating environmental barriers to healthy food choices and active lifestyles—both exceedingly difficult to achieve.*

Because obesity results from chronic consumption of energy (calories) in excess of that used by the body, prevention requires people to balance the energy they consume from food and drinks with the energy expended through metabolic and muscular activity. Although the precise relationship between the diet and activity components of this "equation" is still under investigation,[14,15] it is intuitively obvious that successful prevention strategies—individual and societal—must address both elements.[16]

Guidelines Focus on Individuals

Concern about obesity is not new. By 1952, the American Heart Association had already identified obesity as a cardiac risk factor modifiable through diet and exercise.[17] Subsequently, a number of federal agencies and private organizations devoted to general health promotion or to prevention of chronic conditions for which obesity is a risk factor—coronary heart disease, cancer, stroke, and diabetes—issued guidelines advising Americans to reduce energy intake, raise energy expenditure, or do both to maintain healthy weight (Figure 1). Typically, these guidelines focused on individuals and tended to state the obvious.

From Marion Nestle and Michael F. Jacobson, "Halting the Obesity Epidemic: A Public Health Policy Approach," *Public Health Reports* (January/February 2000).

For example, the otherwise landmark 1977 Senate report on diet and chronic disease prevention, *Dietary Goals for the United States,* omitted any mention of obesity. (The second edition was amended to advise: "To avoid overweight, consume only as much energy [calories] as is expended; if overweight, decrease energy intake and increase energy expenditure."[18]) Overall, the nearly half-century history of such banal recommendations is notable for addressing both physical activity and dietary patterns, but also for lack of creativity, a focus on individual behavior change, and ineffectiveness.

Only rarely did such guidelines deal with factors in society and the environment that might contribute to obesity. Participants in the 1969 White House Conference on Food, Nutrition, and Health recommended a major national effort to reverse the trend toward inactivity in the population through a mass-media campaign focused on milder forms of exercise such as walking or stair-climbing; school physical education programs; and federal funding for community recreation facilities.[19] The 1977 *Dietary Goals* report described certain societal influences on dietary intake, such as television advertising, but made no recommendations for government action beyond education, research, and food labeling.[18]

The most notable exception was the report of a 1977 conference organized by the National Institutes of Health (NIH) to review research and develop recommendations for obesity prevention and management. In one paper, A.J. Stunkard thoroughly reviewed social and environmental influences on obesity.[20] As a result, the conference report included an extraordinarily broad list of proposals for federal, community, and private actions to foster dietary improvements and more active lifestyles. These ranged from coordinated health education and model school programs to changes in regulations for grades of meat, advertising, taxes, and insurance premiums.[21] Some of the proposals cut right to the core of the matter: "Propose that any national health insurance program . . . recognize obesity as a disease and include within its benefits coverage for the treatment of it." "Make nutrition counseling reimbursable under Medicare." and "Fund demonstration projects at the worksite."[22] Perhaps because the recommendations took 23 pages to list, conveyed no sense of priority, would be expensive to implement, but specified no means of funding, they were largely ignored and soon forgotten. Subsequent reports on obesity prevention continued to emphasize individual approaches to decreasing energy intake and increasing energy expenditure without much consideration of the factors in society that act as barriers to such approaches.

National Objectives

Prevention of obesity by individuals and population groups has been an explicit goal of national public health policy since 1980 (see Figure 2). In developing its successive 10-year plans to reduce behavioral risks for disease through specific and measurable health objectives, the US Public Health Service (PHS) said that the government should "lead, catalyze, and provide strategic support" for implementation through collaboration with professional and industry

Figure 1

Examples of Policy Guidelines Published by US Government Agencies and Health Organizations for Prevention of Obesity Through Diet, Exercise, or Both

1952	American Heart Association: *Food for Your Heart*[17]
1965	American Heart Association: *Diet and Heart Disease*
1968	American Heart Association: *Diet and Heart Disease*
1970	White House Conference on Food, Nutrition, and Health[19]
1971	American Diabetes Association: *Principles of Nutrition and Dietary Recommendations*
1974	National Institutes of Health: *Obesity in Perspective*
1974	American Heart Association: *Diet and Coronary Heart Disease*
1977	National Institutes of Health: *Obesity in America*[20,22]
1977	US Senate Select Committee on Nutrition and Human Needs: *Dietary Goals for the United States, 2nd Edition*[18]
1978	American Heart Association: *Diet and Coronary Heart Disease*
1979	US Department of Health, Education, and Welfare: *Healthy People: The Surgeon General's Report on Health Promotion and Disease Prevention*
1979	National Cancer Institute: *Statement on Diet, Nutrition, and Cancer*
1979	American Diabetes Association: *Principles of Nutrition and Dietary Recommendations*
1980	US Department of Agriculture and US Department of Health and Human Services: *Dietary Guidelines for Americans*[24]
1984	National Institutes of Health: *Lowering Blood Cholesterol to Prevent Heart Disease*
1984	American Cancer Society: *Nutrition and Cancer: Cause and Prevention*
1985	National Institutes of Health: *Consensus Development Conference Statement*
1985	US Department of Agriculture and US Department of Health and Human Services: *Dietary Guidelines for Americans, 2nd Edition*
1986	American Heart Association: *Dietary Guidelines for Healthy American Adults*
1986	American Diabetes Association: *Nutritional Recommendations and Principles*
1988	US Department of Health and Human Services: *The Surgeon General's Report on Nutrition and Health*
1988	American Heart Association: *Dietary Guidelines for Healthy American Adults*
1988	National Cancer Institute: *NCI Dietary Guidelines*
1988	National Heart, Lung, and Blood Institute: *National Cholesterol Education Program*
1989	National Research Council: *Diet and Health: Implications for Reducing Chronic Disease Risk*
1990	US Department of Agriculture and US Department of Health and Human Services: *Dietary Guidelines for Americans, 3rd Edition*
1991	American Cancer Society: *Guidelines on Diet, Nutrition, and Cancer*
1993	National Heart, Lung, and Blood Institute: *National Cholesterol Education Program*
1994	American Diabetes Association: *Nutrition Principles for the Management of Diabetes and Related Complications*
1995	US Department of Agriculture and US Department of Health and Human Services: *Dietary Guidelines for Americans, 4th Edition*
1996	American Heart Association: *Dietary Guidelines for Healthy American Adults*
1996	American Diabetes Association: *Nutrition Recommendations and Principles*
1997	American Heart Association: *Guide to Primary Prevention of Cardiovascular Disease*
1997	World Cancer Research Fund and American Institute for Cancer Research: *Food, Nutrition and the Prevention of Cancer: A Global Perspective*
1999	American Heart Association: *Preventive Nutrition: Pediatrics to Geriatrics*

Note: References not indicated are available from the authors on request.

groups.[23] In developing the specific *Promoting Health/Preventing Disease* objectives for obesity prevention and the methods to implement them, PHS suggested that government agencies do such things as work with public and private agencies to distribute copies of the *Dietary Guidelines for Americans*[24] and other educational materials; encourage development of nutrition education and fitness programs through grants to states; and support research on methods to prevent and control obesity among adults and children. Although these obesity objectives were assigned to the Department of Health and Human Services (DHHS), the implementation activities were distributed among multiple agencies within the Department, with no one agency taking lead responsibility. Thus, the Centers for Disease Control and Prevention (CDC) were to encourage adoption of model school curricula, the Food and Drug Administration (FDA) was to develop a mass-media campaign to educate the public about food labels, and NIH was to sponsor workshops and research on obesity. Implementation steps to achieve the physical activity objectives were distributed among at least nine federal agencies.[25] The words used to describe the implementation steps reflected—and continue to reflect—political and funding realities. Government agencies can encourage, publicize, and cooperate with—but usually cannot implement—programs to achieve national obesity objectives.

Nevertheless, evidence of rising rates of obesity in the late 1980s and 1990s[2,13] has focused increasing attention on the need for prevention strategies. In PHS's second 10-year plan, *Healthy People 2000,* the section on physical activity and fitness appears first among the 22 priority areas for behavior change, and the nutrition objectives appear second, emphasizing PHS's view of obesity as a priority public health problem. Among the objectives in these areas, reducing rates of overweight among adults and adolescents appeared second in order only to prevention of cardiovascular disease. *Healthy People 2000* listed specific objectives for promotion of nutrition and physical education in schools, work sites, and communities—public health approaches that would surely create a more favorable environment for prevention of obesity (see Figure 2).[26]

Despite these efforts, the activity levels of Americans appear to have changed little, if at all, from the 1970s to the 1990s.[5,27] Discerning such trends is exceedingly difficult due to the lack of reliable methods for measuring energy expenditure in the population. Moreover, the average caloric intake reported by Americans rose from 1826 kilocalories per day (kcal/d) in 1977–1978 and 1774 kcal/d in 1989–1991[28] to 2002 kcal/d in 1994–1996.[29] No matter how imprecise the data, these trends suggest why average body weights are increasing so significantly. According to data from the 1976–80 and 1988–1994 National Health and Nutrition Examination Surveys, the prevalence of overweight (defined as at or above the 85th percentile of body mass index [BMI] in 1976–1980) rose from 25.4% to 34.9% among American adults, from 24.1% to 33.3% among men and from 26.5% to 36.4% among women; nearly doubled among children ages 6–11 years from 7.6% to 13.7%; and rose from 5.7% to 11.5% among adolescents.[2,4] (The BMI is defined as body weight in kilograms divided by height in meters squared [kg/m^2].) According to the results of telephone surveys conducted by the CDC, the prevalence of obesity (defined as a BMI $\geq$ 30), increased

Figure 2

Principal US Public Health Service Objectives for Reducing the Prevalence of Obesity Through Improved Nutrition and Physical Fitness

Promoting Health/Preventing Disease (1980)[23]

By 1990:

- Reduce the prevalence of significant overweight (>120% ideal weight) among adult men to 10% and among adult women to 17% without nutritional impairment.
- 50% of the overweight population should have adopted weight loss regimens, combining an appropriate balance of diet and physical activity.
- 90% of adults should understand that to lose weight people must either consume foods that contain fewer calories or increase physical activity, or both.

Healthy People 2000 (1990)[26]

By 2000:

- Reduce the prevalence of overweight to no more than 20% of adults and 15% of adolescents.
- Increase to 50% the proportion of overweight people ages 12 and older who have adopted sound dietary practices combined with regular physical activity to attain an appropriate body weight.

Healthy People 2010 (2000)[30]

By 2010:

- Increase to at least 60% the prevalence of healthy weight (body mass index [BMI] 19–25) among adults.
- Reduce to 15% the proportion of adults with BMI $\geq$ 30.
- Reduce to 5% or less the prevalence of obesity in children and adolescents.
- Increase the proportion of schools that teach essential nutrition topics such as balancing food intake and physical activity in at least three grades.
- Increase to at least 85% the proportion of worksites that offer nutrition education and/or weight management programs for employees.
- Increase to at least 75% the proportion of primary care providers who provide or order weight reduction services for patients with cardiovascular disease and diabetes mellitus diagnoses.

The *Healthy People 2010* objectives also address obesity indirectly through specific objectives for increasing moderate and physical activity among children and adults; for encouraging consumption of more healthful diets; for increasing the use of nutrition labels; for reducing sources of unnecessary calories in food products and in restaurant and school meals; for increasing nutrition and physical education in schools; and for improving access to community recreational facilities.[30]

---

from 12% to nearly 18% in just the few years from 1991 to 1998.[2] Trends in prevention and treatment of obesity are also moving in precisely the wrong direction. The proportions of schools offering physical education, overweight people who report dieting and exercising to lose weight, and primary-care physicians who counsel patients about behavioral risk factors for obesity and other conditions have all declined.[7]

In response to these alarming developments, the third PHS 10-year plan, *Healthy People 2010*, continues to emphasize goals related to regular exercise, noting that people with risk factors for coronary heart disease, such as obesity and hypertension, may particularly benefit from physical activity.[30] The first *three* objectives in the nutrition section now focus on increasing the prevalence of healthy weight (BMI 19–25), reducing the prevalence of obesity, and reducing overweight among children and adolescents (Figure 2). But the plan offers little guidance as to how the objectives are expected to be achieved beyond calling for "a concerted public effort" in that direction.[30]

Barriers to Obesity Prevention

Although the impact of obesity on health has been recognized for nearly a half century and its increasing prevalence among adults and children shows no sign of reversal, national action plans consist mostly of wishful thinking and admonitions to individuals rather than public health strategies that could promote more healthful lifestyles (such as those presented by Stunkard in 1977 and later).[20,21] Public health officials need to recognize that when it comes to obesity, our society's environment is "toxic."[31] Unintended consequences of our post-industrial society are deeply rooted cultural, social, and economic factors that actively encourage overeating and sedentary behavior and discourage alterations in these patterns, a situation that calls for more active and comprehensive intervention strategies.

Energy intake   The data indicate that Americans are consuming more calories but are not compensating for them with increased physical activity. If recommendations to consume fewer calories have so little effect, it may be in part because such advice runs counter to the economic imperatives of our food system.[32] While not the sole reason for high caloric intake, massive efforts by food manufacturers and restaurant chains to encourage people to buy their brands must undoubtedly play a role. Promotions, pricing, packaging, and availability all encourage Americans to eat *more* food, not less.

The food industry spends about $11 billion annually on advertising and another $22 billion or so on trade shows, supermarket "slotting fees," incentives, and other consumer promotions.[33] In 1998, promotion costs for popular candy bars were $10 million to $50 million, for soft drinks up to $115.5 million, and for the McDonald's restaurant chain just over a *billion* dollars.[34] Such figures dwarf the National Cancer Institute's $1 million annual investment in the educational component of its 5-A-Day campaign to increase consumption of fruit and vegetables[35] or the $1.5 million budget of the National Heart, Lung, and Blood Institute's National Cholesterol Education Campaign.[36] American children are bombarded daily with dozens of television commercials promoting fast foods, snack foods, and soft drinks.[37] Advertisements for such products are even commonplace in schools, thanks to Channel One, a private venture that provides free video equipment and a daily television "news" program in exchange for mandatory viewing of commercials by students,[38] and school district contracts for exclusive marketing of one or another soft drink in vending machines and sports facilities.[39] Advertising directly affects the food choices of children,[40] who now have far more disposable income than they had several decades ago and far greater influence on their parents' buying habits.[41]

Americans spend about half of their food budget and consume about one-third their daily energy[42] on meals and drinks consumed outside the home, where it is exceedingly difficult to estimate the energy content of the food. About 170,000 fast-food restaurants[43] and three million soft drink vending machines[44] help ensure that Americans are not more than a few steps from immediate sources of relatively non-nutritious foods. As a Coca-Cola Company executive proclaimed, "[T]o build pervasiveness of our products, we're putting ice-cold Coca-Cola classic and our other brands within reach, wherever you look: at the supermarket, the video store, the soccer field, the gas station—everywhere."[45]

Food eaten outside the home, on average, is higher in fat and lower in micronutrients than food prepared at home.[42] Many popular table-service restaurant meals—lunch or dinner—provide 1000 to 2000 kcal each,[46] amounts equivalent to 35% to 100% of a full day's energy requirement for most adults.[47] Restaurants and movie theaters charge just a few cents more for larger-size orders of soft drinks, popcorn, and French fries, and the standard serving sizes of these and other foods have increased greatly in the past decade.[48] For example, in the 1950s, Coca-Cola was packaged only in 6.5-oz bottles; single-serving containers expanded first to 12-oz cans and, more recently, to 20-oz bottles. A 12-oz soft drink provides about 150 kcal, all from sugars, but contains no other nutrients of significance.[49]

Taken together, such changes in the food environment help explain why it requires more and more will power for Americans to maintain an appropriate intake of energy.

Energy expenditure Influencing Americans to increase energy expenditure is as daunting a task as encouraging reductions in energy intake. Twentieth-century labor-saving devices, from automobiles to e-mail, are ubiquitous and have reduced energy needs, as has the shift of a large proportion of the workforce from manual labor to white-collar jobs that require nothing more active than pressing keys on a computer.[50] Wonders of modern civilization such as central heating lessen the energy cost of maintaining body temperature, and air conditioning makes it much more comfortable on hot summer days to stay inside and watch television or play computer games than to engage in outdoor activities. Dangerous neighborhoods—or the perception of danger—discourage people from walking dogs, pushing strollers, playing ball, jogging, or permitting children to play outdoors.[51] Many suburban neighborhoods are structured for the convenience of automobile drivers; they may not have sidewalks and may lack stores, entertainment, or other destinations within walking distance. Meanwhile, the decline in tax support for many public school systems and the need to fulfill competing academic priorities have forced them to relegate physical education to the category of "frill." Many school districts have had to eliminate physical education classes entirely, and fewer and fewer schools offer any opportunity for students to be physically active during the school day.[6] Such barriers make it clear why an attempt to "detoxify" the present environment and create one that fosters healthful activity patterns deserves far more attention than it has received since the 1977 recommendations in *Obesity in America*.[20,22]

Public Health Approaches

In an environment so antagonistic to healthful lifestyles, no quick and easy solution to the problem of obesity should be expected. Meaningful efforts must include the development of government policies and programs that address both the "energy in" and "energy out" components of weight maintenance. Although privately funded campaigns to educate the public and mobilize physicians to combat obesity, such as Shape Up America,[52] are useful adjuncts, they cannot be expected to achieve significant population-wide behavior change. What is needed is *substantial* involvement of and investment by government at all levels. Governmental policies and programs affect many of the environmental determinants of poor diets and sedentary lifestyles. Communities, workplaces, schools, medical centers, and many other venues are subject to federal and other governmental regulations that could be modified to make the environment more conducive to healthful diet and activity patterns. Just as the environmental crisis spurred the public to make a huge financial investment in seeking solutions, so should the obesity epidemic.

In Figure 3, we provide recommendations for a variety of such modifications along with suggestions for new policies targeted to obesity prevention. These recommendations, reflecting the disparate influences on diet and activity, address education, food regulation and advertising, food assistance, health care and the training of health professionals, transportation and urban development, taxation, and the development of federal policy. We offer the suggestions, some of which have been proposed by others,[20,22,53,54] to stimulate discussion of a much wider range of approaches than is typically considered. In doing so, we suggest changes in existing policies and practices[55] that affect health behaviors. We believe these proposals are politically and economically feasible and, collectively, capable of producing a significant effect in helping people to maintain healthy weight. Each of the suggestions could benefit from further discussion and analysis. Here, we comment on just a few of them.

Using media campaigns   Media advertising should be a vital part of any campaign to reduce obesity through promotion of positive changes in behavior, such as eating more fruits, vegetables, and whole grains; switching to lower-fat meat or dairy products; eating fewer hamburgers and steaks; and drinking water instead of soda. Campaigns of this kind can be remarkably effective. For example, the Center for Science in the Public Interest's "1% Or Less" program doubled the market share of low-fat and fat-free milk in several communities through intensive, seven-week paid advertising and public relations campaigns that cost as little as 22 cents per person.[56-58] Those efforts illustrate that advertising can be an affordable, effective method for promoting dietary change—even in the context of media advertising for less nutritious foods. Similar mass-media motivational campaigns could be developed to encourage people to walk, jog, bicycle, and engage in other enjoyable activities that expend energy.

Discouraging TV watching and junk-food advertising   Anti-obesity measures need to address television watching, a major sedentary activity as well as

Figure 3

Reducing the Prevalence of Obesity: Policy Recommendations

Education

- Provide federal funding to state public health departments for mass media health promotion campaigns that emphasize healthful eating and physical activity patterns.
- Require instruction in nutrition and weight management as part of the school curriculum for future health-education teachers.
- Make a plant-based diet the focus of dietary guidance.
- Ban required watching of commercials for foods high in calories, fat, or sugar on school television programs (for example, Channel One).
- Declare and organize an annual National "No-TV" Week.
- Require and fund daily physical education and sports programs in primary and secondary schools, extending the school day if necessary.
- Develop culturally relevant obesity prevention campaigns for high-risk and low-income Americans.
- Promote healthy eating in government cafeterias, Veterans Administration medical centers, military installations, prisons, and other venues.
- Institute campaigns to promote healthy eating and activity patterns among federal and state employees in all departments.

Food labeling and advertising

- Require chain restaurants to provide information about calorie content on menus or menu boards and nutrition labeling on wrappers.
- Require that containers for soft drinks and snacks sold in movie theaters, convenience stores, and other venues bear information about calorie, fat, or sugar content.
- Require nutrition labeling on fresh meat and poultry products.
- Restrict advertising of high-calorie, low-nutrient foods on television shows commonly watched by children or require broadcasters to provide equal time for messages promoting healthy eating and physical activity.
- Require print advertisements to disclose the caloric content of the foods being marketed.

Food assistance programs

- Protect school food programs by eliminating the sale of soft drinks, candy bars, and foods high in calories, fat, or sugar in school buildings.
- Require that any foods that compete with school meals be consistent with federal recommendations for fat, saturated fat, cholesterol, sugar, and sodium content.
- Develop an incentive system to encourage Food Stamp recipients to purchase fruits, vegetables, whole grains, and other healthful foods, such as by earmarking increases in Food Stamp benefits for the purchase of those foods.

Health care and training

- Require medical, nursing, and other health professions curricula to teach the principles and benefits of healthful diet and exercise patterns.
- Require health care providers to learn about behavioral risks for obesity and how to counsel patients about health-promoting behavior change.
- Develop and fund a research agenda focused on behavioral as well as metabolic determinants of weight gain and maintenance, and on the most cost-effective methods for promoting healthful diet and activity patterns.
- Revise Medicaid and Medicare regulations to provide incentives to health care providers for nutrition and obesity counseling and other interventions that meet specified standards of cost and effectiveness.

Transportation and urban development

- Provide funding and other incentives for bicycle paths, recreation centers, swimming pools, parks, and sidewalks.
- Develop and provide guides for cities, zoning authorities, and urban planners on ways to modify zoning requirements, designate downtown areas as pedestrian malls and automobile-free zones, and modify residential neighborhoods, workplaces, and shopping centers to promote physical activity.

Taxes

- Levy city, state, or federal taxes on soft drinks and other foods high in calories, fat, or sugar to fund campaigns to promote good nutrition and physical activity.
- Subsidize the costs of low-calorie nutritious foods, perhaps by raising the costs of selected high-calorie, low-nutrient foods.
- Remove sales taxes on, or provide other incentives for, purchase of exercise equipment.
- Provide tax incentives to encourage employers to provide weight management programs.

Policy development

- Use the National Nutrition Summit to develop a national campaign to prevent obesity.
- Produce a *Surgeon General's Report on Obesity Prevention.*
- Expand the scope of the President's Council on Physical Fitness and Sports to include nutrition and to emphasize obesity prevention.
- Develop a coordinated federal implementation plan for the Healthy People 2010 nutrition and physical activity objectives.

---

one that exposes viewers to countless commercials for high-calorie foods. The average American child between the ages of 8 and 18 spends more than three hours daily watching television and another three or four hours with other media.[59] Television is an increasingly well-established risk factor for obesity and its health consequences in both adults and children.[60,61] At least one study now shows that reducing the number of hours spent watching television or playing video games is a promising approach to preventing obesity in children.[62] Government and private organizations could sponsor an annual "No TV Week" to remind people that life is possible, *even better,* with little or no television and that watching television could well be replaced by physical and social activities that expend more energy. The Department of Education and DHHS could sponsor a national campaign, building on previous work by the nonprofit TV-Free America.[63]

Advertisements for candy, snacks, fast foods, and soft drinks should not be allowed on television shows commonly watched by children younger than age 10. Researchers have shown that younger children do not understand the *concept* of advertising—that it differs from program content and is designed to sell, not inform—and that children of all ages are highly influenced by television commercials to buy or demand the products that they see advertised.[64] It makes no sense for a society to allow private interests to misshape the eating habits of the next generation, and it is time for Congress to repeal the law that blocks the Federal Trade Commission from promulgating industry-wide rules to control advertising during children's television programs.[65]

Promoting physical activity   Federal and state government agencies could do more to make physical activity more attractive and convenient. They could provide incentives to communities to develop safe bicycle paths and jogging trails; to build more public swimming pools, tennis courts, and ball fields; to pass zoning rules favoring sidewalks in residential and commercial areas, traffic-free areas, and traffic patterns that encourage people to walk to school, work, and shopping; and safety protection for streets, parks, and playgrounds. Government could also provide incentives to use mass transit, and disincentives to drive private cars, thereby encouraging people to walk to bus stops and train stations.

Reaching children through the schools   State boards of education and local school boards have an obligation to promote healthful lifestyles. Physical education should again be required, preferably on a daily basis, to encourage students to expend energy and to help them develop lifelong enjoyment of jogging, ball games, swimming, and other low-cost activities. School boards should be encouraged to resist efforts of marketers to sell soda and high-calorie, low-nutrient snack foods in hallways and cafeterias. Congress could support more healthful school meals by insisting that the US Department of Agriculture (USDA) set stricter limits on sales of foods high in energy (calories), fat, and sugar that compete with the sale of balanced breakfasts and lunches.

Adjusting food prices   Price is a factor in food purchases. Lowering by half the prices of fruits and vegetables in vending machines and school cafeterias can result in doubling their sales.[66] The government could adopt policies to decrease the prices of more healthful foods and increase the prices of foods high in energy.[67] Local governments and the media might offer free publicity, awards, or other incentives to restaurants to offer free salads with meals, to charge more for less nutritious foods, and to reduce the prices of more nutritious foods.

Financing Obesity Prevention

The principal barrier to meaningful health-promotion programs is almost always lack of funds, and the educational campaigns and certain other measures we propose would not be inexpensive. But to put such costs in perspective, it is important to understand that the annual costs of direct health care and lost productivity resulting from obesity and its consequences have been estimated at 5.7% of total US health care expenditures, or $52 billion in 1995 dollars.[68] More conservative estimates still suggest that obesity accounts for 1% to 4% of total health care costs.[9] Notwithstanding these enormous costs, Congress and state legislatures provide virtually no funding specifically targeted to anti-obesity measures other than basic research. The $5 million recently granted to the CDC for nutrition and obesity programs represents a small but important step in the right direction.

To compensate for state and federal legislatures' failure to apply general revenues to anti-obesity measures, other commentators have suggested that revenues from taxes on "junk foods" be used to subsidize the costs of more healthful foods.[31] While onerous taxes on commonly purchased products would be highly unpopular and politically unrealistic, small taxes are feasible. Such taxes would likely have little effect on overall sales but could generate sufficient revenues to fund some of the measures that we are suggesting. Legislatures have long levied taxes on products deemed to be unhealthful. Thus, the federal government and states impose taxes on alcoholic beverages and cigarettes; these taxes are supported by large public majorities, especially when the revenues are earmarked for health purposes.[69] Several states currently tax soft drinks and snack foods. In California, for example, soft drinks are the only foods subject to the 7.25% sales tax; we calculate on the basis of population[43] and consumption[70] statistics that this tax alone raises about $200 million per year. A two-cent-per-can tax on soft drinks in Arkansas raises $40 million per year (Personal communication, Tamra Huff, Arkansas Department of Finance and Administration, September 1998). In these and several other states, the tax revenues go into the general treasury. West Virginia, however, uses the revenues from its soft drink tax to support its state medical, dental, and nursing schools, and Tennessee earmarks 21% of the revenues from its tax for cleaning up highway litter.

To fund the television advertisements, physical education teachers, bicycle paths, swimming pools, and other measures that we propose, we suggest that small taxes be levied on several widely used products that are likely to contribute to obesity. We estimate that each of the following hypothetical taxes would generate revenues of about $1 billion per year:

- A 2/3-cent tax per 12 oz on soft drinks.[70]
- A 5% tax on new televisions and video equipment.[43]
- A $65 tax on each new motor vehicle (about 0.3% on a $20,000 car), or an extra penny tax per gallon of gasoline.[43]

A national survey found that 45% of adults would support a one-cent tax on a can of soft drink, pound of potato chips, or pound of butter it the revenues funded a national health education program.[71] Such taxes are too small to raise serious concerns about their regressive nature.

Toward National Action

The USDA and DHHS have announced plans for a National Nutrition Summit, scheduled for May 30–31, 2000. This Summit could catalyze an unprecedented effort to reverse the obesity epidemic. Its focus will be on behavioral factors—especially those that could help prevent overweight and obesity.[72] The Summit provides an ideal opportunity for public and private institutions to initiate the kinds of policies and programs that we are advocating. We believe that the Summit should emphasize ways to improve both government policies and corporate practices that affect individual behavior change.

Government officials could use the Summit to announce actions, including proposed legislation, that their departments will seek to implement (see Figure 3). For example, USDA could announce incentives to encourage Food Stamp recipients to buy more produce, whole grains, and reduced-fat animal products. The Surgeon General could announce a campaign to reduce television watching. Justice Department officials could announce initiatives for reducing inner-city crime to make playing outside safer for children, while the Department of Housing and Urban Development could announce grants for inner-city recreational facilities. The Department of Transportation could announce increased funding to enable states to expand mass transit and provide more bicycle paths. Finally, the futility of current efforts demonstrates the urgent need for research on which to base more effective public health policies. Ending the obesity epidemic will require much greater knowledge of effective diet and activity strategies than is currently available. The research focus must extend beyond genetic, metabolic, and drug development studies to encompass—and emphasize population-based behavioral interventions, policy development, and program evaluation.

Thus, we propose that the measures outlined in Figure 3 be implemented on a trial basis and evaluated for their effectiveness. We do not pretend that these suggestions alone will eliminate obesity from American society, but they will be valuable if they help to produce even small reductions in the rate of obesity, as even modest weight loss confers substantial health and economic benefits.[73] Without such a national commitment and effective new approaches to making the environment more favorable to maintaining healthy weight, we doubt that the current trends can be reversed.

References

1. Infant and adult obesity [editorial]. Lancet 1974;i:17–18.
2. Mokdad AH, Serdula MK, Dietz WH, Bowman BA, Marks JS, Koplan JP. The spread of the obesity epidemic in the United States, 1991–1998. JAMA 1999;282:1519–22.
3. Troiano RP, Flegal KM, Kuczmarski RJ, Campbell SM, Johnson CL. Overweight prevalence and trends for children and adolescents. Arch Pediatr Adolesc Med 1995;149:1085–91.
4. Update: prevalence of overweight among children, adolescents, and adults—United States, 1988–1994. MMWR Morb Mortal Wkly Rep 1997;46:199–202.
5. Must A, Spadano J, Coakley EH, Field AE, Colditz G, Dietz WH. The disease burden associated with overweight and obesity. JAMA 1999;282:1523–9.
6. Allison DB, Fontaine KR, Manson JE, Stevens J, VanItallie TB. Annual deaths attributable to obesity in the United States. JAMA 1999;282: 1530–8.
7. Allison DB, Zannolli R, Narayan KMV. The direct health care costs of obesity in the United States. Am J Public Health 1999;89:1194–9.
8. Rippe JM, Aronne LJ, Gilligan VF, Kumanyika S, Miller S, Owens GM, et al. Public policy statement on obesity and health from the Interdisciplinary Council on Lifestyle and Obesity Management. Nutr Clin Care 1998;1:34–7.
9. Grundy SM. Multifactorial causation of obesity: implications for prevention. Am J Clin Nutr 1998;67(3 Suppl):5365–725.

10. Whitaker RC, Wright JA, Pepe MS, Seidel KD, Dietz WH. Predicting obesity in young adulthood from childhood and parental obesity. N Engl J Med 1997;337:869–73.

11. Methods for voluntary weight loss and control: Technology Assessment Conference statement. Bethesda (MD): National Institutes of Health (US); 1992.

12. Williamson DF. Pharmacotherapy for obesity. JAMA 1999;281:278–80.

13. Expert Panel on the Identification, Evaluation, and Treatment of Overweight in Adults. Clinical guidelines on the identification, evaluation, and treatment of overweight in adults. Bethesda (MD): National Institutes of Health (US); 1998.

14. US Preventive Services Task Force. Guide to clinical preventive services. 2nd ed. Alexandria (VA): International Medical Publishing; 1996.

15. Dalton S. Overweight and weight management. Gaithersburg (MD): Aspen; 1997.

16. Koplan JP, Dietz WH. Caloric imbalance and public health policy. JAMA 1999;282:1579–80.

17. Harvard School of Public Health, Department of Nutrition. Food for your heart: a manual for patient and physician. New York: American Heart Association; 1952.

18. Senate Select Committee on Nutrition and Human Needs (US). Dietary goals for the United States. 2nd ed. Washington: Government Printing Office; 1977.

19. White House Conference on Food, Nutrition, and Health: final report. Washington: Government Printing Office; 1970.

20. Stunkard AJ. Obesity and the social environment: current status, future prospects. In: Bray GA, editor. Obesity in America. Washington: Department of Health, Education, and Welfare (US); 1979. NIH Pub. No.: 79–359.

21. Stunkard A. The social environment and the control of obesity. In: Stunkard AJ, editor. Obesity. Philadelphia: WB Saunders; 1980. p. 438–62.

22. Fullarton JE. Matrix for action: nutrition and dietary practices [appendix]. In: Bray GA, editor. Obesity in America. Washington: Department of Health, Education, and Welfare (US); 1979. p. 241–64. NIH Pub. No.: 79–359.

23. Department of Health and Human Services (US). Promoting health/preventing disease: objectives for the nation. Washington: Government Printing Office; 1980.

24. Department of Agriculture (US) and Department of Health and Human Services (US). Nutrition and your health: dietary guidelines for Americans. Washington: Government Printing Office; 1980.

25. Department of Health and Human Services (US). Promoting health/preventing disease: Public Health Service implementation plans for attaining the objectives for the nation. Public Health Rep 1983; Sept–Oct Suppl.

26. Department of Health and Human Services (US). Healthy People: national health promotion and disease prevention objectives. Washington: Government Printing Office; 1990.

27. Department of Health and Human Services (US). The 1990 Health Objectives for the Nation: a midcourse review. Washington: Office of Disease Prevention and Health Promotion (US); 1986.

28. Life Sciences Research Office, Federation of American Societies for Experimental Biology. Third report on nutrition monitoring in the United States. Vol 2. Prepared for Interagency Board for Nutrition Monitoring and Related Research, US Department of Health and Human Services, US Department of Agriculture. Washington: Government Printing Office; 1995.

29. Department of Agriculture (US). Data Tables: Results from USDA's 1994–96 Continuing Survey of Food Intakes by Individuals and 1994–96 Diet and Health Knowledge Survey, December 1997 [cited 1999 Feb 23]. Available from: URL: http://www.barc.usda.gov/bhnrc/food survey/home.htm.

30. Department of Health and Human Services (US). Healthy People 2010: understanding and improving health. Conference edition. Washington: Government Printing Office; 2000.

31. Battle EK, Brownell KD. Confronting a rising tide of eating disorders and obesity: treatment vs. prevention and policy. Addict Behav 1996;21:755–65.

32. Department of Agriculture, Economic Research Service (US). U.S. Food Expenditures [cited 1999 Dec 11]. Available from: URL: http://www. econ.ag.gov.

33. Gallo AE. The food marketing system in 1996. Agricultural Information Bulletin No. 743. Washington: Department of Agriculture (US); 1998.

34. 44th annual: 100 leading national advertisers. Advertising Age 1999 Sept 27;S1–S46.

35. Gov't & industry launch fruit and vegetable push; but NCI takes back seat. Nutr Week 1992;22(26):1–2.

36. Cleeman JI, Lenfant C. The National Cholesterol Education Program: progress and prospects. JAMA 1998;280:2099–104.

37. Kotz K, Story M. Food advertisements during children's Saturday morning television programming: are they consistent with dietary recommendations? J Am Diet Assoc 1994;94:1296–1300.

38. Hays CL. Channel One's mixed grades in schools. New York Times 1999 Dec 5; Sect. C:1,14–15.

39. Hays CL. Be true to your cola, rah! rah!: battle for soft-drink loyalties moves to public schools. New York Times 1998 Mar 8; Sect. D:1,4.

40. Sylvester GP, Achterberg C, Williams J. Children's television and nutrition: friends or foes. Nutr Today 1995;30(1):6–15.

41. McNeal JU. The kids market: myths and realities. Ithaca (NY): Paramount Market Publishing; 1999.

42. Lin B-H, Frazão E, Guthrie J. Away-from-home foods increasingly important to quality of American diet. Agricultural Information Bulletin No. 749. Washington: Department of Agriculture (US); 1999.

43. Bureau of the Census (US). Statistical abstract of the United States: the national data book: 1997. 117th ed. Washington: Government Printing Office; 1997.

44. Vended bottled drinks. Vending Times 1998;38(9):15,21–2.

45. Annual Report. Atlanta: Coca-Cola Co.; 1997. Available from Coca-Cola Co., One Coca-Cola Plaza, Atlanta GA 30313.

46. Burros M. Losing count of calories as plates fill up. New York Times 1997 Apr 2; Sect. C:1,4.

47. National Research Council. Recommended dietary allowances. 9th rev. ed. Washington: National Academy Press; 1989.

48. Young LR, Nestle M. Portion sizes in dietary assessment: issues and policy implications. Nutr Rev 1995;53:149–58.

49. Jacobson MF. Liquid candy: how soft drinks are harming Americans' health. Washington: Center for Science in the Public Interest; 1998.

50. President's Council on Physical Fitness and Sports (US). Physical activity and health: a report of the Surgeon General. Washington: Department of Health and Human Services (US); 1996.

51. Neighborhood safety and the prevalence of physical inactivity—selected states, 1996. MMWR Morb Mortal Wkly Rep 1999;48:143–6.

52. Welcome to Shape Up America! [cited 1999 Dec 4]. Available from: URL: http://www.shapeup.org.

53. Jeffery RW. Public health approaches to the management of obesity. In: Brownell KD, Fairburn CG, editors. Eating disorders and obesity: a comprehensive handbook. New York: Guilford Press; 1995. p. 558–63.

54. Hirsch J. Obesity prevention initiative. Obes Res 1994;2:569–84.

55. Zepezauer M, Naiman A. Take the rich off welfare. Tucson (AZ): Odonlan Press; 1996.

56. Reger B, Wootan MG, Booth-Butterfield S. Using mass media to promote healthy eating: a community-based demonstration project. Prev Med 1999;29:414–21.

57. Reger B, Wootan MG, Booth-Butterfield S, Smith H. 1% or less: a community-based nutrition campaign. Public Health Rep 1998;113:410–19.

58. Nestle M. Toward more healthful dietary patterns—a matter of policy. Public Health Rep 1998;113;420–3.

59. McClain DL. Where is today's child? probably watching TV. New York Times 1999 Dec 6; Sect. C:18.

60. Anderson RE, Crespo CJ, Bartlett SJ, Cheskin LJ, Pratt M. Relationship of physical activity and television watching with body weight and level of fatness among children: results from the Third National Health and Nutrition Examination Survey. JAMA 1998;279:938–42.

61. Jeffery RW, French SA. Epidemic obesity in the United States: are fast foods and television viewing contributing? Am J Public Health 1998;88:277–80.

62. Robinson TN. Reducing children's television viewing to prevent obesity: a randomized controlled trial. JAMA 1999;282:1561–7.

63. Ryan M. Are you ready for TV-Turnoff Week? Parade 1998 Apr 12;18–19.

64. Fox RF. Harvesting minds: how TV commercials control kids. Westport (CN): Praeger; 1996.

65. Federal Trade Commission Improvements Act of 1980, Pub. L No. 96-252, 94 Stat. 374 (1980).

66. French SA, Story M, Jeffery RW, Snyder P, Eisenberg M, Sidebottom A, Murray D. Pricing strategy to promote fruit and vegetable purchase in high school cafeterias. J Am Diet Assoc 1997;97:1008–10.

67. French SA, Jeffery RW, Story M, Hannan P, Snyder M. A pricing strategy to promote low-fat snack choices through vending machines. Am J Public Health 1997;87:849–51.

68. Wolf AM, Colditz GA. Current estimates of the economic cost of obesity in the United States. Obes Res 1998;6:97–106.

69. Conference Research Center. Special consumer survey report: to tax or not to tax. New York: Conference Board; 1993 Jun.

70. Putnam JJ, Allshouse JE. Food consumption, prices, and expenditures, 1970–97. Statistical Bulletin No. 965. Washington: Department of Agriculture (US); 1999.

71. Bruskin-Goldring Research. Potato chip labels/health programs, January 30–31, 1999. Edison (NJ): Center for Science in the Public Interest; 1999.

72. Department of Agriculture (US) and Department of Health and Human Services (US). National Nutrition Summit: notice of a public meeting to solicit input in the planning of a National Nutrition Summit. Fed Reg 1999;64(Nov 26):66451.

73. Oster G, Thompson D, Edelsberg J, Bird AP, Colditz GA. Lifetime health and economic benefits of weight loss among obese persons. Am J Public Health 1999;89:1536–42.

Michelle Cottle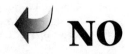 **NO**

Heavy Duty

Kathy Cullinen, head of the Rhode Island Department of Health's Obesity Control Program, spends the first hour or so of our interview doing her best impression of a garden-variety bureaucrat. Soft-spoken and subdued, Cullinen speaks of her small-scale, mostly school-based fat-fighting efforts in a gray, tranquilizing blend of alphabet-soup acronyms (PI, RFP, BRFSS, ASTD) and mind-numbing terms like "needs-assessment" and "incentivize." But as she relaxes and starts talking more expansively about what government *could* do to get citizens in shape—if money and politics were not a consideration—Cullinen's inner revolutionary momentarily claws toward the surface: "Let me give you this wonderful article!" she exhales, popping up from her chair to grab a neatly stapled document from a shelf by the door. "I've been trying to restrain myself, but . . ." Her voice trails off. Handing over the pages, Cullinen appears to have been rendered speechless by her admiration for the ideas within.

The object of Cullinen's ardor is an article dramatically titled "HALTING THE OBESITY EPIDEMIC," from the January/February 2000 issue of *Public Health Reports*. Co-authored by Marion Nestle, the ironically named chair of NYU's Department of Nutrition and Food Studies, and Michael Jacobson, head of the Center for Science in the Public Interest (CSPI), the article offers a public policy blueprint for achieving a Brave New Nonfat World. Proposing everything from junk food taxes to restrictions on soda ads, Nestle and Jacobson argue that public and private health organizations have, for a half-century, foolishly focused anti-obesity efforts on "individual behavior change." "What is needed," they assert, "is *substantial* involvement of and investment by government at all levels." In other words, Uncle Sam needs to start treating your Häagen-Dazs habit like the public health crisis it is.

And slowly, fitfully, he has been. In October 2000 the Centers for Disease Control and Prevention began distributing grants to help states develop anti-obesity programs like Rhode Island's. Legislators in Vermont and California are considering taxing soda and junk food; anti-tax Texas has instead made physical education mandatory in elementary school; and [in 2002] schools in Pennsylvania and Florida sent warning letters home to the parents of overweight kids. Last December the Department of Health and Human Services (HHS) issued "The Surgeon General's Call to Action to Prevent and Decrease Overweight and Obesity," outlining steps communities should take to get in shape. And this April the Internal Revenue Service officially recognized obesity as a disease, ruling that the clinically obese may deduct the cost of their weight-loss treatments.

The reason for all this activity isn't hard to grasp. In 1999 an estimated 61 percent of all adults in the United States were classified as overweight, with nearly 20 percent deemed clinically obese. Moreover, 14 percent of kids and teens are too heavy, putting them at increased risk for health problems once found mostly among adults, such as Type 2 ("adult-onset") diabetes. The surgeon general's office attributes some 300,000 deaths per year to such obesity-linked illnesses as heart disease, diabetes, and cancer. The annual cost of treating these and other fat-related ailments—asthma, arthritis, high blood pressure, gallbladder disease, etc.—tops $117 billion. Accordingly, in recent years fat has increasingly been regarded as a societal rather than a personal problem. Researchers and public health officials contend that we are overweight not simply because of bad habits, bad genes, or bad role models, but because of a bad environment—organized around cars, television, and irresistible bad food. "There are so many pressures on people to be thin and physically fit that if willpower was enough, we'd have the weight problem solved," Kelly Brownell, head of Yale's Center for Eating and Weight Disorders, recently told *USA Today.* "But until the environment changes, it will be impossible to reverse the increasing prevalence of obesity."

Cullinen and her boss, Ann Thacher, chief of health promotion and chronic disease prevention for Rhode Island, could not agree more. "The focus on individual behavior change—like billboard campaigns saying 'Reduce fat in your diet'—has proved ineffective," says Thacher. As a result, the public health community is looking more and more toward "environmental" solutions. These, she explains, could entail everything from encouraging developers to build more inviting staircases (thereby discouraging reliance on elevators), to "incentivizing" the use of public transportation, to encouraging businesses to provide healthful food options and exercise breaks for employees. This sort of "encouragement," of course, would require a wave of new policymaking: new zoning ordinances, new building codes, new education, transportation and public health mandates, and, of course, new taxes. It would also require a fundamental shift in the way people think about food, exercise, entertainment, travel—and pretty much every other aspect of "the American way." For instance, offers Thacher, "you could help people understand that they don't have to drive *everywhere.*"

Some might regard such a massive cultural transformation as impossibly utopian. But Cullinen and Thacher believe it's inevitable, and they take heart from the success of another recent public health crusade: the anti-smoking struggle. "Tobacco has plowed the field for the policy community," says Thacher. As Brownell recently told *USA Today:* "[I]f you look back 30 years ago, you would have said the tobacco industry was massively powerful, and no one would have thought there was any hope for changes. But now you can't smoke in public places, there are sky-high taxes on cigarettes, and states have sued tobacco companies. . . . I think we are at the very beginning of a similar movement with food."

Just a few years back the only people suggesting a parallel between cigarettes and Big Macs were tobacco-industry reps seeking to *discredit* the anti-smoking movement—and their slippery-slope arguments generally elicited jeers. In April 1998, as Congress squabbled over a tobacco bill, a *Washington Post* editorial denounced the fatty-foods analogy as an effort "to change the subject." "Tobacco," the *Post* assured its readers, "is a unique product. Its disastrous effect on public health and the duplicitous history of the industry both make it so. What happens to it is not a threat to other industries."

But the *Post* (among many others) may soon owe those tobacco executives an apology. As early as 1998 Brownell, who is credited with having popularized the "Twinkie tax," caused a stir by informing multiple media outlets, "To me, there is no difference between Ronald McDonald and Joe Camel." By last year the U.S. government was coming around to a similar view. In his obesity "Call to Action," Surgeon General David Satcher cautioned, "Overweight"—anti-fat advocates use the word as a noun as well as an adjective—"and obesity may soon cause as much preventable disease and death as cigarette smoking." Making an oft-cited comparison, the statement noted: "Approximately 300,000 U.S. deaths a year currently are associated with obesity and overweight (compared to more than 400,000 deaths a year associated with cigarette smoking)."

Taking another page from the tobacco playbook, anti-fat advocates deny that eating is purely a matter of personal choice—highlighting fat merchants' aggressive and dishonest sales tactics. Nestle, whose new book *Food Politics* details how the food industry manipulates America's eating habits, explained in a recent phone interview that "where the similarities are really unnerving is in the marketing: The use of targeted messages to children, for example. The use of targeted messages to minorities." The unsuspecting fatties who, under relentless marketing pressure and often at an early age, develop a Hostess habit are—at least in part—victims of forces beyond their control.

But here's where the tobacco-fat analogy begins to fall apart. While the industries' marketing strategies may be similar, and the resulting health costs comparable, the products being marketed are not. Nicotine, as the *Post* rightly implied in its 1998 editorial, is a poisonous, highly addictive substance—addictive in the clinical sense, not in the I-can't-stop-noshing-on-these-Pringles sense. For decades tobacco executives knew this and blatantly lied about it (under oath), even as they worked to hook as many people as possible. McDonald's by contrast may irresponsibly, even intentionally, downplay the unhealthfulness of its fries; but, as even anti-fat warriors admit, those fries are not inherently toxic. And while Keebler tries to entice kids with cartoon pitchmen, no one has accused the company of manipulating the chemistry of Fudge Sticks to ensure clinical addiction.

Most anti-fat warriors admit that their new crusade is trickier than the one against smoking—in no small part because the food industry's argument that any food or drink can be enjoyed in moderation without compromising your health is (though self-interested) basically true. Nonetheless, say anti-fatties, most Americans are either too naïve or too weak to resist the persuasive power of fat merchants. "It's not fair," Nestle told ABC in January. "People are confronted with food in every possible way to eat more. The function of the food industry is to get people to eat more, not less." And, she insisted in our interview, the notion that parents should be responsible for what their kids eat is increasingly unrealistic: "Most parents I know aren't that strong. They're fighting a nine hundred billion dollar a year industry by themselves." Thus, government must level the playing field. CSPI (perhaps the foremost anti-fat organization) has long advocated a restriction on ads for soda and snack food during kids' TV shows. But for better or worse—OK, worse—whipping your target audience into a gotta-have-it frenzy is what advertising is all about. And while using clowns and elves to peddle supercaloric treats to tots may be hardball, it's pretty much par for the course in the jungles of American capitalism. As even Nestle admits, "The seduction of food companies is no different than that of any other companies."

Which is precisely the argument against a government-sponsored war on fat. Does the food industry spend billions each year to make us crave goodies we don't need? Absolutely. So does the fashion industry, the auto industry, and the toy industry. Any number of the products we buy—motorcycles, string bikinis, stiletto heels—can be hazardous to our health when used irresponsibly. There's little doubt that lives and health care dollars would be saved if the government prodded Americans to drop 15 to 50 pounds. We could also reduce skin cancer rates if we taxed flesh-exposing swimsuits and prevent auto accidents if we taxed Corvettes (or teenage drivers). Americans do all kinds of things that are bad for them, and for the most part the government lets us, unless there's a strong likelihood that we will hurt someone other than ourselves.

Which is, incidentally, another important distinction between fatty foods and cigarettes. It's hard to believe the war on tobacco would have gotten out of the barracks were it not for mountains of research demonstrating the health impact of smoking on nonsmokers—innocent bystanders who happened to get in the way of a stray puff in a restaurant or at work. To date, there's no scientific evidence of the dangers of second-hand cholesterol: Watching a co-worker wolf down that Filet-o-Fish may make you want to gag, but it's not going to give you heart disease.

⋘◉⋙

None of this is to say that Americans—especially children—wouldn't benefit from better dietary education. If HHS, state health agencies, or even the American Medical Association want to run public service ads singing the praises of cantaloupe, fantastic. There is also a compelling case that, during school hours, when kids are under government supervision, every effort should be made to provide a healthful environment. Many states are considering prohibiting or restricting vending machines on school grounds. Nestle and CSPI's Jacobson advocate banning junk food ads from the in-class network CHANNEL ONE. And a quick survey of school cafeteria fare—frequently laden with nachos, pizza, burgers, and Tater Tots—suggests that more attention could be paid to the dietary messages we're sending. For that matter, a little classroom time on the ABCs of nutrition and exercise wouldn't hurt either.

But when you move from school to home, and from suggestion to intervention, you quickly enter intellectual quicksand. While anti-tobacco advocates had a clear target, figuring out where to draw the boundary in the fat wars could prove impossibly complicated. As Nestle writes in *Food Politics:* "Unlike the straightforward 'don't smoke' advice, the dietary message can never be 'don't eat.' Instead, it has to be the more complicated and ambiguous 'eat this instead of that,' 'eat this more often than that' and the overall prescription 'eat less.'" The upshot is that it's almost impossible to draw clear, bright lines about which foods merit sanctions such as fat taxes or ad restrictions and which ones don't. One approach is simply to create a broad, amorphous category of "junk food," which is more or less what California did when it created a snack tax in 1991 (aimed primarily at closing its budget gap, not improving health). As a result, California's law was filled with nonsensical distinctions. For instance, Twinkies were taxable; doughnuts weren't. (The following year voters repealed the wildly confusing, highly unpopular measure.) Of course, given the massive economic implications, it's likely that, if implemented nationally, such distinctions would quickly become the focus of intense lobbying—meaning that politics, not merely nutrition, would determine which foods took a hit. To avoid such subjectivity, some anti-fat crusaders have suggested levying taxes according to fat content instead. But that would leave out countless crummy, fattening—yet virtually fat-free—foods (such as Skittles and chocolate syrup), while penalizing relatively healthful foods (think nuts and granola) that are high in fat. At present the anti-fat movement's most popular target seems to be America's soda habit. But a tax that applies to Pepsi ONE and Diet Coke but not to Yoohoo, Gatorade, lemonade, Mocha Frappuccino, or any of the countless sugary fruit "juices" on the market seems decidedly unjust. Now, you could argue—and the anti-fat warriors do—that Diet Coke, while not fattening, has absolutely no nutritional value. But if we're going to expand our list of socially unacceptable products to anything that isn't actively healthy (as opposed to unhealthily fat-promoting), then we are wading deep into Huxleyan territory.

And the quicksand isn't simply intellectual; it's cultural as well. The United States is overwhelmingly fat, but it is not uniformly fat. Poor folks tend to be fatter than rich folks. Minorities tend to be fatter than whites—and not simply because inner-city blacks and Latinos can't afford to eat well. As Thacher and others point out, some of the food traditions woven into Hispanic culture contribute to obesity. In some Latino communities, being plump is still a sign of affluence and is therefore considered desirable. It's one thing for anti-fat warriors to attack a global conglomerate like McDonald's for trying to make people porky; it's quite another to tell an entire community to rethink its culture.

What it comes down to, ultimately, is that our relationships to food are simply too complex for the government to oversee. People eat differently in New Orleans than they do in Berkeley. And they do so, for the most part, because they want to. Sure, we would be a healthier society if everyone ate what they eat in Berkeley. But do we really want to live in a country where the government pressures us to do so? Health is only one measure of a good life, and government is far too crude a mechanism to effectively—or humanely—calibrate its importance for millions of different people. Slippery-slope arguments are usually specious, and until recently the fat-tobacco analogy offered by tobacco execs seemed so as well. But, in fact, we are on the exact slope they claimed, and we are picking up speed. Somewhere, Joe Camel is laughing.

POSTSCRIPT

Should the Government Regulate the Sale, Advertisement, and Distribution of Junk Food?

Americans have been steadily gaining weight over the past 30 years. Children, in particular, have grown heavier for a variety of reasons, including the trend toward less physical activity, more eating away from home, and increased portion sizes. Food manufacturers advertise an increasing array of nonnutritious foods to children while schools offer these foods in the cafeteria. With the success of the antismoking forces, some nutritionists see the government as the answer to the obesity problem. Increased taxes on junk food, warning labels on nonnutritious food packages, and restrictions on advertising have all been discussed as a means of improving the nation's nutritional status. If junk food advertisements were banned from children's television, it is thought that less might be consumed. See "Australian Doctors Call for Ban on Advertising Junk Food to Children," *British Medical Journal* (March 8, 2003); "Congress Protects Those Who Prey on Children," *Knight Ridder/Tribune News Service* (September 21, 1999); and "Oakland Schools Ban Junk Food From Vending Machines," *Nation's Restaurant News* (February 4, 2002).

Other proposals to improve Americans' diets include levying a tax on junk foods such as soft drinks, candy, and sugared cereals. While many states already tax these items if purchased in a restaurant or grocery store, proponents argue that these foods should be taxed regardless of where they are purchased. While this may seem to be a reasonable approach to address the problem, not everyone approves. The food industry, understandably, is not in favor of these measures. See "Restricting 'Junk Foods' in School Is Not the Answer," *Food Technology* (October 2002) and "With 'Fat Tax,' Politicians Will Set Up Camp in Our Fridges," *The Los Angeles Daily Journal* (May 17, 2002). It has even been suggested that the fast-food industry be sued for encouraging obesity. See "Lawyers Poised to Sue US Junk Food Manufacturers," *British Medical Journal* (June 15, 2002) and "Junk Deal: Their Products Cause Heart Disease, Strokes, and Diabetes—Adding Billions to Our Health-Care Bill," *Men's Health* (July–August 2002). Warning labels have also been discussed. Every cigarette pack is sold with a warning label advising smokers that use of the product is hazardous to their health. There are proposals to include similar warnings on junk food packages. See "Junk Food Could Be Sold With Health Warnings," *Campaign* (June 21, 2002).

Should Race Play a Role in the Treatment and Study of Disease?

YES: Esteban González Burchard et al., from "The Importance of Race and Ethnic Background in Biomedical Research and Clinical Practice," *The New England Journal of Medicine* (March 20, 2003)

NO: Richard S. Cooper, Jay S. Kaufman, and Ryk Ward, from "Race and Genomics," *The New England Journal of Medicine* (March 20, 2003)

ISSUE SUMMARY

YES: Physician Esteban González Burchard and his colleagues contend that race should play a role in the treatment and study of disease since there is evidence that the risk of common diseases is determined by race-related genes.

NO: Medical researchers Richard S. Cooper, Jay S. Kaufman, and Ryk Ward argue that the potential for abuse is a reason to disregard race in genetic and medical studies. They also maintain that there is little evidence that the risk of most diseases is linked to race-related genes.

In 1998 former President Bill Clinton committed the country to a goal—eliminating health disparities among racial and ethnic minority populations by the year 2010. The government's plan was to maintain progress on the overall health of Americans while equalizing health care in six areas of priority, which included infant mortality, cancer screening and management, cardiovascular disease, diabetes, HIV/AIDS, and adult and child immunizations against disease. This commitment, known as the Race and Health Initiative, emphasizes key areas of disease management and eradication.

Infant death rates among racial minorities are above the national average. The greatest disparity exists for black Americans, whose infant death rate is more than twice that of white Americans. Cancer and cardiovascular deaths are also higher among racial and ethnic groups, especially among blacks. Diabetes death rates were nearly two and one-half times higher in black and Native American populations and nearly two times higher among Latinos than whites.

Similarly, AIDS has had a disproportionate impact on racial and ethnic minority groups in the United States. Nearly 75 percent of the estimated 40,000 annual HIV infections are among blacks and Latinos. Racial disparities also exist for childhood and adult vaccination rates.

The causes of these differences appear to be a complex mixture of biology, environment, culture, and socioeconomic status. Many racial disparities in health status generally do not reflect biologically determined causes, but rather a groups' living circumstances, access to health care, and cultural factors, such as disenfranchisement with the health care system. There are, however, genetic differences that do affect drug responses and the existence of certain diseases.

Several population-based genetic studies have determined that there are racial differences in the way people metabolize certain medications and respond to treatment. There appear to be many genetic variants affecting drug responses, which should enable health practitioners to prescribe medications and therapies accordingly. Race may play a role in the cause of disease as well. Racially based genetic coding might prove important since some diseases appear in certain groups of people and may be both racially and genetically linked; for example, cystic fibrosis and Tay-Sachs disease.

The subject of medical research and race is, however, related to past abuses and the risk of abuses in the future. Tuskegee, Alabama, will be forever linked in America's memory due to the Tuskegee syphilis study. In the counties surrounding this small southern community, the U.S. Public Health Service ran a 40-year study, from 1932 until 1972, of "untreated syphilis in the male Negro," while telling the men in the study that they were being "treated" for their "bad blood." The outcry over the study, which affected approximately 399 African American men with the disease and 201 controls, led to a lawsuit, Senate hearings, a federal investigation, and new rules about informed consent.

In the following selections, Esteban Gonzàlez Burchard and his colleagues assert that recording a patient's race is the only way in which racially biased health policy and practices may be uncovered. Richard S. Cooper, Jay S. Kaufman, and Ryk Ward counter that the potential for abuse is a reason to disregard race in medical and genetic research.

Esteban González Burchard et al. 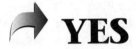 **YES**

The Importance of Race and Ethnic Background in Biomedical Research and Clinical Practice

A debate has recently arisen over the use of racial classification in medicine and biomedical research. In particular, with the completion of a rough draft of the human genome, some have suggested that racial classification may not be useful for biomedical studies, since it reflects "a fairly small number of genes that describe appearance"[1] and "there is no basis in the genetic code for race."[2] In part on the basis of these conclusions, some have argued for the exclusion of racial and ethnic classification from biomedical research.[3] In the United States, race and ethnic background have been used as cause for discrimination, prejudice, marginalization, and even subjugation. Excessive focus on racial or ethnic differences runs the risk of undervaluing the great diversity that exists among persons within groups. However, this risk needs to be weighed against the fact that in epidemiologic and clinical research, racial and ethnic categories are useful for generating and exploring hypotheses about environmental and genetic risk factors, as well as interactions between risk factors, for important medical outcomes. Erecting barriers to the collection of information such as race and ethnic background may provide protection against the aforementioned risks; however, it will simultaneously retard progress in biomedical research and limit the effectiveness of clinical decision making.

Race and Ethnic Background as Geographic and Sociocultural Constructs With Biologic Ramifications

Definitions of race and ethnic background have often been applied inconsistently.[4] The classification scheme used in the 2000 U.S. Census, which is often used in biomedical research, includes five major groups: black or African American, white, Asian, native Hawaiian or other Pacific Islander, and American Indian or Alaska native. In general, this classification scheme emphasizes the geographic region of origin of a person's ancestry.[5] Ethnic background is a broader construct that takes into consideration cultural tradition, common history, religion, and often a shared genetic heritage.

From the perspective of genetics, structure in the human population is determined by patterns of mating and reproduction. Historically, the greatest force influencing genetic differentiation among humans has been geography. Great physical distances and geographic barriers (e.g., high mountains, large deserts, and large bodies of water) have imposed impediments to human communication an interaction and have led to geographically determined endogamous (i.e., within-group) mating patterns resulting in a genetic substructure that largely follows geographic lines. The past two decades of research in population genetics has also shown that the greatest genetic differentiation in the human population occurs between continentally separated groups.

Endogamous mating within continents has given rise to further subdivisions, often corresponding to ethnic groups. This subdivision is again partially attributable to geography but is also associated with social factors, including religion, culture, language, and other sources of group identification. Thus, ethnic groups are genetically differentiated to varying degrees, depending on the extent of reproductive isolation and endogamy, but typically less so than are continentally defined groups.

Considerable debate has focused on whether race and ethnic identity are primarily social or biologic constructs.[6] Unlike a biologic category such as sex, racial and ethnic categories arose primarily through geographic, social, and cultural forces and, as such, are not stagnant, but potentially fluid. Even though these forces are not biologic in nature, racial or ethnic groups do differ from each other genetically, which has biologic implications.

Sociocultural Correlates of Race and Ethnic Background

The racial or ethnic groups described above do not differ from each other solely in terms of genetic makeup, especially in a multiracial and multicultural society such as the United States. Socioeconomic status is strongly correlated with race and ethnic background and is a robust predictor of access to and quality of health care and education, which, in turn, may be associated with differences in the incidence of diseases and the outcomes of those diseases.[7] For example, black Americans with end-stage renal disease are referred for renal transplantation at lower rates than white Americans.[8] Black Americans are also referred for cardiac catheterization less frequently than white Americans.[9] In some cases, these differences may be due to bias on the part of physicians and discriminatory practices in medicine.[10] Nonetheless, racial or ethnic differences in the outcomes of disease sometimes persist even when discrepancies in the use of interventions known to be beneficial are considered. For example, the rate of complications from type 2 diabetes mellitus varies according to racial or ethnic category among members of the same health maintenance organization, despite uniform utilization of outpatient services and after adjustment for levels of education and income, health behavior, and clinical characteristics.[11] The evaluation of whether genetic (as well as nongenetic) differences underlie racial disparities is appropriate in cases in which important racial and ethnic differences persist after socioeconomic status and access to care are properly taken into account.

Evidence of Genetic Differentiation Among Races

There are estimated to be at least 15 million genetic polymorphisms,[12] and an as yet undefined subgroup of these polymorphisms underlie variation in normal and disease traits. The importance of such variation is underscored by the fact that a change of only a single base pair is required to cause many well-known inherited diseases, such as sickle cell disease, or to increase the risk of common disorders, such as Alzheimer's disease. Studies in population genetics have revealed great genetic variation within racial or ethnic subpopulations, but also substantial variation among the five major racial groups, as defined above.[5] This variation has been demonstrated in at least three ways.

First, investigators studying the population genetics of indigenous groups from around the world have constructed ancestral-tree diagrams showing branching relationships among the various indigenous groups. Despite differences in the types of markers used, these studies have been consistent in showing that the human population has major branches corresponding to the major racial groups, with subbranches within each racial group associated with indigenous groups.[13-15]

Second, analysis of genetic clusters has been applied to persons of diverse ancestry, with a focus on genotypes at multiple genetic loci. These analyses have also consistently resulted in the delineation of major genetic clusters that are associated with racial categories.[16-19] The primary difference between the results of these studies and the categories used by the U.S. Census is that South, Central, and West Asians cluster with Europeans and are separate from East Asians.

Third, studies have examined the distribution of differences among racial groups in the frequency of alleles (genetic variants) at both microsatellite and single-nucleotide–polymorphism (SNP) markers, demonstrating a median difference in allele frequency of 15 to 20 percent, with 10 percent of markers showing a difference of 40 percent or more.[5,20,21] Thus, for an allele with a frequency of 20 percent or greater in one racial group, the odds are in favor of seeing the same variant in another racial group. However, variants with a frequency below that level are more likely to be race-specific. This race-specificity of variants is particularly common among Africans, who display greater genetic variability than other racial groups and have a larger number of low-frequency alleles.[17] These results indicate that the frequency of variant alleles underlying disease or normal phenotypes can vary substantially among racial groups, leading to differences in the frequency of the phenotypes themselves. Such differences in frequency are also found among ethnic groups, but these differences are typically not as great. Furthermore, self-defined ancestry is very highly correlated with genetically defined clusters.[5,19]

Genetic Differences in Disease Among Racial and Ethnic Groups

To what degree does genetic variability account for medically important differences in disease outcomes among racial and ethnic groups? The answer depends on the frequency of the genetic variants or alleles (mutations) underlying the susceptibility to the disease. For mendelian disorders, the relevance of race and ethnic background is readily apparent. Mutations that have frequencies of less than 2 percent are nearly always race-specific and, in fact, are often specific to single ethnic groups within a given race. For example, numerous mutations with frequencies in this range occur uniquely in Ashkenazi Jews, French Canadians, the Amish, or European gypsies. This is because such populations descend from a relatively small number of founders and have remained endogamous for a large part of their history. Mutant alleles with frequencies of more than 2 percent but less than 20 percent are typically prevalent within single racial groups but not in other racial groups. For example, hemochromatosis is associated with a mutant allele (C282Y) found in all European groups and at especially high frequency (8 to 10 percent) in northern Europeans, but is virtually absent in nonwhite groups.[22]

"Complex" genetic disorders such as asthma, cancer, diabetes, and atherosclerosis are most likely due to multiple, potentially interacting, genes and environmental factors and are thus more challenging to study. The genetic determinants of the majority of these disorders are currently poorly understood, but the few examples that do exist demonstrate clinically important racial and ethnic differences in gene frequency. For example, factor V Leiden, a genetic variant that confers an increased risk of venous thromboembolic disease, is present in about 5 percent of white people. In contrast, this variant is rarely found in East Asians and Africans (prevalence, ≤1 percent).[23,24] Susceptibility to Crohn's disease is associated with three polymorphic genetic variants in the *CARD15* gene in whites[25]; none of these genetic variants were found in Japanese patients with Crohn's disease.[26] Another important gene that affects a complex trait is *CCR5*—a receptor used by the human immunodeficiency virus (HIV) to enter cells. As many as 25 percent of white people (especially in northern Europe) are heterozygous for the *CCR5−delta32* variant, which is protective against HIV infection and progression, whereas this variant is virtually absent in other groups, thus suggesting racial and ethnic differences in protection against HIV.[27]

Other alleles occur in all ethnic groups but with highly variable frequency. Increasingly, researchers and clinicians are focusing on identifying and studying the genetic variants that influence responses to drugs and the metabolism of drugs (an area of study termed pharmacogenetics). One example is *N*-acetyltransferase 2 (NAT2), an enzyme involved in the detoxification of many carcinogens and the metabolism of many commonly used drugs. Genetic variants of NAT2 result in two phenotypes, slow and rapid acetylators. Population-based studies of NAT2 and its metabolites have shown that the slow-acetylator phenotype ranges in frequency from approximately 14 percent among East Asians to 34 percent among black Americans to 54 percent among whites.[28] Genetic variants of NAT2 are important because they may predict toxic effects of drugs and because they may contribute to racial and ethnic variation in the incidence of environmentally induced cancers.

Racial and Ethnic Differences as Clues to Interactions

Even when all racial and ethnic groups share a genetic variant that causes a disease, studies of different groups may offer important insights. One of the best-known examples of a gene that affects a complex disease is *APOE*. A patient harboring a variant of this gene, *APOE ∈4*, has a substantially increased risk of Alzheimer's disease. *APOE ∈4* is relatively common and is seen in all racial and ethnic groups, albeit at different frequencies, ranging from 9 percent in Japanese populations to 14 percent in white populations to 19 percent in black American populations.[29] However, a recent meta-analysis has demonstrated that the effect of *APOE ∈4* on the risk of Alzheimer's disease varies according to race.[29] Homozygosity for the *∈4* allele increases the risk by a factor of 33 in Japanese populations and by a factor of 15 in white populations, but only by a factor of 6 in black American populations; similarly, heterozygosity for the *∈4* allele increases the risk by a factor of 5.6 in Japanese populations, by a factor of 3.0 in white populations, and by a factor of 1.1 in black American populations. Although the reason for this variation in risk remains unknown, it suggests that there may be genetic or environmental modifiers of this gene. Thus, even when a genetic determinant of a complex disease is present in all racial and ethnic groups, racial and ethnic classification may offer additional important insights.

Racially Admixed Populations

Although studies of population genetics have clustered persons into a small number of groups corresponding roughly to five major racial categories, such classification is not completely discontinuous, because there has been inter-mixing among groups both over the course of history and in recent times. In particular, genetic admixture, or the presence in a population of persons with multiple races or ethnic backgrounds, is well documented in the border regions of continents and may represent genetic gradations (clines)—for example, among East Africans (e.g., Ethiopians)[18] and some central Asian groups.[19] In the United States, mixture among different racial groups has occurred recently, although in the 2000 U.S. Census, the majority of respondents still identified themselves as members of a single racial group. Genetic studies of black Americans have documented a range of 7 to 20 percent white admixture, depending on the geographic location of the population studied.[30] Despite the admixture, black Americans, as a group, are still genetically similar to Africans. Hispanics, the largest and fastest growing minority population in the United States, are an admixed group that includes white and Native American ancestry, as well as African ancestry.[31] The proportions of admixture in this group also vary according to geographic region.

Although the categorization of admixed groups poses special challenges, groups containing persons with varying levels of admixture can also be particularly useful for genetic–epidemiologic studies. For example, Williams et al. studied the association between the degree of white admixture and the incidence of type 2 diabetes mellitus among Pima Indians.[32] They found that the self-reported degree of white admixture (reported as a percentage) was strongly correlated with protection from diabetes in this population. Furthermore, as noted above, information on race or ethnic background can provide important clues to effects of culture, access to care, and bias on the part of caregivers, even in genetically admixed populations. It is also important to recognize that many groups (e.g., most Asian groups) are highly underrepresented both in the population of the United States and in typical surveys of population genetics, relative to their global numbers. Thus, primary categories that are relevant for the current U.S. population might not be optimal for a globally derived sample.

Risks Entailed by Ignoring Race in Biomedical Research and Clinical Practice

Given its controversial social and political history, it may be tempting to abandon the notion of race altogether, particularly if we believe that continued attention to differences among races may perpetuate discrepancies in health status and well-being. Indeed, some have advocated discontinuing the collection of information about race and ethnic background, presumably as a way of protecting minority groups. In California, advocates of this move are pushing for a state law—through the Racial Privacy Initiative[33]—that would prohibit racial classification by the state or other public entities. Although this initiative formally excludes a ban on classification for the purposes of medical research, the abolition of the collection of data on race or ethnic group for all other purposes would eliminate these data from many public data bases on which clinicians and scientists rely in order to make meaningful inferences about the effects of race and ethnic background on health and disease in persons and populations.

We believe that ignoring race and ethnic background would be detrimental to the very populations and persons that this approach allegedly seeks to protect. Information about patients' ethnic or racial group is imperative for the identification, tracking, and investigation of the reasons for racial and ethnic differences in the prevalence and severity of disease and in responses to treatment. This information is also crucial for identifying different risk-factor profiles even when a disease does not occur with dramatically different frequencies in different racial or ethnic groups. Furthermore, knowledge of a person's ancestry may facilitate testing, diagnosis, and treatment when genetic factors are involved. For example, there are already tests to screen for disease-causing mutations that are tailored to specific racial or ethnic groups. Currently, racial and ethnic minorities in the United States are underrepresented in many clinical studies.[34] If investigators ignored race and ethnic background in research studies and persons were sampled randomly, the overwhelming majority of participants in clinical studies in the United States would be white, and minority populations would never be adequately sampled.[5] In cases in which there are important racial and ethnic differences in the causes of disease or other outcomes or in which there are interactions between race or ethnic background and other factors contributing to these outcomes, such patterns would never be discovered, their causes could not be identified, and the appropriate interventions would never be applied in the groups in which they were needed. Despite the fact that the National Institutes of Health requires reporting of all racial or ethnic groups participating in biomedical research, limited progress has been made in the inclusion of minority groups.

Conclusions

There are racial and ethnic differences in the causes, expression, and prevalence of various diseases. The relative importance of bias, culture, socioeconomic status, access to care, and environmental and genetic influences on the development of disease is an empirical question that, in most cases, remains unanswered. Although there are potential social costs associated with linking race or ethnic background with genetics,[35] we believe that these potential costs are outweighed by the benefits in terms of diagnosis and research. Ignoring racial and ethnic differences in medicine and biomedical research will not make them disappear. Rather than ignoring these differences, scientists should continue to use them as starting points for further research. Only by focusing attention on these issues can we hope to understand better the variations among racial and ethnic groups in the prevalence and severity of diseases and in responses to treatment. Such understanding provides the opportunity to develop strategies for the improvement of health outcomes for everyone.

References

1. Lander E. Cracking the code of life. Boston: WGBH, 2001 (transcript).
2. Angier N. Do races differ? Not really, genes show. New York Times. August 22, 2000:F1.
3. Schwartz RS. Racial profiling in medical research. N Engl J Med 2001; 344:1392–3.
4. Sankar P, Cho MK. Genetics: toward a new vocabulary of human genetic variation. Science 2002;298:1337–8.
5. Risch N, Burchard E, Ziv E, Tang H. Categorization of humans in biomedical research: genes, race and disease. Genome Biol 2002;3(7):comment2007.1–comment2007.12.
6. Kaufman JS, Cooper RS. Considerations for use of racial/ethnic classification in etiologic research. Am J Epidemiol 2001;154:291–8.
7. Smedley BD, Stith AY, Nelson AR, eds. Unequal treatment: confronting racial and ethnic disparities in health care. Washington, D.C.: National Academy Press, 2002.

8. Epstein AM, Ayanian JZ, Keogh JH, et al. Racial disparities in access to renal transplantation: clinically appropriate or due to underuse or overuse? N Engl J Med 2000;343:1537–44.

9. Peterson ED, Wright SM, Daley J, Thibault GE. Racial variation in cardiac procedure use and survival following acute myocardial infarction in the Department of Veterans Affairs. JAMA 1994;271:1175–80.

10. Schulman KA, Berlin JA, Harless W, et al. The effect of race and sex on physicians' recommendations for cardiac catheterization. N Engl J Med 1999;340:618–26. [Erratum, N Engl J Med 1999;340:1130.]

11. Karter AJ, Ferrara A, Liu JY, Moffet HH, Ackerson LM, Selby JV. Ethnic disparities in diabetic complications in an insured population. JAMA 2002;287:2519–27.

12. Judson R, Salisbury B, Schneider J, Windemuth A, Stephens JC. How many SNPs does a genome-wide haplotype map require? Pharmacogenomics 2002; 3:379–91.

13. Calafell F, Shuster A, Speed WC, Kidd JR, Kidd KK. Short tandem repeat polymorphism evolution in humans. Eur J Hum Genet 1998;6:38–49.

14. Bowcock AM, Ruiz-Linares A, Tomfohrde J, Minch E, Kidd JR, Cavalli-Sforza LL. High resolution of human evolutionary trees with polymorphic microsatellites. Nature 1994;368:455–7.

15. Bowcock AM, Kidd JR, Mountain JL, et al. Drift, admixture, and selection in human evolution: a study with DNA polymorphisms. Proc Natl Acad Sci U S A 1991;88:839–43.

16. Mountain JL, Cavalli-Sforza LL. Multilocus genotypes, a tree of individuals, and human evolutionary history. Am J Hum Genet 1997;61:705–18.

17. Stephens JC, Schneider JA, Tanguay DA, et al. Haplotype variation and linkage disequilibrium in 313 human genes. Science 2001;293:489–93. [Erratum, Science 2001;293:1048.]

18. Wilson JF, Weale ME, Smith AC, et al. Population genetic structure of variable drug response. Nat Genet 2001;29:265–9.

19. Rosenberg NA, Pritchard JK, Weber JL, et al. Genetic structure of human populations. Science 2002;298:2381–5.

20. Dean M, Stephens JC, Winkler C, et al. Polymorphic admixture typing in human ethnic populations. Am J Hum Genet 1994;55:788–808.

21. Smith MW, Lautenberger JA, Shin HD, et al. Markers for mapping by admixture linkage disequilibrium in African American and Hispanic populations. Am J Hum Genet 2001;69:1080–94.

22. Merryweather-Clarke AT, Pointon JJ, Jouanolle AM, Rochette J, Robson KJ. Geography of HFE C282Y and H63D mutations. Genet Test 2000;4:183–98.

23. Ridker PM, Miletich JP, Hennekens CH, Buring JE. Ethnic distribution of factor V Leiden in 4047 men and women: implications for venous thromboembolism screening. JAMA 1997;277:1305–7.

24. Shen MC, Lin JS, Tsay W. High prevalence of antithrombin III, protein C and protein S deficiency, but no factor V Leiden mutation in venous thrombophilic Chinese patients in Taiwan. Thromb Res 1997;87:377–85.

25. Hugot JP, Chamaillard M, Zouali H, et al. Association of NOD2 leucine-rich repeat variants with susceptibility to Crohn's disease. Nature 2001;411:599–603.

26. Yamazaki K, Takazoe M, Tanaka T, Kazumori T, Nakamura Y. Absence of mutation in the NOD2/CARD15 gene among 483 Japanese patients with Crohn's disease. J Hum Genet 2002;47:469–72.

27. Stephens JC, Reich DE, Goldstein DB, et al. Dating the origin of the CCR5-Delta32 AIDS-resistance allele by the coalescence of haplotypes. Am J Hum Genet 1998;62:1507–15.

28. Yu MC, Skipper PL, Taghizadeh K, et al. Acetylator phenotype, aminobiphenyl-hemoglobin adduct levels, and bladder cancer risk in white, black, and Asian men in Los Angeles, California. J Natl Cancer Inst 1994;86:712–6.

29. Farrer LA, Cupples LA, Haines JL, et al. Effects of age, sex, and ethnicity on the association between apolipoprotein E genotype and Alzheimer disease: a meta-analysis. JAMA 1997;278:1349–56.

30. Parra EJ, Marcini A, Akey J, et al. Estimating African American admixture proportions by use of population-specific alleles. Am J Hum Genet 1998;63:1839–51.

31. Hanis CL, Hewett-Emmett D, Bertin TK, Schull WJ. Origins of U.S. Hispanics: implications for diabetes. Diabetes Care 1991;14:618–27.

32. Williams RC, Long JC, Hanson RL, Sievers ML, Knowler WC. Individual estimates of European genetic admixture associated with lower body-mass index, plasma glucose, and prevalence of type 2 diabetes in Pima Indians. Am J Hum Genet 2000;66:527–38.

33. Racial privacy initiative. Sacramento, Calif.: American Civil Rights Coalition, 2002. (Accessed February 28, 2003, at http://www.racialprivacy.org.)

34. Gifford AL, Cunningham WE, Heslin KC, et al. Participation in research and access to experimental treatments by HIV-infected patients. N Engl J Med 2002;346:1373–82.

35. Foster MW, Sharp RR. Race, ethnicity, and genomics: social classifications as proxies of biological heterogeneity. Genome Res 2002;12:844–50.

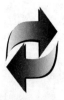

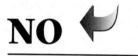

NO

Richard S. Cooper, Jay S. Kaufman, and Ryk Ward

Race and Genomics

Race is a thoroughly contentious topic, as one might expect of an idea that intrudes on the everyday life of so many people. The modern concept of race grew out of the experience of Europeans in naming and organizing the populations encountered in the rapid expansion of their empires.[1] As a way to categorize humans, race has since come to take on a wide range of meanings, mixing social and biologic ingredients in varied proportions. This plasticity has made it a tool that fits equally well in the hands of demagogues who want to justify genocide and eugenics and of health scientists who want to improve surveillance for disease. It is not surprising, therefore, that diametrically opposing views have been voiced about its scientific and social value.[2,3] Indeed, few other concepts used in the conduct of ordinary science are the subject of a passionate debate about whether they actually exist.

Into this storm of controversy rides genomics. With the acknowledgment that race is the product of a marriage of social and biologic influences, it has been proposed that genomics now at least offers the opportunity to put its biologic claims to an objective test.[4] If those claims are validated, race will become a way to choose drug therapy for patients, categorize persons for genetic research, and understand the causes of disease. Genomics, with its technological innovations and authority as "big science," might thereby solve the conundrum of race and bring peace to the warring factions.

Of the many implications that flow from the claim that race categorizes humans, few have more immediate clinical relevance than the choice of drug therapy. Remarkable progress has been made with drugs for cardiovascular disease, and the rapidly evolving patterns of care now include, for the first time, a candidate for "race-specific" therapy.[5] Randomized trials have been interpreted to show that a combination of vasodilators is more effective in treating heart failure in black persons than in white persons[6] and that angiotensin-converting–enzyme (ACE) inhibitors have little efficacy in blacks.[7] The results of the vasodilator trials were inconsistent, however, and never achieved statistical significance for an interaction between treatment and race, the outcome of interest. Moreover, another analysis of the data from the aforementioned ACE-inhibitor trial[7] demonstrated that the original result showing a racial difference

From Richard S. Cooper, Jay S. Kaufman, and Ryk Ward, "Race and Genomics," *The New England Journal of Medicine*, vol. 348, no. 12 (March 20, 2003), pp. 1166–1170. Copyright © 2003 by The Massachusetts Medical Society. All rights reserved. Reprinted by permission.

was unique to the end point that was chosen; in the portion of the study focusing on prevention, the drug had equal efficacy in blacks and in whites in reducing the incidence of the combined end point of death or development of a new onset of heart failure.[8] Similarly, no interaction with race was observed for the relative benefit of ACE inhibitors in preventing heart failure in the Antihypertensive and Lipid-Lowering Treatment to Prevent Heart Attack Trial, supporting the view that the original observation of an effect of race as a type I error.[9]

Promotion of a drug for a race-specific "niche market" could distract physicians from therapies for which unequivocal evidence of benefit already exists. Race-specific therapy draws its rationale from the presumption that the frequencies of genetic variants influencing the efficacy of the drug are substantially different among races. This result is hard to demonstrate for any class of drugs, including those used to treat heart failure. Although a study of polymorphisms in drug-metabolizing enzymes did, in fact, show statistically significant variation in allele frequencies according to race, neither racial categories nor genetic clusters were sufficiently precise to make them clinically useful in guiding the choice of drugs.[10] What is lost in these arguments is the difficulty of translating differences among groups into a test that has adequate predictive value to help with clinical decisions. Race can help to target screening for a disease-associated mutation that is present at a high frequency in one population and is virtually absent in another,[11] but it is impossible for race as we recognize it clinically to provide both perfect sensitivity and specificity for the presence of a DNA-sequence variant. For this reason, race has never been shown to be an adequate proxy for use in choosing a drug; if you really need to know whether a patient has a particular genotype, you will have to do the test to find out.

The availability of high-throughput genotyping creates the opportunity for increasingly sophisticated analyses of the extent to which continental populations vary genetically. Analysis of a large set of multiallelic microsatellite loci has shown that it is possible to cluster persons into population groups with high statistical accuracy.[12] Although clustering persons according to geographic origin has been accomplished most effectively with the use of highly informative, rapidly mutating, microsatellite loci, the use of single-nucleotide polymorphisms (SNPs) or their corresponding haplotypes also results in some degree of classification according to continent.[13]

However, the public health relevance of these data remains controversial. One view holds that the ability to categorize persons according to continental "race" validates the clinical and epidemiologic use of self-reported racial ancestry in terms of the categories of white, black, Asian, Pacific Islander, and Native American used by the U.S. Census.[2] We disagree. The success of microsatellite loci in classifying persons according to continental group depends in part on the effect of population-specific alleles. In neither case is it apparent that such differences have relevance for traits that are important to health. Most population-specific microsatellite alleles are unlikely to be functional; rather, like a last name, they merely help to verify the geographic origin of a person's ancestry. Accumulated small differences in common alleles will yield differences in population risk only if a disease is caused primarily by interactions among multiple loci, and this is both mathematically and biologically implausible.

The same points apply to noncoding SNPs. In addition, coding sequences are highly conserved across groups. Moreover, in cases in which common polymorphisms occur, they are old and tend to be shared.[14] Categorizing people on the basis of differences in allele frequencies is therefore not the same as apportioning the whole of human diversity into medically relevant categories. The more relevant outcome—that the sets of common functional polymorphisms are distributed in discrete racial categories—has not been demonstrated. Furthermore, most population geneticists concur that the bulk of genetic variation (90 to 95 percent) occurs within, not among, continental populations.[12-16] The central observations remain: variation is continuous and discordant with race, systematic variation according to continent is very limited, and there is no evidence that the units of interest for medical genetics correspond to what we call races.

The real effect of the biologic concept of race has always been its implications for common quantitative traits. Marked differences in the rates of cardiovascular diseases, for example, have been held up as examples of how race matters.[17-20] Reframed in genomic terms, it is argued that if "biological is defined by susceptibility to, and natural history of, a chronic disease, then . . . numerous studies . . . have documented biological differences among the races."[2] However, there is no body of evidence to support these broad claims about chronic diseases. Although it is obvious that many genetic diseases vary markedly among populations, those conditions are generally rare. Tay–Sachs disease, cystic fibrosis, and hemoglobinopathies, for example, are absent in many populations but present in others. But for these conditions, continental populations are not the categories of interest: persons of Jewish descent, not "whites," share a risk of Tay–Sachs disease; the frequency of cystic fibrosis varies widely within Europe; and thalassemia occurs in a variety of populations distributed from Italy to Thailand.

Many single-gene disorders have now been defined at the molecular level, and the emerging challenge faced by geneticists is to "make the genome relevant to public health."[21] Defining the molecular underpinnings of common chronic diseases has therefore become the central focus of genetic epidemiology. By extension, some investigators have turned with renewed enthusiasm to race as a tool for categorizing population risk. This approach draws on the practice, of long standing in the public health field in the United States, of granting priority to race or ethnic background as a demographic category—a surveillance practice, it is worth noting, that is virtually unique in the world. At the present time, however, very little is known about the genetic component of diseases of complex causation. Few, if any, well-characterized susceptibility genes have been identified for any of the degenerative conditions that kill at least 5 percent of the population, and we do not even know whether the individual variants are common or rare or whether they affect a protein's structure or its level of expression.

Since we do not know about the genetic variants that predispose persons to common chronic diseases, one might assume that arguments for the existence of genetic predispositions would be made for all population groups equally. The reality is very different. Minority groups, particularly blacks in the

United States, are assumed to be genetically predisposed to virtually all common chronic diseases.[17-20,22-26] Genes are regularly proposed as the cause when no genetic data have been obtained, and the social and biologic factors remain hopelessly confounded.[23-26] Even when molecular data are collected, causal arguments are based on nonsignificant findings or genetic variation that does not have an established association with the disease being studied.[19,20,22] Coincidence is not a plausible explanation of the widespread occurrence of this practice over time and across subdisciplines. The correlation between the use of unsupported genetic inferences and the social standing of a group is glaring evidence of bias and demonstrates how race is used both to categorize and to rank order subpopulations.[27,28]

Not only are the relevant genetic data absent, but the distribution of polygenic phenotypes does not suggest that race is a useful category. Consider as an example height, a continuous trait that is highly heritable in all populations. Does continental race tell us something useful about average height? People who attain both the tallest stature (the Masai) and the shortest (the Biaka) are found in sub-Saharan Africa; Swedish people have traditionally been much taller than Sicilians; and although Japanese people used to be short, the current generation of children in Japan cannot fit in the desks in schools. The concept of race does not summarize this information effectively. If that complexity is multiplied by thousands of traits, which are randomly distributed among groups within continents, one gets an idea of the limitations of race as a classification scheme.

Although the rapid pace of change in genomics makes today's conclusions obsolete tomorrow, some predictions are in order. We can expect genomics increasingly to negate the old-fashioned concept that differences in genetic susceptibility to common diseases are racially distributed. In any common disease, many genes are likely to be involved, and each gene will have many variants. All the current data indicate that susceptibility alleles tend to be old, have moderate-to-small effects, and are shared among many populations. The *APOE* ε4 allele, a well-studied example that contributes to a small extent to individual and potential risk for traits such as heart disease and dementia, is found in virtually all populations, albeit at varying rates.

Recent genomic surveys have also shown that as few as three to five common haplotypes capture the bulk of segregating variation at any specific locus throughout the genome, and those haplotypes are generally represented in the populations of all continents (Fig. 1).[29] Therefore, if susceptibility alleles for chronic diseases are located on common haplotypes, those alleles must be shared by members of all populations. Measuring the net effect of these genetic influences in a given population will require summing the frequencies of these susceptibility alleles in all genomic regions, while taking into account the environmental factors that are either difficult to measure or wholly unknown. Given these daunting epidemiologic challenges, it will be very difficult to calculate the "genetic susceptibility score" for any particular racial category.

This point requires further attention. There is no doubt that there are some important biologic differences among populations, and molecular techniques can help to define what those differences are. Some traits, such as skin

Figure 1

Distribution of Haplotypes According to Continental Population

Across multiple regions of the genome, an average of 5.3 haplotypes were found in samples drawn from the three major geographic populations. As shown in the diagram, the majority of these haplotypes were shared by two or more of the populations. Adapted from Gabriel et al.[29] with the permission of the publisher.

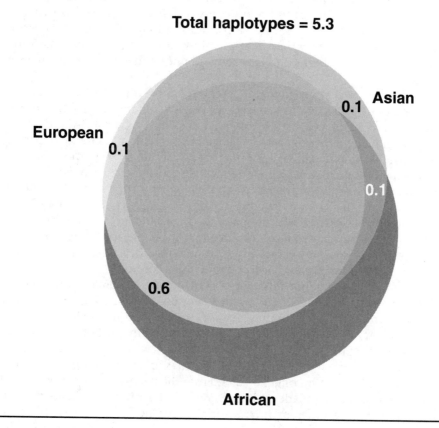

color, vary in a strikingly systematic pattern. The inference does not follow, however, that genetic variation among human populations falls into racial categories or that race, as we currently define it, provides an effective system for summarizing that variation. The confused nature of this debate is apparent when we recognize that although everyone, from geneticists to laypersons, tends to use "race" as if it were a scientific category; with rare exceptions,[15] no one offers a quantifiable definition of what a race is in genetic terms. The free-floating debate that results, while entertaining, has little chance of advancing this field.

What is at stake is a more practical question—namely, has genomics provided evidence that race can act as a surrogate for genetic constitution in medicine or public health? Our answer is no. Race, at the continental level, has not been shown to provide a useful categorization of genetic information about the response to drugs, diagnosis, or causes of disease.

But in the United States, there is substantial variation in health status among major population subgroups. This self-evident truth has been the driving force behind the use of racial or ethnic categories in surveillance for disease. Among persons who are less convinced by the genetic data, variation in environmental exposure is seen as the cause of this phenomenon, and it follows that differences in health occur because privilege and power are unequal in racially stratified societies. The globalization of complex chronic diseases seems to confirm the view that all populations are susceptible and that variation in rates can be understood as the result of differential exposure to environmental causes.

Although we acknowledge the salience of these arguments, the value of continental race as a classification scheme must be questioned in this context much as it was in the context of genetics. For example, persons who could be classified as having "African ancestry" have wide variation in rates of hypertension and diabetes, as do all large continental populations.[30,31] Without the context provided by such variables as the level of education, occupation, type of diet, and place of residence, race as a social category is not a useful predictor of health outcomes. Just as most genetic heterogeneity occurs within populations, there is enormous variation in the patterns of culture-derived behavioral and risk factors. An unintended result of categorizing people according to race can be to foreclose the question of why they have ill health, leaving us blind to the meaning of the more relevant local and individual context.

Race, in the metaphor introduced above, is the product of an arranged marriage between the social and biologic worlds. Although it often seems to travel back and forth between these parallel universes, it maintains a home in both. From the social sphere, race has inherited certain attributes that cannot be alienated from its meaning, no matter how hard we might try. The concept of race has currency in everyday discourse and is an epistemological category independent of the action of geneticists. From the beginning, it has been used not just to organize populations, but to create a classification scheme that explains the meaning inherent in the social order, according to which some groups dominate others.[1,28] There is a tendency for scientists to ignore the messy social implications of what they do. At the extreme, the argument is made that "we just tell the truth about nature," and its negative consequences are political problems that do not concern us. Whether or not such a position is defensible from an ethical point of view, the debate over race cannot be sidestepped so easily. Race already has a meaning. To invoke the authority of genomic science in the debate over the value of race as a category of nature is to accept the social meaning as well.

In the 20th century, physics promised us knowledge of how the universe works, space travel, and the ability to harness the atom as an infinite source of energy. Although vast amounts of knowledge did flow from research in those areas, the consequences in practice were not always benign. The accumulated record of peaceful and nonpeaceful atomic energy subsequently led many physicists to understand more fully that science is a part of society. In this century, biology—especially genomics—has emerged as the beacon of science leading us into the future, where data on the genetic sequence will unlock the secret of life. For genomics to fall in lock step with the socially defined use of race is not a propitious beginning to that journey. The ability to catalogue molecular variants in persons and populations has thrust genetics into a new relationship with society. Interpreting that catalogue within the existing framework of race, as was done in the case of eugenics, violates the principles that give science its unique status as a force outside the social hierarchy, one that does not take sides in factional contests. Racial affiliation draws on deep emotions about group identity and the importance of belonging. The discovery that races exist is not an advance of genomic science into uncharted territory; it is an extension of the atavistic belief that human populations are not just organized, but ordered.

References

1. Montagu A, ed. The concept of race. New York: Free Press of Glencoe, 1964.
2. Risch N, Burchard E, Ziv E, Tang H. Categorization of humans in biomedical research: genes, race and disease. Genome Biol 2002;3(7):comment2007.1–comment2007.12.
3. Muntaner C, Nieto FJ, O'Campo P. The Bell Curve: on race, social class, and epidemiologic research. Am J Epidemiol 1996;144:531–6.
4. Wade N. Race is seen as real guide to track roots of disease. New York Times. July 30, 2002:F1.
5. Franciosa JA, Taylor AL, Cohn JN, et al. African-American Heart Failure Trial (A-HeFT): rationale, design, and methodology. J Card Fail 2002;8:128–35.
6. Carson P, Ziesche S, Johnson G, Cohn JN. Racial differences in response to therapy for heart failure: analysis of the vasodilator-heart failure trials. J Card Fail 1999;5:178–87.
7. Exner DV, Dries DL, Domanski MJ, Cohn JN. Lesser response to angiotensin-converting–enzyme inhibitor therapy in black as compared with white patents with left ventricular dysfunction. N Engl J Med 2001;344:1351–7.
8. Dries DL, Strong M, Cooper RS, Drazner MH. Efficacy of angiotensin-converting enzyme inhibition in reducing progression of asymptomatic left ventricular dysfunction to symptomatic heart failure in black and white patients. J Am Coll Cardiol 2002;40:311–7. [Erratum, J Am Coll Cardiol 2002;40:1019.]
9. The ALLHAT Officers and Coordinators for the ALLHAT Collaborative Research Group. Major outcomes in high-risk hypertensive patients randomized to angiotensin-converting enzyme inhibitor or calcium channel blocker vs diuretic: the Antihypertensive and Lipid-Lowering Treatment to Prevent Heart Attack Trial (ALLHAT). JAMA 2002;288:2981–97. [Erratum, JAMA 2003;289:178.]
10. Wilson JE, Weale ME, Smith AC, et al. Population genetic structure of variable drug response. Nat Genet 2001;29:265–9.
11. Splawski I, Timothy KW, Tateyama M, et al. Variant of SCN5A sodium channel implicated in risk of cardiac arrhythmia. Science 2002;297:1333–6.
12. Rosenberg NA, Pritchard JK, Weber JL, et al. Genetic structure of human populations. Science 2002;298:2381–5.
13. Stephens JC, Schneider JA, Tanguay DA, et al. Haplotype variation and linkage disequilibrium in 313 human genes. Science 2001;293:489–93. [Erratum, Science 2001;293:1048.]
14. Halushka MK, Fan J-B, Bentley K, et al. Patterns of single-nucleotide polymorphisms in candidate genes for blood pressure homeostasis. Nat Genet 1999;22:239–47.

15. Templeton AR. Human races: a genetic and evolutionary perspective. Am Anthropol 1998;100:632–50.

16. Romualdi C, Balding D, Nasidze IS, et al. Patterns of human diversity, within and among continents, inferred from biallelic DNA polymorphisms. Genome Res 2002;12:602–12.

17. Freedman BI. End-stage renal failure in African Americans: insights in kidney disease susceptibility. Nephrol Dial Transplant 2002;17:198–200.

18. Yancy CW. The role of race in heart failure therapy. Curr Cardiol Rep 2002;4:218–25.

19. Hajjar RJ, MacRae CA. Adrenergic-receptor polymorphisms and heart failure. N. Engl J Med 2002;347:1196–9.

20. Henderson SO, Coetzee GA, Ross RK, Yu MC, Henderson BE. Elevated mortality rates from circulatory disease in African American men and women of Los Angeles County, California—a possible genetic susceptibility? Am J Med Sci 2000;320:18–23.

21. The HGP: end of phase 1. Nat Genet 2002;30:125.

22. Kimm SYS, Glynn NW, Aston CE et al. Racial differences in the relation between uncoupling protein genes and resting energy expenditure. Am J Clin Nutr 2002;75:714–9.

23. Robbins AS, Whittemore AS, Thom DH. Differences in socioeconomic status and survival among white and black men with prostate cancer. Am J Epidemiol 2000;151:409–16.

24. Brancati FL, Whelton PK, Kuller LH, Klag MJ. Diabetes mellitus, race, and socioeconomic status: a population-based study. Ann Epidemiol 1996;6:67–73.

25. Brewster LM, Clark JF, van Montfrans GA. Is greater tissue activity of creatine kinase the genetic factor increasing hypertension risk in black people of sub-Saharan African descent? J Hypertens 2000;18:1537–44.

26. Grim CE, Robinson M. Blood pressure variation in blacks: genetic factors. Semin Nephrol 1996;16:83–93.

27. Chase A. The legacy of Malthus: the social costs of the new scientific racism. New York: Alfred A. Knopf, 1977.

28. Gould SJ. The mismeasure of man. Rev. ed. New York: W.W. Norton, 1996.

29. Gabriel SB, Schaffner SF, Nguyen H, et al. The structure of haplotype blocks in the human genome. Science 2002;296:2225–9.

30. Cooper R, Rotimi C, Ataman S, et al. The prevalence of hypertension in seven populations of West African origin. Am J Public Health 1997;87:160–8.

31. Cooper RS, Rotimi CN, Kaufman JS, et al. Prevalence of NIDDM among populations of the African diaspora. Diabetes Care 1997;20:343–8.

POSTSCRIPT

Should Race Play a Role in the Treatment and Study of Disease?

Race continues to be a contentious issue among medical researchers and practitioners especially since the ill-fated Tuskegee syphilis study. Recent discoveries linking gene variants as the cause of disease have also complicated the issue. It appears that a mutation of a single gene is sufficient and necessary to cause some diseases in specific populations and not in others. In more complex illnesses, the role of race is not as clear as other biological, environmental, cultural, social, and economic factors that affect disease. However, the racial disparities in disease incidence and prevalence *are* clear, especially for HIV/AIDS and diabetes. See "Hispanic Children Have Health Risks at Greater Rates," *The Wall Street Journal* (July 3, 2002); "Race, Ethnicity, Culture, and Science: Researchers Should Understand and Justify Their Use of Ethnic Groupings," *British Medical Journal* (July 30, 1994); and "Analyzing Socioeconomic and Racial/Ethnic Patterns in Health and Health Care," *The American Journal of Public Health* (August 1993). Other articles that address the issue of disparity in health care, as opposed to disease incidence, include "National Hispanic Conference Focuses on Disparities in Health Care," *Managed Healthcare Information* (August 26, 2002); "Racial and Ethnic Disparities in the Receipt of Cancer Treatment," *Journal of the National Cancer Institute* (March 6, 2002); and "Racist Health Care?" *Florida Law Review* (July 1996). Finally, numerous articles have been published regarding the role of race in medical research, many focusing on the controversial Tuskegee syphilis study. See "Distrust, Race, and Research," *Archives of Internal Medicine* (November 25, 2002); "The Racial Genetics Paradox in Biomedical Research and Public Health," *Public Health Reports* (September–October 2002); "Cultural Memory and the Tuskegee Syphilis Study," *The Hastings Center Report* (September–October 2001); "Tuskegee: Could It Happen Again?" *Postgraduate Medical Journal* (September 2001); "Experience and Preliminary Results in Human Genome Diversity Research," *Politics and the Life Sciences* (September 1999); "The Meaning of Race in Science—Considerations for Cancer Research: Concerns of Special Populations in the National Cancer Program (Statements From the President's Cancer Panel Meeting, April 9, 1997)," *Cancer* (January 1, 1998); and "Is Research Into Ethnicity and Health Racist, Unsound, or Important Science?" *British Medical Journal* (June 14, 1997).

ISSUE 9

Should Human Cloning
Ever Be Permitted?

YES: John A. Robertson, from "Human Cloning and the Challenge of Regulation," *The New England Journal of Medicine* (July 9, 1998)

NO: George J. Annas, from "Why We Should Ban Human Cloning," *The New England Journal of Medicine* (July 9, 1998)

ISSUE SUMMARY

YES: Attorney John A. Robertson contends there are many benefits to cloning and that a ban on privately funded cloning research is unjustified.

NO: Attorney and medical ethicist George J. Annas argues that cloning devalues people by depriving them of their uniqueness.

The idea that humans may someday be cloned (created from a cell without sexual reproduction) is now closer to reality. In 1996 a Scottish veterinarian named Ian Wilmut was able to produce a sheep by transferring the nucleus of an adult sheep mammary cell into a sheep egg from which the nucleus had been removed. The sheep was named "Dolly," and it possessed the genetic material of only one parent. This experiment increased the prospect of the creation of a new individual genetically identical to an existing or previously living person. Interest in cloning following the birth of Dolly escalated when Richard Seed, a physicist, announced that he would clone humans for a fee. Fear that unregulated cloning of humans would begin before anyone had the chance to evaluate the implications of this new technology sent Congress into action. Legislation to ban cloning was introduced to both houses of Congress. The Bond-Frist bill in the Senate and the Ehlers bill in the House were designed to prohibit or delay cloning indefinitely. This was the first time Congress introduced legislation to stop a single type of medical or scientific research, despite the fact that many medical groups and scientists were opposed to the ban. These bills are currently being reviewed. In addition, some states are now contemplating legislative action of their own. In 1997 Florida considered a law that would have barred the cloning of human DNA, a routine procedure in biomedical research. As of early 1998, 19 European nations have signed a treaty banning cloning.

While most people are comfortable with a moritorium on cloning to allow the implications to be studied, the congressional bills would go beyond restricting the cloning of humans. These bills would end research into what is known as somatic-cell nuclear-transfer technology. This technology involves transferring a human nucleus into a human egg that has had its nucleus removed. Research in this area is believed by some to be instrumental in disease and organ transplantation management. A compromise bill was introduced by Senators Edward Kennedy (D-Massachusetts) and Dianne Feinstein (D-California). This bill would ban the implantation of an embryo developed by the technology into a human uterus in order to create a child but would protect research to clone molecules, cells, and tissues.

Cloning-related research has already been accomplished using laboratory animals. Scientists have simulated models of human disease in cells from mouse embryos and placed these cells into recipient embryos. Some argue that the resulting offspring are valuable tools for studying the roles that genes play in disease. Similar reseach may yield other benefits, including information about the causes of cancer or the mechanics of aging. It is asserted that cloning could also be a source of material for the transplantation of human tissue. The treatment of diseases, such as diabetes or leukemia, and of genetic disorders may significantly improve with the availability of healthy, cloned cells. These cells would less likely be rejected by the body as foreign. Cloning may also help couples who carry genes for serious disorders to have healthy children. Although these benefits are theoretically possible, much research is still needed. A ban on research would not allow us to understand the full benefits of cloning.

Currently, some critics argue that it is immoral to experiment on human embryonic cells. The arguments against this technology are similar to those against abortion. Cloned organs would probably have to develop within human fetuses, which would be aborted when the organs are ready to be harvested. However, many people feel that a fetus is a viable life with rights that need to be protected. It has also been contended that cloning could create serious potential abuses, such as the destruction of embryos and the creation of master races.

In the following selections, John A. Robertson argues that there are many potential benefits of cloning and that the research should only be regulated, not banned. George J. Annas counters that cloning humans would devalue them and deprive them of their uniqueness.

John A. Robertson

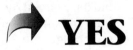 **YES**

Human Cloning and the Challenge of Regulation

The birth of Dolly, the sheep cloned from a mammary cell of an adult ewe, has initiated a public debate about human cloning. Although cloning of humans may never be clinically feasible, discussion of the ethical, legal, and social issues raised is important. Cloning is just one of several techniques potentially available to select, control, or alter the genome of offspring.[1-3] The development of such technology poses an important social challenge: how to ensure that the technology is used to enhance, rather than limit, individual freedom and welfare.

A key ethical question is whether a responsible couple, interested in rearing healthy offspring biologically related to them, might ethically choose to use cloning (or other genetic-selection techniques) for that purpose. The answer should take into account the benefits sought through the use of the techniques and any potential harm to offspring or to other interests.

The most likely uses of cloning would be far removed from the bizarre or horrific scenarios that initially dominated media coverage.[4] Theoretically, cloning would enable rich or powerful persons to clone themselves several times over, and commercial entrepreneurs might hire women to bear clones of sports or entertainment celebrities to be sold to others to rear. But current reproductive techniques can also be abused, and existing laws against selling children would apply to those created by cloning.

There is no reason to think that the ability to clone humans will cause many people to turn to cloning when other methods of reproduction would enable them to have healthy children. Cloning a human being by somatic-cell nuclear transfer, for example, would require a consenting person as a source of DNA, eggs to be enucleated and then fused with the DNA, a woman who would carry and deliver the child, and a person or couple to raise the child. Given this reality, cloning is most likely to be sought by couples who, because of infertility, a high risk of severe genetic disease, or other factors, cannot or do not wish to conceive a child.

Several plausible scenarios can be imagined. Rather than use sperm, egg, or embryo from anonymous donors, couples who are infertile as a result of gametic insufficiency might choose to clone one of the partners. If the husband were the source of the DNA and the wife provided the egg that received the nuclear transfer and then gestated the fetus, they would have a child biologically related to each of them and would not need to rely on anonymous gamete or embryo donation. Of course, many infertile couples might still prefer gamete or embryo donation or adoption. But there is nothing inherently wrong in wishing to be biologically related to one's children, even when this goal cannot be achieved through sexual reproduction.

A second plausible application would be for a couple at high risk of having offspring with a genetic disease.[5] Couples in this situation must now choose whether to risk the birth of an affected child, to undergo prenatal preimplantation diagnosis and abortion or the discarding of embryos, to accept gamete donation, to seek adoption, or to remain childless. If cloning were available, however, some couples, in line with prevailing concepts of kinship, family, and parenting, might strongly prefer to clone one of themselves or another family member. Alternatively, if they already had a healthy child, they might choose to use cloning to create a later-born twin of that child. In the more distant future, it is even possible that the child whose DNA was replicated would not have been born healthy but would have been made healthy by gene therapy after birth.

A third application relates to obtaining tissue or organs for transplantation. A child who needed an organ or tissue transplant might lack a medically suitable donor. Couples in this situation have sometimes conceived a child coitally in the hope that he or she would have the correct tissue type to serve, for example, as a bone marrow donor for an older sibling.[6,7] If the child's disease was not genetic, a couple might prefer to clone the affected child to be sure that the tissue would match.

It might eventually be possible to procure suitable tissue or organs by cloning the source DNA only to the point at which stem cells or other material might be obtained for transplantation, thus avoiding the need to bring a child into the world for the sake of obtaining tissue.[8] Cloning a person's cells up to the embryo stage might provide a source of stem cells or tissue for the person cloned. Cloning might also be used to enable a couple to clone a dead or dying child so as to have that child live on in some closely related form, to obtain sufficient numbers of embryos for transfer and pregnancy, or to eliminate mitochondrial disease.[5]

Most, if not all, of the potential uses of cloning are controversial, usually because of the explicit copying of the genome. As the National Bioethics Advisory Commission noted, in addition to concern about physical safety and eugenics, somatic-cell cloning raises issues of the individuality, autonomy, objectification, and kinship of the resulting children.[5] In other instances, such as the production of embryos to serve as tissue banks, the ethical issue is the sacrifice of embryos created solely for that purpose.

Given the wide leeway now granted couples to use assisted reproduction and prenatal genetic selection in forming families, cloning should not be rejected in all circumstances as unethical or illegitimate. The manipulation of embryos and the use of gamete donors and surrogates are increasingly common. Most fetuses conceived in the United States and Western Europe are now screened for genetic or chromosomal anomalies. Before conception, screening to identify carriers of genetic diseases is widespread.[9] Such practices also deviate from conventional notions of reproduction, kinship, and medical treatment of infertility, yet they are widely accepted.

Despite the similarity of cloning to current practices, however, the dissimilarities should not be overlooked. The aim of most other forms of assisted reproduction is the birth of a child who is a descendant of at least one member of the couple, not an identical twin. Most genetic selection acts negatively to identify and screen out unwanted traits such as genetic disease, not positively to choose or replicate the genome as in somatic-cell cloning.[3] It is not clear, however, why a child's relation to his or her rearing parents must always be that of sexually reproduced descendant when such a relationship is not possible because of infertility or other factors. Indeed, in gamete donation and adoption, although sexual reproduction is involved, a full descendant relation between the child and both rearing parents is lacking. Nor should the difference between negative and positive means of selecting children determine the ethical or social acceptability of cloning or other techniques. In both situations, a deliberate choice is made so that a child is born with one genome rather than another or is not born at all.

Is cloning sufficiently similar to current assisted-reproduction and genetic-selection practices to be treated similarly as a presumptively protected exercise of family or reproductive liberty?[10] Couples who request cloning in the situations I have described are seeking to rear healthy children with whom they will have a genetic or biologic tie, just as couples who conceive their children sexually do. Whether described as "replication" or as "reproduction," the resort to cloning is similar enough in purpose and effects to other reproduction and genetic-selection practices that it should be treated similarly. Therefore, a couple should be free to choose cloning unless there are compelling reasons for thinking that this would create harm that the other procedures would not cause.[10]

The concern of the National Bioethics Advisory Commission about the welfare of the clone reflects two types of fear. The first is that a child with the same nuclear DNA as another person, who is thus that person's later-born identical twin, will be so severely harmed by the identity of nuclear DNA between them that it is morally preferable, if not obligatory, that the child not be born at all.[5] In this case the fear is that the later-born twin will lack individuality or the freedom to create his or her own identity because of confusion or expectations caused by having the same DNA as another person.[5, 11]

This claim does not withstand the close scrutiny that should precede interference with a couple's freedom to bear and rear biologically related children.[10] Having the same genome as another person is not in itself harmful, as widespread experience with monozygotic twins shows. Being a twin does not deny either twin his or her individuality or freedom, and twins often have a special intimacy or closeness that few non-twin siblings can experience.[12] There is no reason to think that being a later-born identical twin resulting from cloning would change the overall assessment of being a twin.

Differences in mitrochondria and the uterine and childhood environment will undercut problems of similarity and minimize the risk of overidentification with the first twin. A clone of Smith may look like Smith, but he or she will not be Smith and will lack many of Smith's phenotypic characteristics. The effects of having similar DNA will also depend on the length of time before the second twin is born, on whether the twins are raised together, on whether they are informed that they are genetic twins, on whether other people are so informed, on the beliefs that the rearing parents have about genetic influence on behavior, and on other factors. Having a previously born twin might in some circumstances also prove to be a source of support or intimacy for the later-born child.

The risk that parents or the child will overly identify the child with the DNA source also seems surmountable. Would the child invariably be expected to match the phenotypic characteristics of the DNA source, thus denying the second twin an "open future" and the freedom to develop his or her own identity?[5,11,13] In response to this question, one must ask whether couples who choose to clone offspring are more likely to want a child who is a mere replica of the DNA source or a child who is unique and valued for more than his or her genes. Couples may use cloning in order to ensure that the biologic child they rear is healthy, to maintain a family connection in the face of gametic infertility, or to obtain matched tissue for transplantation and yet still be responsibly committed to the welfare of their child, including his or her separate identity and interests and right to develop as he or she chooses.

The second type of fear is that parents who choose their child's genome through somatic-cell cloning will view the child as a commodity or an object to serve their own ends.[5] We do not view children born through coital or assisted reproduction as "mere means" just because people reproduce in order to have company in old age, to fulfill what they see as God's will, to prove their virility, to have heirs, to save a relationship, or to serve other selfish purposes.[14] What counts is how a child is treated after birth. Self-interested motives for having children do not prevent parents from loving children for themselves once they are born.

The use of cloning to form families in the situations I have described, though closely related to current assisted-reproduction and genetic-selection practices, does offer unique variations. The novelty of the relation—cloning in lieu of sperm donation, for example, produces a later-born identical twin raised by the older twin and his spouse—will create special psychological and social challenges. Can these challenges be successfully met, so that cloning produces net good for families and society? Given the largely positive experience with assisted-reproduction techniques that initially appeared frightening, cautious optimism is justified. We should be able to develop procedures and guidelines for cloning that will allow us to obtain its benefits while minimizing its problems and dangers.

In the light of these considerations, I would argue that a ban on privately funded cloning research is unjustified and likely to hamper important types of research.[8] A permanent ban on the cloning of human beings, as advocated by the Council of Europe and proposed in Congress, is also unjustified.[15,16] A more limited ban—whether for 5 years, as proposed by the National Bioethics Advisory Commission and enacted in California, or for 10 years, as in the bill of Senator Dianne Feinstein (D-Calif.) and Senator Edward M. Kennedy (D-Mass.) that is now before Congress—is also open to question.[5,17,18] Given the early state of cloning science and the widely shared view that the transfer of cloned embryos to the uterus before the safety and efficacy of the procedure has been established is unethical, few responsible physicians are likely to offer human cloning in the near future.[5] Nor are profit-motivated entrepreneurs, such as Richard Seed, likely to have many customers for their cloning services until the safety of the procedure is demonstrated.[19] A ban on human cloning for a limited period would thus serve largely symbolic purposes. Symbolic legislation, however, often has substantial costs.[20,21] A government-imposed prohibition on privately funded cloning, even for a limited period, should not be enacted unless there is a compelling need. Such a need has not been demonstrated.

Rather than seek to prohibit all uses of human cloning, we should focus our attention on ensuring that cloning is done well. No physician or couple should embark on cloning without careful thought about the novel relational issues and child-rearing responsibilities that will ensue. We need regulations or guidelines to ensure safety and efficacy, fully informed consent and counseling for the couple, the consent of any person who may provide DNA, guarantees of parental rights and duties, and a limit on the number of clones from any single source.[10] It may also be important to restrict cloning to situations where there is a strong likelihood that the couple or individual initiating the procedure will also rear the resulting child. This principle will encourage a stable parenting situation and minimize the chance that cloning entrepreneurs will create clones to be sold to others.[22] As our experience grows, some restrictions on who may serve as a source of DNA for cloning (for example, a ban on cloning one's parents) may also be defensible.[10]

Cloning is important because it is the first of several positive means of genetic selection that may be sought by families seeking to have and rear healthy, biologically related offspring. In the future, mitochondrial transplantation, germ-line gene therapy, genetic enhancement, and other forms of prenatal genetic alteration may be possible.[3,23,24] With each new technique, as with cloning, the key question will be whether it serves important health, reproductive, or family needs and whether its benefits outweigh any likely harm. Cloning illustrates the principle that when legitimate uses of a technique are likely, regulatory policy should avoid prohibition and focus on ensuring that the technique is used responsibly for the good of those directly involved. As genetic knowledge continues to grow, the challenge of regulation will occupy us for some time to come.

References

1. Silver LM. Remaking Eden: cloning and beyond in a brave new world. New York: Avon Books, 1997.

2. Walters L, Palmer JG. The ethics of human gene therapy. New York: Oxford University Press, 1997.
3. Robertson JA. Genetic selection of offspring characteristics. Boston Univ Law Rev 1996; 76:421–82.
4. Begley S. Can we clone humans? Newsweek. March 10, 1997:53–60.
5. Cloning human beings: report and recommendations of the National Bioethics Advisory Commission. Rockville, Md.: National Bioethics Advisory Commission, June 1997.
6. Robertson JA. Children of choice: freedom and the new reproductive technologies. Princeton, N.J.: Princeton University Press. 1994.
7. Kearney W, Caplan AL. Parity for the donation of bone marrow: ethical and policy considerations. In: Blank RH, Bonnicksen Al, eds. Emerging issues in biomedical policy: an annual review. Vol. 1. New York: Columbia University Press, 1992:262–85.
8. Kassirer JP, Rosenthal NA. Should human cloning research be off limits? N Engl J Med 1998; 338:905–6.
9. Holtzman NA. Proceed with caution: predicting genetic risks in the recombinant DNA era. Baltimore: Johns Hopkins University Press, 1989.
10. Robertson JA. Liberty, identity, and human cloning. Texas Law Rev 1998; 77:1371–456.
11. Davis DS. What's wrong with cloning? Jurimetrics 1997;38:83–9.
12. Segal NL. Behavioral aspects of intergenerational human cloning: what twins tell us. Jurimetrics 1997;38:57–68.
13. Jonas H. Philosophical essays: from ancient creed to technological man. Englewood Cliffs, N.J.: Prentice-Hall, 1974:161.
14. Heyd D. Genethics: moral issues in the creation of people. Berkeley: University of California·Press, 1992.
15. Council of Europe. Draft additional protocol to the Convention on Human Rights and Biomedicine on the prohibition of cloning human beings with explanatory report and Parliamentary Assembly opinion (adopted September 22, 1997). XXXVI International Legal Materials 1415 (1997).
16. Human Cloning Prohibition Act, H.R. 923, S.1601 (March 5, 1997).
17. Act of Oct. 4, 1997, ch. 688, 1997 Cal. Legis. Serv. 3790 (West, WESTLAW through 1997 Sess.).
18. Prohibition on Cloning of Human Beings Act, S.1602, 105th Cong. (1998).
19. Stolberg SG. A small spark ignites debate on laws on cloning humans. New York Times, January 19, 1998:A1.
20. Gusfield J. Symbolic crusade: status politics and the American temperance movement. Urbana: University of Illinois Press, 1963.
21. Wolf SM. Ban cloning? Why NBAC is wrong. Hastings Cent Rep 1997;27(5):12.
22. Wilson JG. The paradox of cloning. The Weekly Standard. May 26, 1997:23–7.
23. Zhang J, Grifo J, Blaszczyk A, et al. In vitro maturation of human preovulatory oocytes recontrructed by germinal visicle transfer. Fertil Steril 1997;68:Suppl:S1. abstract.
24. Bonnicksen AL. Transplanting nuclei between human eggs: implications for germ-line genetics. Politics and the Life Sciences. March 1998:3–10.

George J. Annas 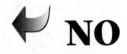 **NO**

Why We Should Ban Human Cloning

In February the U.S. Senate voted 54 to 42 against bringing an anticloning bill directly to the floor for a vote.[1] During the debate, more than 16 scientific and medical organizations, including the American Society of Reproductive Medicine and the Federation of American Societies for Experimental Biology, and 27 Nobel prize-winning scientists, agreed that there should be a moratorium on the creation of a human being by somatic nuclear transplants. What the groups objected to was legislation that went beyond this prohibition to include cloning human cells, genes, and tissues. An alternative proposal was introduced by Senator Edward M. Kennedy (D-Mass.) and Senator Dianne Feinstein (D-Calif.) and modeled on a 1997 proposal by President Bill Clinton and his National Bioethics Advisory Commission. It would, in line with the views of all of these scientific groups, outlaw attempts to produce a child but permit all other forms of cloning research.[2,3] Because the issue is intimately involved with research with embryos and abortion politics, in many ways the congressional debates over human cloning are a replay of past debates on fetal-tissue transplants[4] and research using human embryos.[5] Nonetheless, the virtually unanimous scientific consensus on the advisability of a legislative ban or voluntary moratorium on the attempt to create a human child by cloning justifies deeper discussion of the issue than it has received so far.

It has been more than a year since embryologist Ian Wilmut and his colleagues announced to the world that they had cloned a sheep.[6] No one has yet duplicated their work, raising serious questions about whether Dolly the sheep was cloned from a stem cell or a fetal cell, rather than a fully differentiated cell.[7] For my purposes, the success or failure of Wilmut's experiment is not the issue. Public attention to somatic-cell nuclear cloning presents an opportunity to consider the broader issues of public regulation of human research and the meaning of human reproduction.

Cloning and Imagination

In the 1970s, human cloning was a centerpiece issue in bioethical debates in the United States.[8,9] In 1978, a House committee held a hearing on human cloning

From George J. Annas, "Why We Should Ban Human Cloning," *The New England Journal of Medicine,* vol. 339, no. 2 (July 9, 1998), pp. 118–125. Copyright © 1998 by The Massachusetts Medical Society. All rights reserved. Reprinted by permission.

in response to the publication of David Rorvik's *In His Image: The Cloning of a Man*.[10] All the scientists who testified assured the committee that the supposed account of the cloning of a human being was fictional and that the techniques described in the book could not work. The chief point the scientists wanted to make, however, was that they did not want any laws enacted that might affect their research. In the words of one, "There is no need for any form of regulation, and it could only in the long run have a harmful effect."[11] The book was an elaborate fable, but it presented a valuable opportunity to discuss the ethical implications of cloning. The failure to see it as a fable was a failure of imagination. We normally do not look to novels for scientific knowledge, but they provide more: insights into life itself.[12]

This failure of imagination has been witnessed repeatedly, most recently in 1997, when President Clinton asked the National Bioethics Advisory Commission to make recommendations about human cloning. Although acknowledging in their report that human cloning has always seemed the stuff of science fiction rather than science, the group did not commission any background papers on how fiction informs the debate. Even a cursory reading of books like Aldous Huxley's *Brave New World,* Ira Levin's *The Boys from Brazil,* and Fay Weldon's *The Cloning of Joanna May,* for example, would have saved much time and needless debate. Literary treatments of cloning inform us that cloning is an evolutionary dead end that can only replicate what already exists but cannot improve it; that exact replication of a human is not possible; that cloning is not inherently about infertile couples or twins, but about a technique that can produce an indefinite number of genetic duplicates; that clones must be accorded the same human rights as persons that we grant any other human; and that personal identity, human dignity, and parental responsibility are at the core of the debate about human cloning.

We might also have gained a better appreciation of our responsibilities to our children had we examined fiction more closely. The reporter who described Wilmut as "Dolly's laboratory father,"[13] for example, probably could not have done a better job of conjuring up images of Mary Shelley's *Frankenstein* if he had tried. Frankenstein was also his creature's father and god; the creature told him, "I ought to be thy Adam." As in the case of Dolly, the "spark of life" was infused into the creature by an electric current. Shelley's great novel explores virtually all the noncommercial elements of today's debate.

The naming of the world's first cloned mammal also has great significance. The sole survivor of 277 cloned embryos (or "fused couplets"), the clone could have been named after its sequence in this group (for example, C-137), but this would only have emphasized its character as a laboratory product. In stark contrast, the name Dolly (provided for the public and not used in the scientific report in *Nature,* in which she is identified as 6LL3) suggests a unique individual. Victor Frankenstein, of course, never named his creature, thereby repudiating any parental responsibility. The creature himself evolved into a monster when he was rejected not only by Frankenstein, but by society as well. Naming the world's first mammal clone Dolly was meant to distance her from the Frankenstein myth both by making her something she is not (a doll) and by accepting "parental" responsibility for her.

Unlike Shelley's world, the future envisioned in Huxley's *Brave New World,* in which all humans are created by cloning through embryo splitting and conditioned to join a specified worker group, was always unlikely. There are much more efficient ways of creating killers or terrorists (or even soldiers and workers) than through cloning. Physical and psychological conditioning can turn teenagers into terrorists in a matter of months, so there is no need to wait 18 to 20 years for the clones to grow up and be trained themselves. Cloning has no real military or paramilitary uses. Even clones of Adolf Hitler would have been very different people because they would have grown up in a radically altered world environment.

Cloning and Reproduction

Even though virtually all scientists oppose it, a minority of free-marketers and bioethicists have suggested that there might nonetheless be some good reasons to clone a human. But virtually all these suggestions themselves expose the central problem of cloning: the devaluing of persons by depriving them of their uniqueness. One common example suggested is cloning a dying or recently deceased child if this is what the grieving parents want. A fictional cover story in the March 1998 issue of *Wired,* for example, tells the story of the world's first clone.[14] She is cloned from the DNA of a dead two-week-old infant, who died from a mitochondrial defect that is later "cured" by cloning with an enucleated donor egg. The closer one gets to the embryo stage, the more cloning a child looks like the much less problematic method of cloning by "twinning" or embryo splitting. And proponents of cloning tend to want to "naturalize" and "normalize" asexual replication by arguing that it is just like having "natural" twins.

Embryo splitting might be justified if only a few embryos could be produced by an infertile couple and all were implanted at the same time (since this does not involve replicating an existing and known genome). But scenarios of cloning by nuclear transfer have involved older children, and the only reason to clone an existing human is to create a genetic replica. Using the bodies of children to replicate them encourages all of us to devalue children and treat them as interchangeable commodities. For example, thanks to cloning, the death of a child need no longer be a singular human tragedy but, rather, can be an opportunity to try to replicate the no longer priceless (or irreplaceable) dead child. No one should have such dominion over a child (even a dead or dying child) as to use his or her genes to create the child's child.

Cloning would also radically alter what it means to be human by replicating a living or dead human being asexually to produce a person with a single genetic parent. The danger is that through human cloning we will lose something vital to our humanity, the uniqueness (and therefore the value and dignity) of every human. Cloning represents the height of genetic reductionism and genetic determinism.

Population geneticist R. C. Lewontin has challenged my position that the first human clone would also be the first human with a single genetic parent by arguing that, instead, "a child by cloning has a full set of chromosomes like anyone else, half of which were derived from a mother and half from a father. It happens that these chromosomes were passed through another individual, the cloning donor, on the way to the child. That donor is certainly not the child's 'parent' in any biological sense, but simply an earlier offspring of the original parents."[15] Lewontin takes genetic reductionism to perhaps its logical extreme. People become no more than containers of their parents' genes, and their parents have the right to treat them not as individual human beings, but rather as human embryos—entities that can be split and replicated at their whim without any consideration of the child's choice or welfare. Children (even adult children), according to Lewontin's view, have no say in whether they are replicated or not, because it is their parents, not they, who are reproducing. This radical redefinition of reproduction and parenthood, and the denial of the choice to procreate or not, turns out to be an even stronger argument against cloning children than its biologic novelty. Of course, we could require the consent of adults to be cloned—but why should we, if they are not becoming parents?

Related human rights and human dignity would also prohibit using cloned children as organ sources for their father or mother original. Nor is there any constitutional right to be cloned in the United States that is triggered by marriage to someone with whom an adult cannot reproduce sexually, because there is no tradition of asexual replication and because permitting asexual replication is not necessary to safeguard any existing conception of ordered liberty (rights fundamental to ordered liberty are the rights the Supreme Court sees as essential to individual liberty in our society).

Although it is possible to imagine some scenarios in which cloning could be used for the treatment of infertility, the use of cloning simply provides parents another choice for choice's sake, not out of necessity. Moreover, in a fundamental sense, cloning cannot be a treatment for infertility. This replication technique changes the very concept of infertility itself, since all humans have somatic cells that could be used for asexual replication and therefore no one would be unable to replicate himself or herself asexually. In vitro fertilization, on the other hand, simply provides a technological way for otherwise infertile humans to reproduce sexually.

John Robertson argues that adults have a right to procreate in any way they can, and that the interests of the children cannot be taken into account because the resulting children cannot be harmed (since without cloning the children would not exist at all).[16] But this argument amounts to a tautology. It applies equally to everyone alive; none of us would exist had it not been for the precise and unpredictable time when the father's sperm and the mother's egg met. This biologic fact, however, does not justify a conclusion that our parents had no obligations to us as their future children. If it did, it would be equally acceptable, from the child's perspective, to be gestated in a great ape, or even a cow, or to be composed of a mixture of ape genes and human genes.

The primary reason for banning the cloning of living or dead humans was articulated by the philosopher Hans Jonas in the early 1970s. He correctly noted that it does not matter that creating an exact duplicate of an existing person is impossible. What matters is that the person is chosen to be cloned because of some characteristic or characteristics he or she possesses (which, it is hoped, would also be possessed by the genetic copy or clone). Jonas argued that cloning is always a crime against the clone, the crime of depriving the clone of his or her "existential right to certain subjective terms of being"—particularly, the "right to ignorance" of facts about his or her origin that are likely to be "paralyzing for the spontaneity of becoming himself" or herself.[17] This advance knowledge of what another has or has not accomplished with the clone's genome destroys the clone's "condition for authentic growth" in seeking to answer the fundamental question of all beings, "Who am I?" Jonas continues: "The ethical command here entering the enlarged stage of our powers is: never to violate the right to that ignorance which is a condition of authentic action; or: to respect the right of each human life to find its own way and be a surprise to itself."[17]

Jonas is correct. His rationale, of course, applies only to a "delayed genetic twin" or "serial twin" created from an existing human, not to genetically identical twins born at the same time, including those created by cloning with use of embryo splitting. Even if one does not agree with him, however, it is hypocritical to argue that a cloning technique that limits the liberty and choices of the resulting child or children can be justified on the grounds that cloning expands the liberty and choices of would-be cloners.[18]

Moratoriums and Bans on Human Cloning

Members of the National Bioethics Advisory Commission could not agree on much, but they did conclude that any current attempt to clone a human being should be prohibited by basic ethical principles that ban putting human subjects at substantial risk without their informed consent. But danger itself will not prevent scientists and physicians from performing first-of-their-kind experiments—from implanting a baboon's heart in a human baby to using a permanent artificial heart in an adult—and cloning techniques may be both safer and more efficient in the future. We must identify a mechanism that can both prevent premature experimentation and permit reasonable experimentation when the facts change.

The mechanism I favor is a broad-based regulatory agency to oversee human experimentation in the areas of genetic engineering, research with human embryos, xenografts, artificial organs, and other potentially dangerous boundary-crossing experiments.[19] Any such national regulatory agency must be composed almost exclusively of nonresearchers and nonphysicians so it can reflect public values, not parochial concerns. Currently, the operative American ethic seems to be that if any possible case can be imagined in which a new technology might be useful, it should not be prohibited, no matter what harm might result. One of the most important procedural steps Congress should take in setting up a federal agency to regulate human experimentation would be to put the burden of proof on those who propose to undertake novel experiments (including cloning) that risk harm and call deeply held social values into question.

This shift in the burden of proof is critical if society is to have an influence over science.[20] Without it, social control is not possible. This model applies the precautionary principle of international environmental law to cloning and other potentially harmful biomedical experiments involving humans. The principle requires governments to protect the public health and the environment from realistic threats of irreversible harm or catastrophic consequences even in the absence of clear evidence of harm.[21] Under this principle, proponents of human cloning would have the burden of proving that there was some compelling contravailing need to benefit either current or future generations before such an experiment was permitted (for example, if the entire species were to become sterile). Thus, regulators would not have the burden of proving that there was some compelling reason not to approve it. This regulatory scheme would depend on at least a de facto, if not a de jure, ban or moratorium on such experiments and a mechanism such as my proposed regulatory agency that could lift the ban. The suggestion that the Food and Drug Administration (FDA) can substitute for such an agency is fanciful. The FDA has no jurisdiction over either the practice of medicine or human replication and is far too narrowly constituted to represent the public in this area. Some see human cloning as inevitable and uncontrollable. [22,23] Control will be difficult, and it will ultimately require close international cooperation. But this is no reason not to try—any more than a recognition that controlling terrorism or biologic weapons is difficult and uncertain justifies making no attempt at control.

On the recommendation of the National Bioethics Advisory Commission, the White House sent proposed anticloning legislation to Congress in June 1997. The Clinton proposal receded into obscurity until early 1998, when a Chicago physicist, Richard Seed, made national news by announcing that he intended to raise funds to clone a human. Because Seed acted like a prototypical "mad scientist," his proposal was greeted with almost universal condemnation.[24] Like the 1978 Rorvik hoax, however, it provided another opportunity for public discussion of cloning and prompted a more refined version of the Clinton proposal: the Feinstein–Kennedy bill. We can (and should) take advantage of this opportunity to distinguish the cloning of cells and tissues from the cloning of human beings by somatic nuclear transplantation[25] and to permit the former while prohibiting the latter. We should also take the opportunity to fill in the regulatory lacuna that permits any individual scientist to act first and consider the human consequences later, and we should use the controversy over cloning as an opportunity to begin an international dialogue on human experimentation.

References

1. U.S. Senate. 144 Cong. Rec. S561–S580, S607–S608 (1998).
2. S.1611 (Feinstein–Kennedy Prohibition on Cloning of Human Beings Act of 1998).
3. Cloning human beings: report and recommendations of the National Bioethics Advisory Commission. Rockville, Md.: National Bioethics Advisory Commission, June, 1997.
4. Annas GJ, Elias S. The politics of transplantation of human fetal tissue. N Engl J Med 1989; 320:1079–82.

5. Annas GJ, Caplan A, Elias S. The politics of human embryo research—avoiding ethical gridlock. N Engl J Med 1996;334:1329–32.
6. Wilmut I, Schnieke AE, McWhir J, Kind AJ, Campbell KH. Viable offspring derived from fetal and adult mammalian cells. Nature 1997; 385:810–3.
7. Butler D. Dolly researcher plans further experiments after challenges. Nature 1998;391:825–6.
8. Lederberg J. Experimental genetics and human evolution. Am Naturalist 1996; 100:519–31.
9. Watson JD. Moving toward the clonal man. Atlantic Monthly. May 1971:50–3.
10. Rorvik DM. In his image: the cloning of a man. Philadelphia: J.B. Lippincott, 1978.
11. Development in cell biology and genetics, cloning. Hearings before the Subcommittee on Health and the Environment of the Committee on Interstate and Foreign Commerce of the U.S. House of Representatives, 95th Congress, 2d Session, May 31, 1978.
12. Chomsky N. Language and problems of knowledge: the Managua lectures. Cambridge, Mass.: MIT Press, 1988.
13. Montalbano W. Cloned sheep is star, but not sole project, at institute. Los Angeles Times. February 25, 1997:A7.
14. Kadrey R. Carbon copy: meet the first human clone. Wired. March 1998:146–50.
15. Lewontin RC. Confusion over cloning. New York Review of Books. October 23, 1997:20–3.
16. Robertson JA. Children of choice: Freedom and the new reproductive technologies. Princeton, N.J.: Princeton University Press, 1994:169.
17. Jonas H. Philosophical essays: From ancient creed to technological man. Englewood Cliffs, N.J.: Prentice-Hall, 1974:162–3.
18. Annas GJ. Some choice: law, medicine and the market. New York: Oxford University Press, 1998:14–5.
19. Annas GJ. Regulatory models for human embryo cloning: the free market, professional guidelines, and government restrictions. Kennedy Inst Ethics J 1994; 4:235–49.
20. Hearings before the U.S. Senate Subcommittee on Public Health and Safety, 105th Congress, 1st Session, March 12, 1997. (Or see: http://www-busph.bu.edu/depts/lw/clonetest.htm.)
21. Cross FD. Paradoxical perils of the precautionary principle. Washington Lee Law Rev 1996; 53:851–925.
22. Kolata GB. Clone: the road to Dolly, and the path ahead. New York: W. Morrow, 1998.
23. Silver LM. Remaking Eden: cloning and beyond in a brave new world. New York: Avon Books, 1997.
24. Knox RA. A Chicagoan plans to offer cloning of humans. Boston Globe. January 7, 1998:A3.
25. Kassirer JP, Rosenthal NA. Should human cloning research be off limits? N Engl J Med 1998; 338:905–6.

POSTSCRIPT

Should Human Cloning
Ever Be Permitted?

Early in 1998 Senator Christopher Bond (R-Missouri) debated the issue of human cloning. He stated that "science has given us partial-birth abortions and Dr. Kevorkian's assisted suicide. We should say no to these scientific advances and no to the cloning of human embryos." Senator Bond, as well as other politicians and activists, are treating the issue of cloning as similar to the abortion issue. Congress agrees and has banned human cloning. See "After Heated Debate, U.S. House Votes Again to Ban Cloning," *The Chronicle of Higher Education* (March 14, 2003). Some argue that cloning could result in the production of made-to-order humans and organ farming for money. The Bond-Frist bill and the Ehlers bill, submitted to Congress, call for a total ban on cloning and on research involving somatic-cell nuclear transfer. The monitoring required to enforce the ban could necessitate intruding into scientific labs and policing the intent of researchers. There are also concerns that the ban is to be imposed by Congress, not a scientific regulatory body. This brings cloning into a political rather than a scientific arena.

Are there ways to prevent potential abuses of cloning without banning all research involving somatic-cell nuclear transfer? Discussions about restricting research were held in the 1970s, when recombinant DNA technology was first introduced. Rather than ban this technology, scientists and representatives of the government and the public developed stringent voluntary standards and guidelines to regulate it. Since that time, the technology has yielded significant benefits in medicine and health. Although many scientists have announced a self-imposed five-year moritorium on the cloning of human beings, they have argued that research involving the use of somatic-cell nuclear transfer should continue. They state that this research could result in cures for cancer and other diseases and offer infertile couples another option to have a child. Articles that contain arguments in favor of continuing this research include "Rein in the Extremists: European Parliament's Vote to Stop Stem Cells Being Harvested From Embryos and Ban Therapeutic Cloning Has Spread Dismay Among Many Biomedical Researchers," *New Scientist* (April 19, 2003); "Fetal Positions," *Mother Jones* (May/June 1998); and "Animal Cloning Technology Applied to Disease," *World Disease Weekly Plus* (May 11, 1998). In "Cooling Down Over Cloning," *Lancet* (January 17, 1998), the importance of carefully considered and informed decisions about cloning is discussed. E. V. Kontorovich, in "Asexual Revolution," *National Review* (March 9, 1998), asserts that even if cloning could actually improve human health, it should be rejected. See also "The Moral Case Against Cloning for Biomedical Research," *Issues in Law & Medicine* (Spring 2003).

On the Internet . . .

Web of Addictions

The Web of Addictions site is dedicated to providing accurate information about the use of alcohol and other drugs. The site was developed to provide data about drug abuse and to provide a resource for teachers, students, and others who need factual information about the subject.

http://www.well.com/user/woa/

The American Institute of Stress

This American Institute of Stress site details ways to identify and manage stress effectively. It offers soothing music and several useful links.

http://www.stress.org

Ethics in Medicine: Spirituality and Medicine

This Ethics in Medicine Web site provides insight into the physician's involvement in his or her patient's spiritual beliefs. Topics discussed include taking a "spiritual history" of the patient, the importance of attending to spirituality in medicine, and what role the physician's personal beliefs should play in the physician-patient relationship.

http://eduserv.hscer.washington.edu/bioethics/
topics/spirit.html

PART 3

Mind/Body Relationship

*H*umans have long sought to extend life, eliminate disease, and prevent sickness. In modern times, people depend on technology to develop creative and innovative ways to improve health. However, as cures for AIDS, cancer, and heart disease continue to elude scientists and doctors, many people question whether or not modern medicine has reached a plateau in improving health. As a result, over the last decade, an emphasis has been placed on prevention as a way to improve health. Managing stress and using prayer are ways many individuals attempt to prevent and control illness. The issue of whether or not addiction is a brain disease as opposed to a controllable behavior is also addressed in this part.

- Should Addiction to Drugs Be Labeled a Brain Disease?

- Is Stress Responsible for Disease?

- Can Spirituality Overcome Disease?

ISSUE 10

Should Addiction to Drugs Be Labeled a Brain Disease?

YES: Alan I. Leshner, from "Addiction Is a Brain Disease," *Issues in Science and Technology* (Spring 2001)

NO: Sally L. Satel, from "The Fallacies of No-Fault Addiction," *The Public Interest* (Winter 1999)

ISSUE SUMMARY

YES: Alan I. Leshner, director of the National Institute on Drug Abuse at the National Institutes of Health, states that addiction to drugs and alcohol is not a behavioral condition but a treatable disease.

NO: Psychiatrist Sally L. Satel counters that labeling addiction as a chronic and relapsing brain disease is propaganda. Satel asserts that most addicts are the instigators of their own addiction.

There are many different theories as to why some individuals become addicted to alcohol or other drugs. Historically, drug dependency has been viewed as either a disease or a moral failing. In more recent years, other theories of addiction have been developed, including behavioral, genetic, sociocultural, and psychological theories.

The view that drug addiction and alcoholism are moral failings maintains that abusing drugs is voluntary behavior. Users choose to overindulge in such a way that they create suffering for themselves and others. American history is marked by repeated and failed governmental efforts to control this abuse by eliminating drug and alcohol use with legal sanctions, such as the enactment of Prohibition in the late 1920s and the punishment of alcoholics and drug users via jail sentences and fines. However, there seem to be several contradictions to this behavioral model of addiction. Addiction may be a complex condition that is caused by multiple factors, including environment and biology. It is not totally clear that abusing drugs is voluntary behavior. From a historical perspective, punishing alcoholics and drug addicts has been ineffective.

In the United States today, the primary theory for understanding the causes of addiction is the disease model rather than the moral model. Borrowing from the modern mental health movement, the idea of addiction as a disease has been promoted by mental health advocates. Diseases such as bipolar disorder and schizophrenia are defined as the result of brain abnormalities rather than as the result of environmental factors or poor parenting. Likewise, addiction is seen as not a moral weakness but rather a brain disorder that can be treated. In 1995 the National Institute of Drug Addiction (NIDA) supported the idea that drug addiction was a type of brain disorder. Following NIDA's support, the concept of addiction as a brain disease has become more widely accepted.

This model has been advocated by the medical and alcohol treatment communities as well as by self-help groups such as Alcoholics Anonymous and Narcotics Anonymous. The disease model implies that addiction is not the result of voluntary behavior or a lack of self-control; it is caused by biological factors that are treatable. While there are somewhat different interpretations of this theory, it generally refers to addiction as an organic brain syndrome with biological and genetic origins rather than voluntary and behavioral origins.

Alan I. Leshner states that taking drugs causes changes in neurons in the central nervous system, and this compels the individual to use drugs. These neurological changes, which are not reversible, force addicts to continue to take drugs. Sally L. Satel counters that most addicts are not innocent victims of chronic disease, instead they are individuals who are responsible for their illness and recovery.

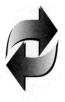

Alan I. Leshner

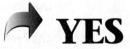 **YES**

Addiction Is a Brain Disease

The United States is stuck in its drug abuse metaphors and in polarized arguments about them. Everyone has an opinion. One side insists that we must control supply, the other that we must reduce demand. People see addiction as either a disease or as a failure of will. None of this bumpersticker analysis moves us forward. The truth is that we will make progress in dealing with drug issues only when our national discourse and our strategies are as complex and comprehensive as the problem itself.

A core concept that has been evolving with scientific advances over the past decade is that drug addiction is a brain disease that develops over time as a result of the initially voluntary behavior of using drugs. The consequence is virtually uncontrollable compulsive drug craving, seeking, and use that interferes with, if not destroys, an individual's functioning in the family and in society. This medical condition demands formal treatment.

We now know in great detail the brain mechanisms through which drugs acutely modify mood, memory, perception, and emotional states. Using drugs repeatedly over time changes brain structure and function in fundamental and long-lasting ways that can persist long after the individual stops using them. Addiction comes about through an array of neuroadaptive changes and the laying down and strengthening of new memory connections in various circuits in the brain. We do not yet know all the relevant mechanisms, but the evidence suggests that those long-lasting brain changes are responsible for the distortions of cognitive and emotional functioning that characterize addicts, particularly including the compulsion to use drugs that is the essence of addiction. It is as if drugs have highjacked the brain's natural motivational control circuits, resulting in drug use becoming the sole, or at least the top, motivational priority for the individual. Thus, the majority of the biomedical community now considers addiction, in its essence, to be a brain disease: a condition caused by persistent changes in brain structure and function.

This brain-based view of addiction has generated substantial controversy, particularly among people who seem able to think only in polarized ways. Many people erroneously still believe that biological and behavioral explanations are alternative or competing ways to understand phenomena, when in fact they are complementary and integratable. Modem science has taught that it is much too simplistic to set biology in opposition to behavior or to pit willpower against brain chemistry. Addiction involves inseparable biological and behavioral components. It is the quintessential biobehavioral disorder.

Many people also erroneously still believe that drug addiction is simply a failure of will or of strength of character. Research contradicts that position. However, the recognition that addiction is a brain disease does not mean that the addict is simply a hapless victim. Addiction begins with the voluntary behavior of using drugs, and addicts must participate in and take some significant responsibility for their recovery. Thus, having this brain disease does not absolve the addict of responsibility for his or her behavior, but it does explain why an addict cannot simply stop using drugs by sheer force of will alone. It also dictates a much more sophisticated approach to dealing with the array of problems surrounding drug abuse and addiction in our society.

The Essence of Addiction

The entire concept of addiction has suffered greatly from imprecision and misconception. In fact, if it were possible, it would be best to start all over with some new, more neutral term. The confusion comes about in part because of a now archaic distinction between whether specific drugs are "physically" or "psychologically" addicting. The distinction historically revolved around whether or not dramatic physical withdrawal symptoms occur when an individual stops taking a drug; what we in the field now call "physical dependence."

However, 20 years of scientific research has taught that focusing on this physical versus psychological distinction is off the mark and a distraction from the real issues. From both clinical and policy perspectives, it actually does not matter very much what physical withdrawal symptoms occur. Physical dependence is not that important, because even the dramatic withdrawal symptoms of heroin and alcohol addiction can now be easily managed with appropriate medications. Even more important, many of the most dangerous and addicting drugs, including methamphetamine and crack cocaine, do not produce very severe physical dependence symptoms upon withdrawal.

What really matters most is whether or not a drug causes what we now know to be the essence of addiction: uncontrollable, compulsive drug craving, seeking, and use, even in the face of negative health and social consequences. This is the crux of how the Institute of Medicine, the American Psychiatric Association, and the American Medical Association define addiction and how we all should use the term. It is really only this compulsive quality of addiction that matters in the long run to the addict and to his or her family and that should matter to society as a whole. Compulsive craving that overwhelms all other motivations is the root cause of the massive health and social problems associated with drug addiction. In updating our national discourse on drug abuse, we should keep in mind this simple definition: Addiction is a brain disease expressed in the form of compulsive behavior. Both developing and recovering from it depend on biology, behavior, and social context.

It is also important to correct the common misimpression that drug use, abuse, and addiction are points on a single continuum along which one slides back and forth over time, moving from user to addict, then back to occasional user, then back to addict. Clinical observation and more formal research studies support the view that, once addicted, the individual has moved into a different state of being. It is as if a threshold has been crossed. Very few people appear able to successfully return to occasional use after having been truly addicted. Unfortunately, we do not yet have a clear biological or behavioral marker of that transition from voluntary drug use to addiction. However, a body of scientific evidence is rapidly developing that points to an array of cellular and molecular changes in specific brain circuits. Moreover, many of these brain changes are common to all chemical addictions, and some also are typical of other compulsive behaviors such as pathological overeating.

Addiction should be understood as a chronic recurring illness. Although some addicts do gain full control over their drug use after a single treatment episode, many have relapses. Repeated treatments become necessary to increase the intervals between and diminish the intensity of relapses, until the individual achieves abstinence.

The complexity of this brain disease is not atypical, because virtually no brain diseases are simply biological in nature and expression. All, including stroke, Alzheimer's disease, schizophrenia, and clinical depression, include some behavioral and social aspects. What may make addiction seem unique among brain diseases, however, is that it does begin with a clearly voluntary behavior—the initial decision to use drugs. Moreover, not everyone who ever uses drugs goes on to become addicted. Individuals differ substantially in how easily and quickly they become addicted and in their preferences for particular substances. Consistent with the biobehavioral nature of addiction, these individual differences result from a combination of environmental and biological, particularly genetic, factors. In fact, estimates are that between 50 and 70 percent of the variability in susceptibility to becoming addicted can be accounted for by genetic factors.

Over time the addict loses substantial control over his or her initially voluntary behavior, and it becomes compulsive. For many people these behaviors are truly uncontrollable, just like the behavioral expression of any other brain disease. Schizophrenics cannot control their hallucinations and delusions. Parkinson's patients cannot control their trembling. Clinically depressed patients cannot voluntarily control their moods. Thus, once one is addicted, the characteristics of the illness—and the treatment approaches—are not that different from most other brain diseases. No matter how one develops an illness, once one has it, one is in the diseased state and needs treatment.

Moreover, voluntary behavior patterns are, of course, involved in the etiology and progression of many other illnesses, albeit not all brain diseases. Examples abound, including hypertension, arteriosclerosis and other cardiovascular diseases, diabetes, and forms of cancer in which the onset is heavily influenced by the individual's eating, exercise, smoking, and other behaviors.

Addictive behaviors do have special characteristics related to the social contexts in which they originate. All of the environmental cues surrounding initial drug use and development of the addiction actually become "conditioned" to that drug use and are thus critical to the development and expression of addiction. Environmental cues are paired in time with an individual's initial drug use experiences and, through classical conditioning, take on conditioned stimulus properties. When those cues are present at a later time, they elicit anticipation of a drug experience and thus generate tremendous drug craving. Cue-induced craving is one of the most frequent causes of drug use relapses, even after long periods of abstinence, independently of whether drugs are available.

The salience of environmental or contextual cues helps explain why reentry to one's community can be so difficult for addicts leaving the controlled environments of treatment or correctional settings and why aftercare is so essential to successful recovery. The person who became addicted in the home environment is constantly exposed to the cues conditioned to his or her initial drug use, such as the neighborhood where he or she hung out, drug-using buddies, or the lamppost where he or she bought drugs. Simple exposure to those cues automatically triggers craving and can lead rapidly to relapses. This is one reason why someone who apparently overcame drug cravings while in prison or residential treatment could quickly revert to drug use upon returning home. In fact, one of the major goals of drug addiction treatment is to teach addicts how to deal with the cravings caused by inevitable exposure to these conditioned cues.

Implications

Understanding addiction as a brain disease has broad and significant implications for the public perception of addicts and their families, for addiction treatment practice, and for some aspects of public policy. On the other hand, this biomedical view of addiction does not speak directly to and is unlikely to bear significantly on many other issues, including specific strategies for controlling the supply of drugs and whether initial drug use should be legal or not. Moreover, the brain disease model of addiction does not address the question of whether specific drugs of abuse can also be potential medicines. Examples abound of drugs that can be both highly addicting and extremely effective medicines. The best-known example is the appropriate use of morphine as a treatment for pain. Nevertheless, a number of practical lessons can be drawn from the scientific understanding of addiction.

It is no wonder addicts cannot simply quit on their own. They have an illness that requires biomedical treatment. People often assume that because addiction begins with a voluntary behavior and is expressed in the form of excess behavior, people should just be able to quit by force of will alone. However, it is essential to understand when dealing with addicts that we are dealing with individuals whose brains have been altered by drug use. They need drug addiction treatment. We know that, contrary to common belief, very few addicts actually do just stop on their own. Observing that there are very few heroin addicts in their

50 or 60s, people frequently ask what happened to those who were heroin addicts 30 years ago, assuming that they must have quit on their own. However, longitudinal studies find that only a very small fraction actually quit on their own. The rest have either been successfully treated, are currently in maintenance treatment, or (for about half) are dead. Consider the example of smoking cigarettes: Various studies have found that between 3 and 7 percent of people who try to quit on their own each year actually succeed. Science has at last convinced the public that depression is not just a lot of sadness; that depressed individuals are in a different brain state and thus require treatment to get their symptoms under control. The same is true for schizophrenic patients. It is time to recognize that this is also the case for addicts.

The role of personal responsibility is undiminished but clarified.   Does having a brain disease mean that people who are addicted no longer have any responsibility for their behavior or that they are simply victims of their own genetics and brain chemistry? Of course not. Addiction begins with the voluntary behavior of drug use, and although genetic characteristics may predispose individuals to be more or less susceptible to becoming addicted, genes do not doom one to become an addict. This is one major reason why efforts to prevent drug use are so vital to any comprehensive strategy to deal with the nation's drug problems. Initial drug use is a voluntary, and therefore preventable, behavior.

Moreover, as with any illness, behavior becomes a critical part of recovery. At a minimum, one must comply with the treatment regimen, which is harder than it sounds. Treatment compliance is the biggest cause of relapses for all chronic illnesses, including asthma, diabetes, hypertension, and addiction. Moreover, treatment compliance rates are no worse for addiction than for these other illnesses, ranging from 30 to 50 percent. Thus, for drug addiction as well as for other chronic diseases, the individual's motivation and behavior are clearly important parts of success in treatment and recovery.

Implications for treatment approaches and treatment expectations.   Maintaining this comprehensive biobehavioral understanding of addiction also speaks to what needs to be provided in drug treatment programs. Again, we must be careful not to pit biology against behavior. The National Institute on Drug Abuse's recently published Principles of Effective Drug Addiction Treatment provides a detailed discussion of how we must treat all aspects of the individual, not just the biological component or the behavioral component. As with other brain diseases such as schizophrenia and depression, the data show that the best drug addiction treatment approaches attend to the entire individual, combining the use of medications, behavioral therapies, and attention to necessary social services and rehabilitation. These might include such services as family therapy to enable the patient to return to successful family life, mental health services, education and vocational training, and housing services.

That does not mean, of course, that all individuals need all components of treatment and all rehabilitation services. Another principle of effective addiction treatment is that the array of services included in an individual's treatment plan must be matched to his or her particular set of needs. Moreover, since those needs will surely change over the course of recovery, the array of services provided will need to be continually reassessed and adjusted.

What to do with addicted criminal offenders.   One obvious conclusion is that we need to stop simplistically viewing criminal justice and health approaches as incompatible opposites. The practical reality is that crime and drug addiction often occur in tandem: Between 50 and 70 percent of arrestees are addicted to illegal drugs. Few citizens would be willing to relinquish criminal justice system control over individuals, whether they are addicted or not, who have committed crimes against others. Moreover, extensive real-life experience shows that if we simply incarcerate addicted offenders without treating them, their return to both drug use and criminality is virtually guaranteed.

A growing body of scientific evidence points to a much more rational and effective blended public health/public safety approach to dealing with the addicted offender. Simply summarized, the data show that if addicted offenders are provided with well-structured drug treatment while under criminal justice control, their recidivism rates can be reduced by 50 to 60 percent for subsequent drug use and by more than 40 percent for further criminal behavior. Moreover, entry into drug treatment need not be completely voluntary in order for it to work. In fact, studies suggest that increased pressure to stay in treatment—whether from the legal system or from family members or employers—actually increases the amount of time patients remain in treatment and improves their treatment outcomes.

Findings such as these are the underpinning of a very important trend in drug control strategies now being implemented in the United States and many foreign countries. For example, some 40 percent of prisons and jails in this country now claim to provide some form of drug treatment to their addicted inmates, although we do not know the quality of the treatment provided. Diversion to drug treatment programs as an alternative to incarceration is gaining popularity across the United States. The widely applauded growth in drug treatment courts over the past five years—to more than 400—is another successful example of the blending of public health and public safety approaches. These drug courts use a combination of criminal justice sanctions and drug use monitoring and treatment tools to manage addicted offenders.

Updating the Discussion

Understanding drug abuse and addiction in all their complexity demands that we rise above simplistic polarized thinking about drug issues. Addiction is both a public health and a public safety issue, not one or the other. We must deal with both the supply and the demand issues with equal vigor. Drug abuse and addiction are about both biology and behavior. One can have a disease and not be a hapless victim of it.

We also need to abandon our attraction to simplistic metaphors that only distract us from developing appropriate strategies. I, for one, will be in some ways sorry to see the War on Drugs metaphor go away, but go away it must. At some level, the notion of waging war is as appropriate for the illness of addiction as it is for our War on Cancer, which simply means bringing all forces to bear on the problem in a focused and energized way. But, sadly, this concept has been badly distorted and misused over time, and the War on Drugs never became what it should have been: the War on Drug Abuse and Addiction. Moreover, worrying about whether we are winning or losing this war has deteriorated to using simplistic and inappropriate measures such as counting drug addicts. In the end, it has only fueled discord. The War on Drugs metaphor has done nothing to advance the real conceptual challenges that need to be worked through.

I hope, though, that we will all resist the temptation to replace it with another catchy phrase that inevitably will devolve into a search for quick or easy-seeming solutions to our drug problems. We do not rely on simple metaphors or strategies to deal with our other major national problems such as education, health care, or national security. We are, after all, trying to solve truly monumental, multidimensional problems on a national or even international scale. To devalue them to the level of slogans does our public an injustice and dooms us to failure.

Understanding the health aspects of addiction is in no way incompatible with the need to control the supply of drugs. In fact, a public health approach to stemming an epidemic or spread of a disease always focuses comprehensively on the agent, the vector, and the host. In the case of drugs of abuse, the agent is the drug, the host is the abuser or addict, and the vector for transmitting the illness is clearly the drug suppliers and dealers that keep the agent flowing so readily. Prevention and treatment are the strategies to help protect the host. But just as we must deal with the flies and mosquitoes that spread infectious diseases, we must directly address all the vectors in the drug-supply system.

In order to be truly effective, the blended public health/public safety approaches advocated here must be implemented at all levels of society—local, state, and national. All drug problems are ultimately local in character and impact, since they differ so much across geographic settings and cultural contexts, and the most effective solutions are implemented at the local level. Each community must work through its own locally appropriate antidrug implementation strategies, and those strategies must be just as comprehensive and science-based as those instituted at the state or national level.

The message from the now very broad and deep array of scientific evidence is absolutely clear. If we as a society ever hope to make any real progress in dealing with our drug problems, we are going to have to rise above moral outrage that addicts have "done it to themselves" and develop strategies that are as sophisticated and as complex as the problem itself. Whether addicts are "victims" or not, once addicted they must be seen as "brain disease patients."

Moreover, although our national traditions do argue for compassion for those who are sick, no matter how they contracted their illnesses, I recognize that many addicts have disrupted not only their own lives but those of their families and their broader communities, and thus do not easily generate compassion. However, no matter how one may feel about addicts and their behavioral histories, an extensive body of scientific evidence shows that approaching addiction as a treatable illness is extremely cost-effective, both financially and in terms of broader societal impacts such as family violence, crime, and other forms of social upheaval. Thus, it is clearly in everyone's interest to get past the hurt and indignation and slow the drain of drugs on society by enhancing drug use prevention efforts and providing treatment to all who need it.

Sally L. Satel

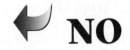

The Fallacies of No-Fault Addiction

On November 20, 1995, more than one hundred substance-abuse experts gathered in Chantilly, Virginia for a meeting organized by the government's top research agency on drug abuse. One topic for discussion was whether the agency, the National Institute on Drug Abuse (NIDA), which is part of the National Institutes of Health, should declare drug addiction a disease of the brain. Overwhelmingly, the assembled academics, public-health workers, and state officials declared that it should.

At the time, the answer was a controversial one, but, in the three years since, the notion of addiction as a brain disease has become widely accepted, thanks to a full-blown public education campaign by NIDA. Waged in editorial board rooms, town-hall gatherings, Capitol Hill briefings and hearings, the campaign reached its climax last spring [1999] when media personality Bill Moyers catapulted the brain-disease concept into millions of living rooms with a five-part PBS special called "Moyers on Addiction: Close to Home." Using imaging technology, Moyers showed viewers eye-catching pictures of addicts' brains. The cocaine-damaged parts of the brain were "lit up"—an "image of desire" was how one of the researchers on Moyers' special described it.

These dramatic visuals lend scientific credibility to NIDA's position. But politicians—and, in particular, President Clinton's drug czar, General Barry Mc-Caffrey, who has begun reciting the brain-disease rhetoric—should resist this medicalized portrait. First, it reduces a complex human activity to a slice of damaged brain tissue. Second, and more importantly, it vastly underplays the paradoxically voluntary nature of addictive behavior. As a colleague said: "We could examine brains all day and by whatever sophisticated means we want, but we would never label someone a drug addict unless he acted like one."

No-Fault Addiction

The idea of a "no-fault" disease did not originate at NIDA. For the last decade or so it was vigorously promoted by mental-health advocates working to transform the public's understanding of severe mental illness. Diseases like schizophrenia and manic depressive illness, they properly said, were products of a defective brain, not bad parenting. Until the early 1980s, when accumulated neuroscientific discoveries showed, irrefutably, that schizophrenia was marked by measurable abnormalities of brain structure and function, remnants of the psychiatric profession and much of the public were still inclined to blame parents for their children's mental illness.

NIDA borrowed the brain-disease notion from the modern mental-health movement, understandably hoping to reap similar benefits—greater acceptance of its efforts and of its own constituent sufferers, that is, addicts. By focusing exclusively on the brain, NIDA ironically diminishes the importance of its own research portfolio, which devotes an ample section to behavioral interventions. It may well be that researchers will someday be able to map the changes in brain physiology that accompany behavioral changes during recovery. Nevertheless, it is crucial to recognize that the human substrate upon which behavioral treatments work, first and foremost, is the will.

Some of those experts that met in Chantilly would say that emphasizing the role of will, or choice, is just an excuse to criminalize addiction. Clinical experience in treating addicts, however, suggests that such an orientation provides therapeutic grounds for optimism. It means that the addict is capable of self-control—a much more encouraging conclusion than one could ever draw from a brain-bound, involuntary model of addiction.

What Does Brain Disease Mean?

A recent article in the journal *Science,* "Addiction is a Brain Disease, and It Matters," authored by NIDA director Alan I. Leshner, summarizes the evidence that long-term exposure to drugs produces addiction: Taking drugs elicits changes in neurons in the central nervous system that compel the individual to take drugs. Because these changes are presumed to be irreversible, the addict is perpetually at risk for relapse.

> Virtually all drugs of abuse have common effects, either directly or indirectly, on a single pathway deep within the brain. . . . Activation of this pathway appears to be a common element in what keeps drug users taking drugs. . . . The addicted brain is distinctly different from the non-addicted brain, as manifested by changes in metabolic activity, receptor availability, gene expression and responsiveness to environmental cues. . . . That addiction is tied to changes in brain structure and function is what makes it, fundamentally, a brain disease.

Others are less dogmatic. Harvard biochemist Bertha Madras acknowledges a virtual library of documented, replicable brain changes with drug exposure, but she also points out that there have been no scientific studies correlating them with behavior. This missing connection, upon which the addiction-as-a-brain-disease argument clearly depends, has prompted some very unsympathetic reactions. John P. Seibyl, a psychiatrist and nuclear radiologist at Yale University School of Medicine, has called the notion of predicting behavior from brain pathology "modern phrenology."

Not even Alcoholics Anonymous, the institution most responsible for popularizing the disease concept of addiction, supports the idea that drug-induced brain changes determine an addict's behavior. AA employs disease as a metaphor for loss of control. And even though AA assumes that inability to stop drinking, once started, is biologically driven, it does not allow this to overshadow AA's central belief that addiction is a symptom of a spiritual defect, and can thus be overcome through the practice of honesty, humility, and acceptance.

The brain-disease advocates, of course, operate by an entirely different frame of reference. To them, "addiction" means taking drugs compulsively because the brain, having already been changed by drugs, orders the user to do so. As Moyers put it on "Meet the Press," drugs "hijack the brain . . . relapse is normal." The brain-disease advocates assume a correlation between drug-taking behavior and brain-scan appearance, though one has yet to be clearly demonstrated, and speculate, based on preliminary evidence, that pathological changes persist for years. A physiological diagnosis, to stretch the meaning of that word, should of course yield a medicinal prescription. So, brain-disease advocates seem confident, despite evidence to the contrary, that a neuroscience of addiction will give rise to pharmaceutical remedies. Meanwhile, the search for a cocaine medication, having begun with such high hopes, has come up empty. And there is good reason to wonder if this enterprise will ever bear fruit. Even the widely used medication for heroin addiction—methadone—is only partly helpful in curtailing drug use. It fails to remedy the underlying anguish for which drugs like heroin and cocaine are the desperate remedy.

Addicted to Politics

The dispute over whether addiction is a brain disease isn't merely a dispute among doctors. It is, for many reasons, political. The efforts of NIDA do not simply aim to medicalize addiction, presumably a medical concern, but to destigmatize the addict, clearly a sociopolitical concern. This is also the agenda of the newly formed group, Physician Leadership on National Drug Policy. "Concerted efforts to eliminate stigma" should result in substance abuse being "accorded parity with other chronic, relapsing conditions insofar as access to care, treatment benefits and clinical outcomes are concerned," a statement from the Leadership group says. These sentiments have been echoed by the Institute of Medicine, a quasi-governmental body that is part of the National Academy of Sciences. "Addiction . . . is not well understood by the public and policy makers. Overcoming problems of stigma and misunderstanding will require educating the public, health educators, policymakers and clinicians, highlighting progress made, and recruiting talented researchers into the field."

Indeed, the politics of drug addiction have begun to strain the logic of drug-addiction experts. In their *Lancet* article, "Myths About the Treatment of Addiction," researchers Charles O'Brien and Thomas McLellan state that relapse to drugs is an inherent aspect of addiction and should not be viewed as a treatment failure. They sensibly point out that in long-term conditions—for example, asthma, diabetes, and hypertension—relapse is often the result of the patient's poor compliance with proper diet, exercise, and medication. But then they jump to the conclusion that since the relapse of some addicts follows from poor compliance too, addiction is like any other disease. This is incorrect. Asthmatics and diabetics who resist doctor's orders share certain characteristics with addicts. But asthmatics and diabetics can also deteriorate spontaneously on the basis of unprovoked, unavoidable primary, physical reasons alone; relapse to addiction, by contrast, invariably represents a voluntary act in conscious defiance of "doctor's orders." The bottom line is that conditions like asthma and diabetes are not developed through voluntary behavior. An asthmatic does not choose to be short of breath. Addicts, however, choose to use drugs.

Analogies aside, calling addiction a chronic and relapsing disease is simply wrong. Treatment-outcome studies do support the claim, but data from the large Epidemiologic Catchment Area (ECA) study, funded by the National Institute of Mental Health, show that in the general population remission from drug dependence (addiction) and drug abuse is the norm. Contra publicist Bill Moyers and researchers O'Brien and McLellan, relapse is not. According to ECA criteria for remission—defined as no symptoms for the year just prior to the interview— 59 percent of roughly 1,300 respondents who met lifetime criteria were free of drug problems. The average duration of remission was 2.7 years, and the mean duration of illness was 6.1 years with most cases lasting no more than 8 years.

Yet, if NIDA and other public-health groups can change how the public views addiction, tangible political gains will follow. Such groups aim at securing more treatment and services for addicts, expanded insurance coverage, and increased funding for addiction research. These are not unreasonable aims insofar as substandard quality of care, limited access to care, and understudied research questions remain serious problems. But the knee-jerk reflex to decry stigma has been naively borrowed from the mental-health community. Stigma deters unwanted behaviors, and it enforces societal norms. Destigmatizing addicts (recasting them as chronic illness sufferers) threatens one of the most promising venues for anti-addiction efforts: the criminal justice system. The courts and probation services can impose sanctions that greatly enhance retention and prevent relapse. (More about this later.)

A Medical Cure for Addiction?

One of NIDA's major goals has been the development of a cocaine medication by the turn of the century. . . . [N]o magic bullet is in sight. To date, over 40 pharmaceuticals have been studied in randomized controlled trials in humans for cocaine abuse or dependence. Some of these were intended to block craving, others to substitute for cocaine itself, but none have yet been found even minimally effective. The NIDA director has downgraded predictions about the curative power of medication, promoting it as potentially "complementary" to behavioral therapy.

The basic problem with putative anticraving medications is their lack of specificity. Instead of deploying a surgical strike on the neuronal site of cocaine yearning, these medications end up blunting motivation in general and may also depress mood. Likewise, experiments with cocaine-like substances have proven frustrating. Instead of suppressing the urge to use the drug, they tend to work like an appetizer, producing physical sensations and emotional memories reminiscent of cocaine itself, triggering a hunger for it.

If a selective medication could be developed, it might be especially helpful to cocaine addicts who have abstained for a time but who experience sudden spontaneous bursts of craving for cocaine, a feeling that is often reported as alien, coming "out of nowhere," and uncoupled from a true desire to use cocaine. Such craving may be triggered by environmental cues (e.g., passing through the neighborhood where the addict used to get high). Generally, the addict learns his idiosyncratic cues, avoids them, and arms himself with exercises and strategies (e.g., immediately calling a 12-step sponsor) that help him fight the urge. It is always conceivable that a medication could help in terms of suppressing the jolt of desire and, ultimately, uncoupling the cue from the conditioned response.

Another pharmacological approach to cocaine addiction has been immunization against the drug's effect. In late 1995, scientists reported the promising effects of a cocaine vaccine in rats. The animals were inoculated with an artificial cocaine-like substance that triggered the production of antibodies to cocaine. When actual cocaine was administered, the antibodies attached to the molecules of cocaine, reducing the amount of free drug available in the bloodstream to enter the brain.

The vaccine is still being developed for use in humans, but the principle behind its presumed effect is already being exploited by an available anti-heroin medication called naltrexone. Naltrexone blocks opiate molecules at the site of attachment to receptors on the neuron. This way, an addict who administers heroin feels no effect. Uncoupling the desired response (getting high) from the action intended to produce it (shooting up) is called "extinction," and, according to behaviorist theory, the subject will eventually stop administering a drug if he no longer achieves an effect. Though naltrexone is effective, most heroin addicts reject it in favor of methadone's calming effect.

Optimism surrounding the pharmaceutical approach to drug dependence stems, in fact, from the qualified success of methadone, an opioid painkiller developed by German chemists during World War II. It was first tested in 1964 as a substitute for heroin in the United States, and now about 19 percent of the nation's estimated 600,000 heroin addicts are enrolled in methadone-maintenance clinics. Numerous studies have documented the socioeconomic benefits of methadone: significant reductions in crime, overdoses, unemployment, and, in some regions, HIV.

Unlike heroin, which needs to be administered every four to eight hours to prevent withdrawal symptoms, methadone requires only daily dosing. "Successful methadone users are invisible," the director of the Beth Israel Medical Center in New York City told the *New York Times.* Between 5 percent and 20 percent remain on the medication for over 10 years, and many are indeed invisible. An example mentioned in the *Times* article is Jimmie Maxwell, an 80-year-old jazz trumpet player who has stayed clean for the past 32 years by taking methadone every day. Unfortunately, people like Maxwell, who lead an optimal life and are otherwise drug-free, represent perhaps 5 percent to 7 percent of methadone patients. Moreover, patients in methadone maintenance are frequently not drug-free; as many as 35 percent to 60 percent also use cocaine or other illicit drugs or black-market sedatives. During a six-year follow-up, D. Dwayne Simpson of the Institute of Behavioral Research at Texas Christian University found over half of all patients were readmitted to their agency at some point.

This should come as little surprise. Methadone will only prevent withdrawal symptoms and the related physiological hunger for heroin, but it alone can't medicate the psychic deficits that led to addiction, such as deep-seated inabilities to tolerate boredom, depression, stress, anger, loneliness. The addict who initiated heavy drug use in his teens hasn't even completed the maturational tasks of adolescence, let alone prepared himself psychologically to solve the secondary layer of troubles that accumulated over years of drug use: family problems, educational deficiencies, disease, personal and economic losses. Only a fraction of heroin addicts become fully productive on methadone alone.

The biological view of addiction conceals an established fact of enormous and pressing clinical relevance: The course of addictive behavior can be influenced by the very consequences of the drug taking itself. Indeed, when the addict reacts to aversive sequelae of drug use—economic, health, legal, and personal—by eventually quitting drugs, reducing use, changing his pattern of use or getting help, he does so voluntarily. Rather than being the inevitable, involuntary product of a diseased brain, the course addiction follows may represent the essence of a free will. Consequences can inspire a change in voluntary behavior, irrespective of its predictability or biological underpinnings. Involuntary behavior cannot be changed by its consequences. A review of the clinical features of addiction will help illustrate the mix of voluntary and involuntary behaviors associated with addiction, belying the claim that addiction is a brain disease.

Harnessing the Will to Stay Clean

It is especially common for heroin-dependent individuals to become immune to the euphoric effect of the drug yet still seek the drug to keep from going into withdrawal. Upon cessation of heroin, a predictable pattern of gross physiological symptoms appears. The same is true of cessation of other opioid drugs including Demerol, morphine, Percocet, codeine, as well as alcohol. To picture this one only need recall actor Jack Lemmon in the movie, *Days of Wine and Roses,* his body wracked with tremors, sweating, anxious, desperate for a drink after running out of whisky. Or Frank Sinatra in *Man with the Golden Arm,* the heroin addict suffering painful muscle cramps and powerful cravings for heroin after his last fix wore off.

Unlike heroin and alcohol, cocaine does not produce such serious physical withdrawal symptoms. The heavy cocaine addict typically uses the drug in a driven, repetitive manner for 24 to 72 hours straight. Cocaine wears off very quickly and, as it fades, the yearning for more is overpowering. Each fresh hit quells the intense craving. The process winds down only when the addict becomes exhausted, runs out of money, or becomes paranoid, a potential effect of cocaine and other stimulants, such as methamphetamine. He then "crashes" into a phase of agitated depression and hunger followed by sleep for 12 to 36 hours. Within hours to days after awakening, he experiences powerful urges to use the drug again, and the cycle resumes.

A regular user in the midst of a cocaine binge or experiencing heroin withdrawal cannot readily stop using if drugs are available. He is presumably in the "brain-disease" state, when use is most compulsive, neuronal disruption most intense. True, even purposeful behavior can occur in this state—for example, the attempt, sometimes violent, to get money or drugs is highly goal-directed. But, at the same time, addicts in such an urgent state will ignore their screaming babies, frantically gouge themselves with dirty needles, and ruin families, careers, and reputations.

Nonetheless, most addicts have broken the cycle many times. Either they decide to go "cold turkey" or end up doing so, unintentionally, by running out of drugs or money or landing in jail. Some heroin addicts admit themselves to the hospital to detoxify because they want to quit, others to reduce the cost of their habit, knowing they'll be more sensitive to the effects of heroin afterward. This latter trip to the hospital, while motivated by an effort to pursue drug use more efficiently, is nonetheless a purposeful move that, under other circumstances, might be taken by the addict to re-exert control.

In the days between binges, cocaine addicts make many deliberate choices including (potentially) the choice to stop using. Heroin-dependent individuals, by comparison, use the drug several times a day but can be quite functional in all respects as long as they have stable access to some form of opiate drug in order to prevent withdrawal symptoms. Certainly, some addicts may "nod off" in abandoned buildings, true to stereotype, if they consume more opiate than the amount to which their body has developed tolerance, but others can be "actively engaged in activities and relationships," according to ethnographers Edward Preble and John J. Casey, Jr. "The brief moments of euphoria after each administration constitute a small fraction of their daily lives. The rest of the time they are aggressively pursuing a career . . . hustling."

According to the Office of National Drug Control Policy, as many as 46 percent of drug users not in treatment reported exclusively legal sources of income, and 42 percent reported both legal and illegal. The National Institute of Justice found that between 33 percent and 67 percent of arrested drug users indicate "full and part time work" as their main source of income. It is reasonable to assume that individuals who are most heavily involved in drug use participate least in the legitimate economy. Nonetheless, the fact that many committed drug users do have jobs shows that addiction does not necessarily preclude purposeful activity.

The temporal architecture of an addict's routine reveals periods in which the individual is capable of reflection and deliberate behavior. During the course of a heroin addict's day, for example, he may feel rather calm, and his thoughts might be quite lucid, if he is confident of access to drugs and if he is using it in doses adequate to prevent withdrawal symptoms, but not large enough to sedate. Likewise, there are periods within a cocaine addict's week when he is neither engaged in a binge nor wracked with intense craving for the drug. During such moments, does anyone believe the addict is the victim of a brain disease?

Society's Expectations

Thus, when properly "fixed," the heroin addict might rationally decide to enter a detoxification program or enter a methadone-maintenance program. And between binges the cocaine addict could decide to enter a treatment program or move across town away from the visual cues and the personal associations that provoke craving. Yes, the addict can do such things. But if asked to do so at any given moment, will he?

Probably not. Even those who wish most passionately for a better life may fear coping without drugs. It gets worse: The addict may believe a better life is just not possible. Yet, chances are that some would say "yes" to the possibility of overcoming their addiction. And this can be encouraged behaviorally through rewards and punishments. For example, society could decide to make some necessities—welfare payments, employment, public housing, or child custody—contingent on abstinence. A systematic plan that closes absolutely all avenues of support to those who can't or won't stop using drugs—allowing them only elective treatment or, once arrested for nonviolent drug-related crime, court-ordered treatment—would be too radical, unfair even.

For one thing, the treatment system—especially residential treatment for both voluntary and criminally coerced addicts—would need to be greatly expanded to accommodate those who did not curtail use under pressure alone. Moral objections to refusing addicts access to many public goods and services—or, better, administering small punishments or rewards contingent on performance—would need to be overcome. According to a behavioral model of addiction, it is not unethical. Society can and should legitimately place expectations and demands on addicts because their "brain disease" is not a persistent state. Furthermore, experimental evidence shows that addicts can control drug taking.

In his book, *Heavy Drinking: The Myth of Alcoholism as a Disease*, philosopher Herbert Fingarette cites numerous independent investigations conducted under controlled conditions showing the degree to which alcoholics are capable of regulating themselves. Researchers found, for example, that the amount of alcohol consumed was related to its cost and the effort required to obtain it. Once offered small payments, subjects were able to refuse freely available alcohol. And, after drinking an initial "priming" dose, the amount of alcohol subsequently consumed was inversely proportionate to size of the payment. Other experiments showed that the drinkers' beliefs and attitudes about alcohol influenced how much they consumed. This is potentially very significant to drug addiction; for example, the demand for heroin and cocaine is elastic, responding to price.

The story of the returning Vietnam servicemen is a revealing natural experiment that "changed our views of heroin" according to epidemiologist Lee Robins and colleagues who wrote the now classic paper on the subject, "Vietnam Veterans Three Years After Vietnam." They found that only 14 percent of men who were dependent on heroin in Vietnam—and who failed a publicized urine test at departure because they did not stop using—resumed regular heroin use back home. The rest had access to heroin, and had even used some occasionally, but what made them decide to stop for good, Robins found, was the "sordid" culture surrounding heroin use, the drug's price, and fear of arrest.

Enlightened Coercion

Behavioral therapies are not then the problem; they make the most practical and theoretical sense. The literature consistently shows that an addict who completes a treatment program—any program—either stops or markedly reduces his use of drugs after discharge. The problem is that only a small number of participants finish their programs. Estimates of attendance beyond 52 weeks, the generally accepted minimum duration for treatment, range from 8 percent to 20 percent of patients entering any of the three most common types of programs: outpatient counseling, methadone maintenance, and residential treatment.

How best to instill "motivation" is a perennial topic among clinicians; at least one form of psychotherapy has been developed for that explicit purpose. But routinely neglected by most mainstream addiction experts is the powerful yet counter-intuitive fact that patients who enter treatment involuntarily under court order will fare as well, sometimes even better, than those who enroll voluntarily. Numerous studies support this. Large government-funded studies spanning three decades—the Drug Abuse Reporting Program (1970s), Treatment Outcome Prospective Study (1980s), and the Drug Abuse Treatment Outcome Study (1990s)—all found that the longer a person stays in treatment the better his outcome. Not surprisingly, those under legal supervision stay longer than their voluntary counterparts.

The best-studied population of coerced addicts was part of California's Civil Addict Program (CAP), started in 1962. During its most active years, in the 1970s, the program was impressively successful. It required addicts to be treated in a residential setting for two years and then closely supervised by specially trained parole officers for another five. These officers had small caseloads, performed weekly urine tests, and had the authority to return individuals to forced treatment if they resumed drug use. Most of the addicts were remanded to CAP for nonviolent drug-related crimes, but some were sent because their addictions were so severe they were unable to care for themselves. This latter group was civilly committed in much the same way that the gravely disabled mentally ill are often institutionalized.

The success came after a difficult start. During the first 18 months, many California judges, unfamiliar with the new procedures, released patients on a writ of habeus corpus almost immediately after they had been committed. This judicial blunder, however, allowed M. Douglas Anglin, director of UCLA's Drug Abuse Research Center, and his colleagues to conduct an extensive evaluation of nearly 1,000 addicts, comparing those who received compulsory treatment with those who were mistakenly freed. The two groups were otherwise comparable with respect to drug use and demographics. The researchers found that

22 percent of the addicts who were committed reverted to heroin use and crime, less than half the rate for the prematurely released group. Other large-scale studies, including the 1984 Treatment Outcome Prospective Study and the 1988 Drug Abuse Reporting Program, also show that drug use and criminal behavior decline more among those receiving compulsory treatment than among the voluntary patients.

Though still legally on the books, CAP has become moribund. The practice of court-ordered residential treatment continues, but parole and probation officers today are not nearly as scrupulous in supervising their charges as were their CAP counterparts. Among the exceptions is a program developed by the Brooklyn District Attorney called Drug Treatment Alternative-to-Prison (DTAP). It is the first prosecution-run program in the country to divert prison-bound drug offenders to residential treatment.

The program targets drug-addicted felons with prior nonviolent convictions who have been arrested for sales to undercover agents. Defendants who accept the program have their prosecution deferred if they enter the 15 to 24 month program. Charges are dismissed upon successful completion of the program. The program's one-year retention rate of 57 percent is markedly superior to the 13 percent to 25 percent rate typically seen in standard residential treatment. Recidivism to crime at 6, 12, and 24 months after program completion is consistently half that of DTAP-eligible defendants who were regularly prosecuted and sent to prison.

The Success of Drug Courts

In addition to coercing criminally involved addicts to undergo residential treatment, the criminal justice system is in an excellent position to use sanctions as leverage for compliance with outpatient treatment. Since 1989, it has been doing so through "drug courts." These specialized courts offer nonviolent defendants the possibility of a dismissed charge if they plead guilty and if they agree to be diverted to a heavily monitored drug-treatment program overseen by the drug-court judge. During regularly scheduled status hearings, the judge holds the defendant publicly accountable for his progress by taking into account dirty or missed urine tests and cooperation with the treatment program. Successes are rewarded and violations are sanctioned immediately, though in a graduated fashion, starting with small impositions that become increasingly aversive if further infractions occur. Ideally, the sanctions become incentives to compliance; repeated failure results in incarceration.

Early data on over 80 drug courts show an average retention rate of 71 percent (defined as the sum of all participants who have completed drug-court programs and those who are still in programs). Even the lowest rate of 31 percent exceeds the average retention rate of about 10 percent to 15 percent (at the one-year mark) for noncriminal addicts in public-sector treatment programs. One study conducted by the Urban Institute was specifically designed to examine the influence of sanctions on offenders in the District of Columbia drug court. In the first option—the "sanctions track"—urines were obtained twice weekly, and the defendant was subject to increasingly severe penalties (e.g., a day or more in jail) for missing or dirty urines. The second, or "treatment track," was an intensive treatment program lasting several hours a day, but it didn't impose sanctions frequently or reliably. And finally, the control group had urine tests twice a week, but there were no predictable consequences for missed or dirty urines.

Researchers found that treatment-track participants were twice as likely to be drug free in the month before sentencing as those in the standard track (27 percent versus 12 percent), while sanctions-track participants, subject to frequent urine testing and known consequences for violations, were three times as likely (37 percent versus 12 percent) to be free of drugs. The certainty of consequences was psychologically powerful to the participants. As senior researcher Adele Harrell learned in her focus groups, study participants credited their ability to stay clean to the "swiftness of the penalties—they had to report to court immediately for a test failure—and their fairness."

And the longer participants stayed in drug court, the better they fared. According to information maintained by the Drug Court Clearinghouse at American University, the differences in re-arrest rates were significant. Up to this point, drug courts operational for 18 months or more reported a completion rate of 48 percent. Depending upon the characteristics and degree of social dysfunction of the graduates, re-arrest—for drug crimes, primarily—was 4 percent within one year of graduation. Even among those who never finished the program (about one in three fail to complete) re-arrest one year after enrollment ranged from 5 percent to 28 percent. Contrast this with the 26 percent to 40 percent re-arrest rate among traditionally adjudicated individuals convicted of drug possession who will commit another offense within one year, according to the Bureau of Justice Statistics.

These examples show how law enforcement brings addicts into a treatment system, enhances the probability that they will stay, and imposes sanctions for poor compliance with treatment. (The Urban Institute study even forces one to question whether treatment is invariably necessary, so long as sanctions are in place.) They also highlight the folly of dividing addicts into two camps—"bad people" for the criminal justice system to dispose of and "chronic illness sufferers" for medical professionals to treat. If the brain-disease model transforms every addict into a "sufferer," then we would be hard pressed to justify the use of coercion to change behavior. Thus the brain-disease model fails to accommodate one of the most productive collaborations in the history of antidrug efforts.

Taking Control

Labeling addiction a chronic and relapsing brain disease is mere propaganda. By downplaying the volitional dimension of addiction, the brain-disease model detracts from the great promise of strategies and therapies that rely on sanctions and rewards to shape self-control. And by reinforcing a dichotomy between punitive and clinical approaches to addiction, the brain-disease model devalues the enormous contribution of criminal justice to combating addiction. The fact that many, perhaps most, addicts are in control of their actions and appetites for circumscribed periods of time shows that they are not perpetually helpless victims of chronic disease. They are the instigators of their own addiction, just as they can be the agents of their own recovery.

POSTSCRIPT

Should Addiction to Drugs Be Labeled a Brain Disease?

To some, one of the most valuable aspects of labeling addiction a disease is that it removes alcohol and drug use from the moral realm. Many believe that addiction sufferers should be treated and helped rather than scorned and punished. Although the moral model of addiction has by no means disappeared in the United States, today more resources are directed toward rehabilitation than toward punishment. Increasingly, it is being recognized and understood that fines, blaming the victim, and imprisonment do little to curb alcohol and drug addiction in society.

Several recent studies support the hypothesis that addiction to drugs and alcohol is a brain disease and should be treated as such. See "Drug Addiction and Its Underlying Neurobiological Basis," *Science* (November 9, 2001); "Frontal Cortex," *American Journal of Psychiatry* (October 2002); "Addiction Is a Disease," *Psychiatric Times* (October 1, 2002); "Drug Tolerance, Central to Addiction, Responds to Learned Cues," *Pain & Central Nervous System Week* (August 5, 2002); "Drug Addiction and the Hippocampus," *Science* (November 9, 2001); "The Unsatisfied Mind: Are Reward Centers in Your Brain Wired for Substance Abuse?" *Discover* (November 2001); "Cocaine Craving Persists After Drug Use Stops," *Health & Medicine Week* (August 13, 2001); "Seeing Drugs as a Choice or as a Brain Anomaly," *The New York Times* (June 24, 2000); and "Addiction Is a Brain Disease, and It Matters," *Bench & Bar* (January 2000).

Critics argue, however, that this belief either underemphasizes or ignores the impact of self-control, learned behaviors, and many other factors that lead to alcohol and drug abuse. Furthermore, most treatment programs in the United States are based on the concept of addiction as a brain disease, and most are considered to be generally ineffective when judged by their high relapse rates. See "Addiction and Responsibility," *Social Research* (Fall 2001); "Does Motivation to Change Mediate the Effect of DSM-IV Substance Use Disorders on Treatment Utilization and Substance," *Addictive Behaviors* (March–April 2002); and "Playing With Fire—Why People Engage in Risky Behavior: Various Hypotheses Focus on Personality, Age, Parenting, and Biology," *The Scientist* (January 27, 2003).

It appears that the causes of addiction are complex. Brain, mind, and behavioral specialists are rethinking the whole notion of addiction. With input from neuroscience, biology, pharmacology, psychology, and genetics, many are questioning assumptions and identifying some common characteristics among addicts that will, it is hoped, improve treatment outcomes and even prevent people from using drugs in the first place.

ISSUE 11

Is Stress Responsible for Disease?

YES: Editors of *Harvard Health Letter,* from "Can Stress Make You Sick?" *Harvard Health Letter* (April 1998)

NO: Christopher Caldwell, from "The Use and Abuse of Stress," *The Weekly Standard* (June 2, 1997)

ISSUE SUMMARY

YES: The editors of the *Harvard Health Letter* maintain that there is evidence that individuals who are chronically stressed possess an increased risk of cancer and heart disease.

NO: Writer Christopher Caldwell argues that no one, including doctors, can come to an agreement on what stress is, so stress can not be blamed as the cause of disease.

In the 1930s Dr. Hans Selye, a stress researcher, asserted that the physical symptoms activated by stress can protect the body but can also cause disease and damage. Selye wrote that "it is immaterial whether the agent or situation we face is pleasant or unpleasant; all that counts is the intensity of the demand for adjustment and adaption." Stressful experiences include major life events such as divorce, trauma, or the birth of a child, and day-to-day events such as traffic jams, deadlines, or lost keys. The effects of chronic stress may be increased by drugs, a poor diet, and lack of exercise. Selye also described the response to stressors as a three-stage general adaptation syndrome. The three stages are alarm, resistance, and exhaustion. During the alarm stage the body's systems release the hormones cortisol and epinephrine, which enable the body to meet challenges caused by stress. In the resistance stage the body adapts to the challenge of stress by increasing strength and endurance. During the final stage, exhaustion, the body's psychological and physical energy is depleted and rest is necessary. If the body does not rest and the stress continues, illness may follow.

Several researchers have attempted to identify causes of stress, or specific factors that increase the likelihood of stress-related illness. In the early 1960s physicians Thomas Holmes and Richard Rahe developed a scale that identified certain stressful life events, both positive and negative. Individuals who scored high on the scale, the researchers determined, were more likely to become ill. In 1974 two California doctors, Meyer Friedman and Ray Rosenman, correlated people with hurried, hostile personalities to higher instances of stress-related heart disease. They maintained that people who have more easygoing and relaxed personalities are less likely to develop stress-related heart problems. A third stress theory, "psychological hardiness," was developed in the late 1970s. According to researcher Suzanne Kobasa, people who react positively to stress are less likely to develop illnesses since they possess psychological hardiness that helps them withstand the rigors of stress exposure. Kobasa defined hardiness as having a sense of challege when confronted with new events, a commitment to one's work, and a sense of control over one's environment, particularly the workplace.

Some argue that although an understanding of the causes of stress is important, understanding the physical and emotional harm that can result from exposure to stress is equally important. Assertions have been made that many physical symptoms such as high blood pressure, headaches, and irritable bowel syndrome have been linked to stress. Pregnant women exposed to severe stress may deliver a low-birth-weight or premature baby. Specific illnesses have also been linked to stress exposure. These include heart disease, certain cancers, and the common cold. Reported among the behavioral and emotional reactions to stress are anxiety, burnout, substance abuse, and nervousness.

People have always been exposed to stress. Early men and women faced physical stress daily in an effort to avoid dangerous animals, ensure enough food, and cope with harmful weather patterns. Modern humans experience different kinds of stressful events, such as job burnout, financial problems, and difficult interpersonal situations. It is argued that because modern life can be so hectic, it is easy to blame many illnesses and negative behaviors on stressful events.

To control stress, support groups, classes, and worksite health programs have been developed. These programs help individuals manage stress through a variety of methods, including relaxation techniques, meditation, and biofeedback. A technique called "stress inoculation training" consists of three phases: conceptualization, skill acquisition, and application and follow-through. Other programs teach time management to minimize the effects of stressful and debilitating deadlines. Some programs encourage exercise and nutritious eating to maintain a healthy body, which can better withstand stress. While many people have positive feelings about these programs and feel less stressed, the evidence linking stress management programs and disease reduction is not always clear. Is exposure to stress a legitimate concern that needs to be managed, or is it an inevitable part of life?

In the following articles, the editors of the *Harvard Health Letter* contend that emotions are tied to health. They also maintain that researchers who study stress and health conclude that many illnesses are related to problems with the body's reaction to stress. Christopher Caldwell argues that stress is a part of life and that too many individuals believe that exposure to stress has made them sick.

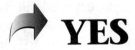 **YES**

Can Stress Make You Sick?

Many people may recall reading newspaper accounts last year of a study which found that people with a wide variety of social ties were much less likely to catch colds than those who had limited contacts with friends, relatives, neighbors, and business associates.

The investigation, which was published in June 1997 in the Journal of the American Medical Association, revealed that a lack of diverse social contacts was a stronger risk factor for colds than smoking, low vitamin C intake, or elevated stress hormones.

The Carnegie Mellon University researchers who conducted the study say that interacting with a broad array of individuals likely tempers a person's physical response to stressful situations. Although it remains unproven, the investigators suspect that social support may somehow boost immune function.

Age-Old Thinking

The idea that emotions are tied to health is not a new one. Before Hippocrates (500 B.C.) and until contemporary times, doctors believed that "the passions" played a role in causing disease. Modern scientists have had little reason to revisit this antiquated notion—until recently. As they have gained a greater understanding of the way the body functions at the cellular level, they have made the surprising discovery that certain molecules transmit signals between the nervous and immune systems.

Meanwhile, animal studies have demonstrated that impairing communication between the two systems—either by genetic engineering or with drugs—is associated with a susceptibility to inflammatory diseases, thyroid problems, and arthritis. Such research may one day explain why there are so many variations in people's vulnerability to infections, autoimmune disorders, and even cancer.

Most human research on stress and health has looked at the link between emotions, hypertension, and heart disease. A growing and convincing body of data suggest that chronic anger, anxiety, loneliness, or depression can be lethal to people with coronary artery disease. There is also some evidence that physically healthy people who experience frequent blow-ups, who are chronically depressed, or who are constantly anxious may be setting the stage for future heart disease.

Researchers point to the fact that some heart attacks are triggered by the sudden clumping together of blood platelets—one of the body's reactions to the evolutionary "fight or flight" response—which is evoked by fear or anger. When these emotions run high, platelets become stickier as the body prepares itself to stanch a potential wound.

Investigators who study the effects of stress on health believe that heart disease is only one of many ills that may ultimately be linked to disturbances of the flight or flight reaction.

An Ongoing Struggle

Everyone experiences stress in one form or another. There is the acute stress of a traumatic event, such as the death or illness of a loved one or the loss of a job, or the day-to-day wear and tear from sitting in traffic jams, feeling angry or isolated, or constantly worrying about work, finances, or relationships.

When the brain perceives stress—either from an internal or external trigger—the flight or flight response kicks in. Initially, this reaction stimulates the release of two stress hormones: adrenalin, which is produced by the adrenal glands near the kidneys, and corticotrophin-releasing hormone (CRH), from nerve cells in the hypothalamus, at the base of the brain. CRH then travels to the pituitary gland, where it causes the release of adrenocorticotrophic hormone (ACTH); this triggers the production of cortisol by the adrenal gland.

In response, blood platelets aggregate, immune cells activate, blood sugar rushes to muscles to give them energy, the heart and breathing rate quickens, and blood pressure rises. Cortisol, a steroid hormone which at first sustains the stress response, later slows it down so the body can return to normal functioning.

Sometimes, however, this feedback loop goes awry. If stress hormones fail to turn off once the challenge has passed or if a person is subjected to chronic stress, cortisol and other hormones can get out of whack. Instead of providing protection, they may suppress the immune system by interfering with the regular repair and maintenance functions of the body, leaving people open to infections and disease.

A Heavy Burden

In a report published in the January 15, 1998, issue of the New England Journal of Medicine, Bruce S. McEwen, a neuroscientist at Rockefeller University, uses the term allostatic load to refer to the long-term physical effects of the body's response to stress. Allostasis is derived from the Greek word that means "to achieve stability through change." However, the price our bodies pay for accommodating to stressful changes may be high; some people develop a hyperactivity or hypoactivity of the normal stress response.

Too little production of stress hormones can be just as harmful as too much, because it may trigger the secretion of other substances that compensate for the loss. For example, if cortisol does not increase in response to stress, inflammatory cytokines (signals), which are regulated by cortisol, will rise.

On the other hand, too much cortisol can predispose a person to infection, bone loss, muscle weakening, and increased insulin production. Women with a history of depression tend to have higher cortisol levels and lower bone mineral density than those who are not depressed. And studies on aging animals and humans suggest that chronic exposure to stress hormones may accelerate changes in the brain that lead to memory loss.

No one knows why stress hormones don't turn off in some people when the stressful event has passed. It is also unclear why some individuals lose the ability to produce stress hormones when they need them.

The Rockefeller researchers believe that regular, moderate exercise is probably the best way to counteract the deleterious effects of stress. Physical activity can reduce insulin levels raised by excessive cortisol secretion and also lowers blood pressure and the heart's resting rate. People who exercise regularly may find that they can more easily give up overeating or excessive alcohol consumption, which they had previously used to quell stress.

The Cancer Connection

There is some, but less conclusive, evidence that stress may somehow be linked to cancer. Over the past decade, studies have suggested that emotional support not only enhances the lives of cancer patients but also prolongs life. In a 1989 investigation, Stanford University researchers found that women with metastatic breast cancer who participated in support groups survived an average of 18 months longer than those who did not.

In January 1998, a published report by Ohio State University researchers indicated that breast cancer patients with high levels of anxiety about their disease experienced a 20%–30% reduction in the effectiveness of their natural killer (NK) cells compared to those with low levels of stress. NK cells fight infection and cancer.

Previous research has found that cancer patients who say they feel emotionally supported have highly active NK cells; experts speculate that emotional support boosts the activity of these white blood cells by decreasing stress.

However, only a few studies have ever looked at whether reducing stress can actually improve immune function and thus slow the progression of cancer. Now, several such investigations are under way. One, by the same Ohio State University researchers, is measuring baseline levels of NK activity and other cellular reactions in 235 women with metastatic breast cancer who will undergo surgery. After their operations, one group will attend support groups for a year and learn ongoing coping skills; the other will not attend such sessions. Stress levels, immune and endocrine response, and cancer recurrence will be compared to the women's baseline measurements after five years.

The study will shed new light on the 1989 Stanford investigation, which was designed only to examine the impact of particular kinds of emotional support on quality of life; the investigators had not intended to look at survival rates and did not measure immune responses or tumor growth.

However, the same Stanford researchers are now in the process of replicating their previous study, but this time they are monitoring cortisol levels, NK cell activity, cancer recurrence, and survival rates. The final results are expected to be published in about two years.

The Jury Is Out

It's important to keep in mind that no one has yet proven that reducing stress alters immune function in a way that influences cancer. In fact, the hypothesis itself is controversial: scientists don't fully understand the ways in which immune responses affect the progression of cancer.

And although the Ohio State and Stanford groups will track several indicators that predict a person's prognosis, such as whether cancer has spread to lymph nodes, they can't account for all factors that may alter the outcome. For example, researchers will not know if some of the participants' previous chemotherapy treatments suppressed immune function. Finally, it's possible that support groups have no effect on immune response; they may bolster health simply because they encourage participants to comply with drug or dietary regimens. Nevertheless, research suggests that people with or without the stress of illness enjoy better health and a better quality of life when they get emotional support through a network of friends, relatives, and associates or through structured groups.

When experts recommend that people reduce stress in their lives, it doesn't necessarily mean that you need to leave the city for the country, quit your job, or make other dramatic changes to avoid an early grave. It may simply mean exercising more, expanding your social circle, reaching out to others, joining a support group, or putting traffic jams in perspective.

Researchers who study stress and health suspect that many ills are linked to problems with the body's "fight or flight" reaction.

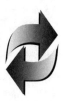

Christopher Caldwell　　　　　　　　　　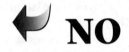 **NO**

The Use and Abuse of Stress

Springfield, Massachusetts, home of the Merriam-Webster's Dictionary, has long been proud of its annual spelling bee. But in the first week of May, Springfield superintendent of schools Peter Negroni canceled the event forever, on the grounds that "the bee provided too much stress and too few rewards." He announced that henceforth the school system would replace it with Scrabble.

The local newspaper applauded, as well it might. For the problem Negroni cited—stress—is now viewed as a society-wide scourge, and efforts to battle it are expensive and intense. According to the journal of the Society for the Advancement of Management, stress is the cause of as many as 90 percent of all job-related doctors' visits, is responsible for over half the sick days American workers take, and is the culprit in up to 80 percent of on-the-job accidents. The total cost to American companies: up to $300 billion a year.

Companies now call for outside "stress audits," courts throughout the world are increasingly indulgent of stress-based awards, and "stress management" has become a multi-billion-dollar industry. A survey by stress expert Kenneth R. Pelletier found that stress-management plans are by far the leading priority for corporate health programs, cited four times as often as the next closest concern (cardiac care). What should alarm us, and lead us to distrust all of the statistics cited above, is that no one—not the doctors who study it, not the plaintiffs who claim it, not even the "stress-management consultants" who have become the ethicists of the stress trade—can come to any agreement on what stress *is*.

It's not that the medical study of stress is bogus and newfangled; quite the contrary. Hippocrates spoke of something like stress (*pónos*). Our current understanding of the problem has its beginnings with doctors Walter Bradford Cannon and Hans Selye, who, working separately between the wars, uncovered the syndrome Selye would name "stress." Cannon investigated the "fight-or-flight" response—the way in which the human body produces adrenaline and other hormones in response to outside stimuli. When activated, these hormones sharpen the attention, speed up the heart, and prepare the body for action. But the response also depletes the immune system and temporarily halts the normal function of certain of the body's regulatory networks. Cannon and

Selye speculated that, in the 20th century, the fight-or-flight response was not being evoked at rare moments of extreme need, as it presumably was when pre-historic man had to outrun a lion, but that it had become a chronic condition. The irony was that 20th-century man, awash in conveniences and more di-vorced from nature than ever before, lived in a state of constant, or at least over-frequent, bodily vigilance that was causing his body to squander its whole bank account of self-protective resources.

Cannon and Selye were medical researchers, but their followers turned their research into an amalgam of social theory and psychiatric dogma. Now, it seems, practically *everything* causes stress. According to the Society for the Advancement of Management,

> causes of workplace stress include: schedules and deadlines, fear of failure, inadequate support, problems with the boss, job ambiguity, role conflict, change, new technology, work overload or underload, repetitive work, ex-cess rules and regulations, lack of participation in decisions, poor interper-sonal relationships, career development factors (obsolescence, under/over promotion, organizational structure, organizational leadership, culture), and poor working conditions that include the climate, overcrowding, poli-tics, and communication problems.

(Sorry—did someone say "the climate"?) As if that weren't enough to worry about, *success* on the job—or the "success syndrome," as stress-management con-sultants put it—affects one in five managers, and can cause "apathy, irritability, uninvolvement in projects, decline in productivity, marital problems, and exces-sive drinking or smoking." Stress-management candidates include people dying of AIDS, hot-tempered adolescents, people scared of surgery, binge drinkers, un-dergraduates with exam anxiety, athletes who choke, vaguely defined "Type A personalities," and on and on.

The comprehensive nature of the stress theory is the first indication that we're in the presence of a racket. Stress-related lawsuits and claims are booming in courts across the country. Under the 1970 Occupational Safety and Health Act, companies are responsible for "all diseases arising out of and in the course of employment," and that is now taken to include stress. The National Institute for Occupational Safety and Health considers stress one of the 10 leading occu-pational diseases. Recent rulings on the Americans with Disabilities Act make it likely that that act, too, will be used to buttress stress-related claims. The U.S. Court of Appeals for the 6th Circuit recently ruled that a factory employee in Michigan could collect for a heart attack suffered on the factory floor and caused, he said, by the stress-inducing incompetence of one of his fellow work-ers and the unpleasant noise at work.

For all its American roots, stress is a global issue, at least in any country where people have grown impatient with modern life. Sweden's incredibly gen-erous 1991 Work Environment Act makes it the responsibility of employers to make sure "that the employee is not exposed to physical *or mental* loads which may lead to ill health or accidents." One British citizen got a settlement for the stress of being stuck in an elevator. British papers have been in a panic about stress since 1994, when the social worker John Walker received £175,000 for being "severely mentally wounded" by the stress at work. More recently, the Scottish social worker Janet Ballantyne received a settlement of £66,000 for the stress caused by her "outspoken and abrasive" boss. (It's interesting that both these British stress collectors hail from UNISON, the same left-wing union of underpaid social workers. As one London businessman told the London *Times,* "I've yet to see a damages claim brought by a City stockbroker.")

Clearly, if we're looking for a synonym for stress it would be something like "modern life," and the current anti-stress activism is an ethical and political critique of it. University of Chicago anthropologist Richard Shweder thinks that stress is merely a synonym for unhappiness, much as people a century ago talked of angst and ennui. Others see it as similar to the 19th-century fad ailment of hysteria. But it is more than that, for unlike its forebears, stress is linked to treatments and to states and corporations that mandate them. As University of Montreal psychologist Ethel Roskies puts it, "The most distinctive characteristic of stress management as a treatment is its universality; there is no one for whom treatment is apparently unneeded or inappropriate." According to Roskies, "Essentially, the diagnosis of a clinical stress problem has less to do with the etiology or severity of the problem itself than with the prediction of its responsiveness to the teaching of coping skills."

That means that stress can degenerate into a hunt for problems to fit preexisting (and lucrative) solutions. Some commonsense techniques for stress reduction appear to work. Meditation, biofeedback, hypnosis, "visulization therapy," and relaxation coaching show results. But other techniques appear so commonsensical as to be laughable: Stress consultant Ray Shelton has said his Awareness-Attitude-Action model relies in part on "avoiding excess coffee and junk food." And treatments can veer into charlatanism: "acupressure," "meridian energy flow," and something called "trampoline therapy." The *Washington Post*'s Liza Mundy attended a Fred Pryor motivational seminar designed to fight stress and learned little more than that she ought to keep a "smile file" of happy thoughts and "take time out to just be." European American Bank, meanwhile, reportedly invited Jesse "Two Owls" Teasley of the Oglala Sioux tribe to talk about *tai chi*—not, to the best of anyone's knowledge, an American Indian cultural product.

The very idea of stress management, its opponents suggest, instills "learned helplessness"—the assumption that people don't have enough internal resources to quiet the storm within their own minds. Stress thus becomes the close relative of the "Twinkie Defense." If self-help methods don't work, then obviously society has the obligation to protect us from our own adrenaline.

The great pop-psych expression of this attitude is the Social Readjustment Rating Scale, devised by two psychologists in 1967. It ranks stressful events using a point system. Death of a spouse is 100, pregnancy is 40, problems with the law is 29, etc. If your tally rises above 150 points, you have a 50 percent possibility of suffering stress.

The effect of such a scale is to muddy all *moral* claims—the notion that maybe you ought to feel bad if you do something wrong. By assuming that a tragedy, like the death of a spouse, can be ranked on the same scale as a pregnancy makes the very idea of stress itself arbitrary. Is it worse than initiating a divorce or changing your diet? Where does "having an incompetent co-worker" (the problem that allegedly caused a heart attack) fit in?

The current conception of "stress" is a way of micromanaging fairness. It's just *unfair* that someone's stress rating should rise above 150 points, and there's no reason it should! If a guy gets up to 300 points and flies off the handle, who can blame him? The goal of the Social Readjustment Rating System is to quantify moral, physical, and spiritual well-being so that they can be redistributed, as money and goods are in a socialist society.

Stress is now the preserve of those unacknowledged legislators of the world: social workers and other members of the caring professions. It is they, not the wider public, who decide the stress agenda. While 74 percent of corporate managers in one survey felt that the responsibility for stress management "should lie with the individual rather than the organization," institutional stress professionals continue to extend their reach and their agenda. That agenda is, not to put too fine a point on it, pro-feminist, anti-competitive, and inclined to see a racist under every bed.

The classic idea of stress has been easily adapted to a feminized America. Much of the initial research on stress had to do with men; the fact that they were undeniably more susceptible to stress-related heart attacks made it likely they suffered more stress. But recent research, all of it sociological and psychological rather than medical, has sought to put women at center-stage. The prevailing theory is that "juggling work and home" *must* make women's lives more stressful than men's, whether or not there's any evidence to back it up. Too little attention has been paid, say the stress enthusiasts, to women's stress, brought about by the fact that women have been "socialized to care for others."

From heart attacks to the woes of caring for others—yet again we see, even inside the world of stress management, a great leveling taking place. These days, women are increasingly considered the true victims of stress. Take NBC's "Stressed Out in America," a series of spots that ran on the network's weekend *Today* show throughout the month of April. "It's estimated that—get this— 75 percent of all doctor visits are due to stress-related disorders," said host Jodi Applegate. "Now there's evidence to suggest that women may be more prone to stress than men." Participants consistently favored stereotypical female coping mechanisms to stereotypical male ones. Take Xavier Amador of Columbia University: "Really what we mean is it's important to talk about how you feel, and— and the worst thing you can do if you're stressed out is to keep it inside and carry it with you." Then Amador talked about the importance of using "I" statements: "It's very important that you talk about how you feel, not what the other person is doing. So, if you're stressed out, you come home, the dishes aren't done, don't say, 'You don't do the dishes, why didn't you do the dishes?' Say, '*I* would really appreciate it.'"

The who-does-the-dishes example hardly came out of thin air. Indeed, one commonplace assertion in the world of stress management is that stress in men is caused by their being too aggressive, while stress in women is caused by women's being too passive. Says Dr. Redford Williams, director of the Behavioral Medicine Research Center at Duke, "You should just cool out. Let it go."

But what if the situation is amenable to change? "That means you should really swing into action . . . and for women that often means being assertive."

The agenda of the stress industry also includes race. The most notorious recent example was a study by Harvard epidemiologists Nancy Krieger and Stephen Sidney on "Racial Discrimination and Blood Pressure," which appeared in last October's *American Journal of Public Health.* Blacks die on average seven years earlier than whites, from cancer, heart attacks, and a variety of diseases to which they have a higher propensity. The two researchers asked for responses about exposure to racial discrimination and plotted the results against high-blood-pressure statistics. There was no statistically significant relationship; in fact, those blacks who had faced zero episodes of discrimination had higher blood pressure than those who had faced one or more. But Krieger and Sidney assumed a relationship anyway, on the grounds that those with the highest blood pressure were probably *underreporting* the number of racist incidents they'd been exposed to, and that they were thus merely victims of "internalized oppression."

High stress, in the categories of race and gender, is seen as merely a stand-in for virtue. That's not the case with stress in the category of achievement—and the contrast is instructive. We all know about how dangerous it is to be a "Type A," shorthand for "Type A behavior syndrome," which researchers define as "characterized by competitive drive, impatience, hostility, and rapid speech and motor movements." For years, doctors and stress researchers have found a correlation between those behavioral qualities and a high incidence of coronary heart disease.

If, for physicians, the Type A is merely a cardiac-ward candidate who deserves attention, for stress professionals he's the vice president in the penthouse with the five secretaries and the attitude. An unmistakable note of righteous discipline, even divine wrath, can be heard in their discussions of Type A personalities. In their view, for Type As, excessive work is an "obsessive-compulsive disorder." NBC's "Stressed Out in America" suggested that Type As who are always nervously looking for the shortest line in a supermarket should instead seek out the *longest* one.

Here as elsewhere, "stress" is frequently an explicit indictment of competitiveness, and this means an implicit indictment of the economic status quo. Karen Nussbaum, the director of the working women's department at the AFL-CIO, told a *Newsday* reporter that "companies that really want to relieve stress should be more concerned with redistributing work, paying a decent wage, and creating a family-friendly environment." Stress thus serves as the ultimate pretext for gripes about the need for economic reorganization.

As a medical matter, the study of stress is an effort to examine the problem that the human animal lives under conditions of modernity to which his system has not adapted. It is a serious issue that deserves serious study. But that is not why America has become so addicted to talk about stress. "Stress" is a smoke screen—a cover for what is, at root, a political and moral movement aimed at fixing "inappropriate" ways of responding to modernity. Its agenda is large enough and its rationale vague enough that it ought to be drawing more skeptical interest, and meeting more resistance.

POSTSCRIPT

Is Stress Responsible for Disease?

Some physicians maintain that stress can make people sick. Some estimate that close to two-thirds of all physician visits are related to negative stress. In the early 1990s Sheldon Cohen, a professor at Carnegie Mellon University, conducted a study that showed the relationship between stress and the common cold. He measured the stress levels of nearly 400 men and women and then exposed them to cold viruses. Almost half of the subjects under the most stress became ill compared to 27 percent of the least stressed. The kind of stress that was most likely to increase the probability of developing a cold was related to extended conflict in personal relationships. Stress does not cause colds, but researchers hypothesize that it makes us more susceptible to cold viruses by negatively affecting the immune system. Similar studies have indicated that stress may play a major role in headaches, gastrointestinal distress, asthma, and skin disorders. Stress may even play a role in the aging process. A recent study found that cortisol, the major human stress hormone, can increase mental deterioration in healthy people. These findings appear in "Cortisol Levels During Human Aging Predict Hippocampal Atrophy and Memory Deficits," *Nature Neuroscience* (May 1998). More recent studies on this issue can be found in "Adrenal Hormone and Cortisol Stress Reactions Were Lowered by Some GI Drugs," *Pain & Central Nervous System Week* (March 3, 2003); "Reactivity and Regulation in Cortisol and Behavioral Responses to Stress," *Child Development* (March–April 2003); and "Higher Cortisol Flags Stress in Academic Doctors," *Family Practice News* (February 1, 2003).

However, we are all exposed to stressful situations. According to Christopher Caldwell, stress is blamed for too much that goes wrong in our lives. The definition of stress is too comprehensive, making "stress management" a multibillion-dollar industry. Caldwell asserts that a more skeptical examination of the definition of stress is necessary. Further readings on the stress-illness relationship include "Stress and Atherosclerosis," *Harvard Health Letter* (February 1998); "Fight or Flight—Or Sit Tight?" *Consumer Reports on Health* (February 1998); "Protective and Damaging Effects of Stress Mediators," *The New England Journal of Medicine* (January 15, 1998); "How Stress Can Make You Sick," *Current Health* (November 1997); "Stressed Out and Sick From It," *Redbook* (March 1997); and "Depression, Stress, and the Heart: Evidence Is Accumulating That Psychosocial Factors, in Particular Depression, Contribute to Coronary Artery Disease," *Heart* (November 2002).

ISSUE 12

Can Spirituality Overcome Illness?

YES: Herbert Benson and Marg Stark, from *Timeless Healing: The Power and Biology of Belief* (Scribner, 1996)

NO: William B. Lindley, from "Prayer and Healing," *Truth Seeker* (vol. 122, no. 2, 1995)

ISSUE SUMMARY

YES: Herbert Benson, an associate professor of medicine at Harvard Medical School, and journalist Marg Stark contend that faith and spirituality will enhance and prolong life.

NO: William B. Lindley, associate editor of *Truth Seeker*, counters that there is no scientific way to determine that spirituality can heal.

Practitioners of holistic medicine believe that people must take responsibility for their own health by practicing healthy behaviors and maintaining positive attitudes instead of relying on health providers. They also believe that physical disease has behavioral, psychological, and spiritual components. These spiritual components can be explained by the relationship between beliefs, mental attitude, and the immune system. Until recently, few studies existed to prove a relationship between spirituality—a feeling of connectedness to the greater self—and health.

Much of modern medicine has spent the past century ridding itself of mysticism and relying on science. Twenty years ago, no legitimate physician would have dared to study the effects of spirituality on disease. Recently, however, at the California Pacific Medical Center in San Francisco, California, Elisabeth Targ, clinical director of psychosocial oncology research, has recruited 20 faith healers to determine if prayer can affect the outcome of disease. Targ states that her preliminary results are encouraging. In addition to Targ's study, other research has shown that religion and spirituality can help determine health and well-being. According to a 1995 investigation at Dartmouth College, one of the strongest predictors of success after open-heart surgery was the level of comfort patients derived from religion and spirituality. Other recent studies have linked health with church attendance, religious commitment, and spirituality. There are, however, other studies that have not been as successful; a recent one involving the effects of prayer on alcoholics found no relationship.

Can spirituality or prayer in relation to health and healing be explained scientifically? Prayer or a sense of spirituality may function in a similar manner as stress management or relaxation. Spirituality or prayer may cause the release of hormones that help lower blood pressure or produce other benefits. Although science may never be able to exactly determine the benefits of spirituality, it does appear to help some people.

In the following selections, Herbert Benson and Marg Stark state that spirituality can have a significant influence over the body. William B. Lindley argues that people do not become ill because their mental states, psyches, or attitudes negatively affect their biological systems.

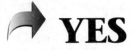
Timeless Healing: The Power and Biology of Belief

At one time or another, I'm sure nearly everyone experiences extraordinary and magical events, the converging of time and circumstance so logic-defiant that one cannot help but feel these events were divinely directed. It could be a chance reunion with a long-lost friend, a life change that comes at precisely the time you need it, or an image you see in a cloud formation. It could be a clergyperson's sermon that seems eerily relevant to the problems you've been facing, something as dramatic as hearing a voice speak to you inspirationally or as quiet as a bliss that envelops you suddenly. Whatever the form, the more the incident means to us, the more we attach sacred status to it in our lives. We shake our heads, asking, "What are the chances?" all the while feeling a profound reverberation within that perhaps life is not random, that perhaps these are tangible signs that a mystical force contours our life.

But it's possible that the reverberation you feel within when an experience you deem magical or spiritual occurs may not be just emotional but physical as well. Not only did my research—and that of my colleagues—reveal that 25% of people feel more spiritual as the result of the elicitation of the relaxation response, but it showed that those same people have fewer medical symptoms than do those who reported no increase in spirituality from the elicitation.

I decided to call the combined force of these internal influences the *faith factor*—remembered wellness and the elicitation of the relaxation response. But it became clear that a person's religious convictions or life philosophy enhanced the average effects of the relaxation response in three ways: (1) People who chose an appropriate focus, that which drew upon their deepest philosophic or religious convictions, were more apt to adhere to the elicitation routine, looking forward to it and enjoying it; (2) affirmative beliefs of any kind brought forth remembered wellness, reviving top-down, nerve-cell firing patterns in the brain that were associated with wellness; (3) when present, faith in an eternal or life-transcending force seemed to make the fullest use of remembered wellness because it is a supremely soothing belief, disconnecting unhealthy logic and worries.

I already knew that eliciting the relaxation response could "disconnect" everyday thoughts and worries, calming people's bodies and minds more quickly and to a degree otherwise unachievable. It appeared that beliefs added to the response transported the mind/body even more dramatically, quieting worries and fears significantly better than the relaxation response alone. And I speculated that religious faith was more influential than other affirmative beliefs.

I want to emphasize that the benefits of the faith factor are not the exclusive domain of the devout. People don't have to have a professed belief in God to reap the psychological and physical rewards of the faith factor. With lead investigator Dr. Jared D. Kass, a professor at Lesley College Graduate School of Arts and Sciences in Cambridge, MA, my colleagues and I developed a questionnaire to quantify and describe the spiritual feelings that accompanied the relaxation response, to document their frequency and potential health effects.

Based on the survey responses, we calculated "spirituality scores." But because virtually all of our survey respondents reported a "belief in God," this statement could not be used to differentiate people. It was the more amorphous feeling of spirituality that could be linked to better psychological and physical well-being. However, there is one group that does seem more likely to have spiritual encounters. Indeed, women had higher spirituality scores than men, for reasons we don't yet understand.

As subjective as remembered wellness is, there are some definitive things I can say about incorporating healing beliefs and faith into your life. These are some of the principles and practical lessons I've drawn from my long medical quest for lasting truths. I hope they prove helpful to you:

Let faith, the ultimate belief, heal you   According to medical research, faith in God is good for us, and this benefit is not exclusive to one denomination or theology. You can believe in God in a quiet, introspective way or declare your convictions out loud to the world—either way, you'll still reap the physiologic rewards.

For many reasons, religious activity and churchgoing are also healthy. Religious groups encourage all kinds of health-affirming activities—fellowship and socializing perhaps first among them, but also prayer, volunteerism, familiar rituals and music. Prayer, in particular, appears to be therapeutic, the specifics of which science will continue to explore.

Trust your instincts more often   People describe the process of finding out what is important to them, of tapping into their beliefs, in very different ways, sometimes calling it "soul-searching," "mulling it over," "listening to one's heart," "going inside of one's self," "praying," or "sleeping on it." Some people act on instincts or common sense; others find a truth or intuition emerges slowly. But most people know when something "feels right." Most people have a kind of internal radar that occasionally calls out to them.

The next time you're faced with a major decision, medical or otherwise, ask yourself, "What would I do if the choice were entirely up to me?" I'm not suggesting that you make decisions based on this factor alone, but at least let belief be a player. Honor your convictions and perceptions enough to make them a part of a hearty intellectual argument.

Let your instincts guide you. Follow them up with research. Put your health in good, trustworthy hands. Let your health have time to correct itself. Invest remembered wellness and a reasonable application of self-care, medications and surgery for maximum health returns.

Practice and apply self-care regularly Work with your doctor, and with unconventional practitioners if you so choose, to learn self-care habits. I consider self-care anything an individual can do, independent of doctors or healers, to enhance his or her health. This includes mind/body reactions such as remembered wellness, the relaxation response and the faith factor. It also embraces good nutrition, exercise and other means of stress management.

I use the term "self-care" because it puts the onus on you, it shifts the emphasis from your role as passive patient to active participant—a shift that medicine has not always encouraged. However, I caution against becoming self-absorbed in self-care. Don't become fixated on your health or on the avoidance of aging, illness or death. Make your daily elicitation of the relaxation response, your jog or your salad at lunch a no-brainer, which you do not analyze or overthink. Simply delight in the event itself.

It's almost always valuable to seek the assistance of your physician to determine the difference between a condition that will benefit from self-care exclusively and one that requires drugs or procedures to treat. Learning about your body is an evolutionary process. You'll work toward a more independent attitude. Become acquainted with the warning signs of heart attacks, strokes, cancer and other life-threatening diseases. Over time, you'll develop a sense of what symptoms are important—those that are extreme or don't go away.

How influential can a coordinated contingent of self-care habits be? We honestly don't know, but *Prevention* advisor Dean Ornish, MD, president of the Preventive Medicine Research Institute in Sausalito, CA, found that heart disease could not only be relieved but reversed when patients made significant changes in diet, exercise and stress management. Our two programs will soon be compared in a groundbreaking research project sponsored by the Commonwealth of Massachusetts Group Insurance Commission and the John Hancock Insurance Company. In this comparison, patients with heart disease will be divided between our two clinics in hopes that we can gauge the adherence to and results of various self-care components and other treatments.

Beware of people with all the answers Be careful of any physician, nontraditional healer, spiritual guide, mind/body guru, or any adviser who claims to have all the answers or wants others to think so. Besides love and sex, writers and lecturers today take up few topics with as much evangelistic zeal as health and spirituality. It is no small task shielding these very personal matters from unhealthy speculation and overanalysis, but start with tuning out overly confident or all-knowing mentors and guides. Value your emotions and intuitions the same way your brain does; don't let someone manipulate your wiring for his or her gain.

Mind/body medicine should remind us of the precious nature of our minds, and of the importance of critiquing the messages we allow to become actualized in our brains/bodies.

Whether or not you believe in God, I believe that we are all wired to crave meaning in life, to assign profound power and sacredness to human experiences, and sometimes even to lend "god" status or "godliness" to humans and human endeavors. Be wary of this tendency, because it may rob spiritual life of its grandeur and of the wonderful transcendent qualities that cannot be accessed entirely by human intellect, and because it makes us very susceptible to human manipulation. Not only is your body a temple, but your mind is an architect, busy transforming the ideas you feed it. Protect it from those who exploit the power of remembered wellness for personal gain.

Remember that the 'nocebo' is equally powerful   Unfortunately, remembered wellness has a flip side. It can have negative side effects, called the *nocebo* (as opposed to placebo). Our agitated minds may inappropriately trigger the fight-or-flight response in the body. Similarly, automatic negative thoughts, bad moods and compulsive worrying eventually take up physical residence in our bodies. Extreme examples of the nocebo effect include voodoo death, belief-engendered death, mass psychogenic illness, false memories and "memories" of alien abductions. People who dwell on worst-case scenarios, who exaggerate risks, or who project doubt and undue worry keep the nocebo effect busy in their physiologies. They signal their brains to send help when no physical sickness is present, persuading the body to get sick when there is no biologic reason sickness should occur.

Remember that immortality is impossible   While it's healthy to listen to your heart, it's also harmful to deny or duck the truth. No one lives forever. No matter how well-versed you become in mind/body medicine, no matter how far medical progress may be able to set back the clock, death is, like illness and pain, an unfortunate but natural fact of life.

I must sound as if I'm talking in circles, first telling you not to let a diagnosis define you, then warning you not to fall prey to denial. Nonetheless, some lecturers and New Age entrepreneurs imply that all disease is curable and that we can avoid death and aging if we only believe. These salespeople do great harm to people by fostering guilt, and they damage the field of mind/body medicine, which is legitimately trying to establish its findings and change the way Western medicine is practiced. No evidence exists that death can be denied its eventual toll.

Indeed, fear of death can bring out the worst in people, but the realization that death is an inevitable, natural occurrence can also propel healthy, impassioned living.

Living well, exercising and eating appropriately, seeing doctors when you need to but not overrelying on the medical system—these are all proven buffers against disease and illness.

Believe in something good   Even though we do not necessarily need all the pills and procedures that conventional medicine and unconventional medicine give us, these medicinal symbols retain an aura of effectiveness and often appease our desire for action. While we must learn to use medicine more appropriately for the conditions it can help, and to wean ourselves from excessive spending on unnecessary therapies, we'll often need some catalysts for belief, even if belief is really the healer.

So remember the vigor from the time you felt healthiest in your life. Remember the blessing your mother said to you before you left for school, the smell of incense at church, or the tranquility you felt picking up stones from the beach on Cape Cod. Remember the time the penicillin vanquished your ear infection, or the time the surgeon removed the splinter from deep in your foot and your pain immediately ceased. Remember how full-throated you sang in the choir or how long you stayed on the dance floor of a nightclub. Remember the doctor who really cared about you or the chaplain who prayed with you in the hospital. Remember the way you felt when you made love to your husband or wife, and the way you felt when your daughter or son was born.

Then let go, and believe. You've read all about your physiology, you've surrounded yourself with good caregivers who help you take a moderate, balanced approach to your health and health care. Now it's time to enjoy your endowment, this wiring for faith that makes the power of remembered wellness so enduring.

Believe in something good if you can. Or even better, believe in something better than anything you can fathom. Because for us mortals, this is very profound medicine.

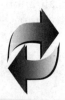

NO ↵

Prayer and Healing

I was raised in Christian Science. That gives me somewhat of an inside perspective on prayer and healing. However, the Christian Science experience is far from typical. The "Scientific Statement of Being" begins: "There is no life, truth, intelligence nor substance in matter." Most Christians who offer prayers of petition for the healing of an illness believe that their bodies are real and the illness is real, but they want supernatural intervention, the sort of thing Jesus is reported to have done in the gospels. Christian Science, interpreting Jesus' work quite differently insists that reality lies elsewhere. The analogue to prayer is "knowing the truth." Christian Science insists that miracles are not "supernatural, but divinely natural."

As I grew up and matter made more sense to me, I drifted away from Christian Science. Then I began hearing about natural, nonmiraculous analogues to what I had been taught: psychosomatic diseases and cures, the placebo effect, and, more recently, the neurochemical connections between mood and the immune system. These, along with "spontaneous remission" of cancers, were attempts to explain "miracles" without invoking the supernatural or the paranormal. (Note that "spontaneous" (natural), and "God did it" (supernatural), are "explanations" that explain nothing. There's no "how.") Believers in miracles—evangelicals, Christian Scientists, miscellaneous New Agers, and so forth—continue as before.

Prayer and Healing

Healing Words by Larry Dossey, M.D., is a book devoted to prayer and healing, and its author believes firmly that prayer (communication with "the Absolute") brings about beneficial effects that are real and substantial and supernatural or paranormal in character. However, when he raises the question, "What is prayer?", the answer is so far-ranging that all sorts of things that would not ordinarily be considered prayer are included. He rejects the Christian concept of prayer! Of course he doesn't use such strong language as "reject," preferring slippery words like "redefine," "tentative" and "reevaluate." He has a chart contrasting the "traditional Western model" with the "modern" model of prayer.

Probably over 95% of the prayers for healing that are made in the United States would be of the "old" model, which Dossey considers obsolete. Interestingly enough, Christian Science prayer would fall under the 5% that he would approve of.

Even though Dossey seems to think little of traditional prayer, his citations of many experiments that allegedly demonstrate the efficacy of prayer do not indicate whether the style of prayer was traditional or otherwise. (He clearly expresses his opinion that all kinds work, some better than others.) The experiments are broken down into various categories of what was prayed over—barley seeds(!), mice, people, etc.—but not into categories of what kind of prayer was made.

Sometimes Dossey seems to be unaware of the implications of what he says. For example, he quotes psychologist Lawrence LeShan to the effect that healing through prayer is effective in perhaps 15 to 20% of cases and that nobody can tell in advance which cases will have happy outcomes. Somewhat disheartened by this, Dossey goes on to claim that prayer works anyway. Then he mentions the "bizarre," "perverted" use of prayer by high school football teams in Texas, where, of course, they offer up highly unsportsmanlike prayers for victory. Such prayers obviously "work" 50% of the time. (We might cut this to 48% or so for tie games.) Thus one can conclude that prayer for victory in football is three times as efficacious as prayer for healing!

The Problems of Prayer

Dossey wisely reminds us that if all prayers for healing led to success, population growth would be even more catastrophic than it is; 100% success rates for other kinds of prayer could have other horrible long-term effects. (Billy Graham put it a little differently: "God answers all prayers; sometimes the answer is 'no.'") However, once this is admitted—and note that it flatly contradicts Jesus' promise in Matthew 7:7,8: "Ask, and it will be given you; search, and you will find; knock, and the door will be opened for you. For everyone who asks receives, and everyone who searches finds, and for everyone who knocks, the door will be opened"—the result is indistinguishable from that of no prayer at all.

Another problem is the intent of the person praying. Others who have faced the incoherent attempts to define prayer have said that the essence of prayer, whether there be a Supreme Being or not, is that the person praying must intend, or want, or be praying for, a particular happy ending to the current crisis. However, Dossey rejects the concept of intent. He states: "For reasons I shall discuss later, never once did I pray for specific outcomes—for cancers to go away, for heart attacks to be healed, for diabetes to vanish." He reports on an interesting group, Spindrift, that provides many "proofs" that prayer works. This group had a number of Christian Scientists in it. (One was a Christian Science practitioner whose "license" was revoked after The First Church of Christ, Scientist found out what he was up to.) Spindrift took up the question of directed vs. undirected prayer, and found that the undirected prayer worked somewhat better. Most of the other experiments by other groups, for example, with barley seeds, were directed—the intent to have the seeds flourish was in the minds of the people who prayed over them.

Prayer Experiments

Let's take a closer look at those experiments. There is a long list of them. The compiler is Daniel J. Benor, M.D. He published his survey in the journal *Complementary Medical Research* in 1990. The activity is called "spiritual healing," and this is defined as "the intentional influence of one or more people upon another living system without utilizing known physical means of intervention." (Note how this differs from the Spindrift effort cited above and from Dossey's preference for nondirected prayer.) Of 131 trials, five involved water, with three showing "significant results," but what was being prayed for in the water cases is not mentioned. There were ten trials of "enzymes," including trypsin, dopamine, and noradrenaline. (Are these enzymes? I think not.) There were seven trials on fungi and yeasts, with some prayers being for, some against, the prosperous growth of the culture. Similarly for the ten trials on bacteria, mainly E. coli and salmonella. Cells in vitro (tube or glass dish) were prayed over, including four trials on snail pacemaker cells. There were 19 trials on plants and seeds, including five on the above-mentioned barley seeds. Three of these involved different kinds of person praying: one with neurotic depression, one with psychotic depression, and one with a green thumb. As you might guess, the last showed the strongest beneficial effect. Other plants and seeds prayed over include: rye grass, wheat seeds, radish seeds, mung beans, potatoes and corn. The prayer trials on animals include 14 on anesthetized mice, with a variety of experimental conditions and effects sought. Humans were also prayed over for a total of 38 of the 131 trials. Some of the conditions prayed over are obviously psychosomatic, some less so. Clearly there is an enthusiastic "spiritual healing research" community doing many things we wouldn't ordinarily think of.

Something I was unable to find in all this is any breakdown by religion of the person praying. Christians would consider it vital to ask whether the words "In Jesus' name we pray, amen" were spoken. If they weren't, the Christians would be extremely skeptical of the efficacy of the prayers. If they were confronted by overwhelming evidence that a non-Christian prayer was highly effective, they would suspect Satanism and look for evidence of it. Similarly perhaps for Muslims. Catholics might accept evidence of efficacy of prayers invoking the Trinity while being skeptical of those with Protestant prayer tags. Regrettably, the 131 trials provide us with no information along these lines.

Another missing factor that I regret is a detailed skeptical review of the experimental methodology of some of the more impressive trials. The Committee for the Scientific Investigation of Claims of the Paranormal seems to be silent in this area. While they have offered some criticism of Therapeutic Touch, they seem to be silent on the question of religious prayer healing, except in "revivals," where some noteworthy frauds have been exposed. This is part of a pattern. Most of the subjects discussed in the *Skeptical Inquirer* are New Age phenomena, such as crop circles, UFOs, pyramid power, astrology, and so on.

CSICOP seems to be leaving Christianity alone, at least for the time being. Dossey's book cries for skeptical attention. As in the other cases, such attention would have to be very painstaking, time-consuming, and expensive.

Meanwhile, prayers for healing continue, some effectively utilizing known psychosomatic processes, others producing remarkable placebo effects (the same thing, except that we don't know what's happening), and many more where supernatural claims are made, as well as those disappointing cases where God seems to have said "no."

POSTSCRIPT

Can Spirituality Overcome Illness?

 $\mathbf{C}$ an we influence the course of our own illnesses? Can emotions, stress management, and prayer prevent or cure disease? Benson, who developed the "relaxation response," thinks there is a strong link between religious commitment and good health. He contends that people do not have to have a professed belief in God to reap the psychological and physical rewards of the "faith factor." Benson defined the faith factor as the combined force of the relaxation response and the placebo effect.

Dr. Bernard Siegel, writing in his bestseller *Love, Medicine and Miracles* (Harper & Row, 1986), argues that there are no "incurable diseases, only incurable people" and that illness is a personality flaw. In "Welcome to the Mind/Body Revolution," *Psychology Today* (July/August 1993), author Marc Barash further discusses how the mind and immune system influence each other. The *American Journal of Public Health* (1997) published a literature review entitled "The Spiritual Dimension of Health: A Review," which discussed many aspects of spirituality and health.

In *You Don't Have to Die: Unraveling the AIDS Myth* (Burton Goldberg Group, 1994), a chapter entitled "Mind-Body Medicine" discusses the body's innate healing capabilities and the role of self-responsibility in the healing process. A long-term AIDS survivor who traveled the country interviewing other long-term survivors found that the one thing they all shared was the belief that AIDS was survivable. They all also accepted the reality of their diagnosis but refused to see their condition as a death sentence.

Readings that address these issues include "Spirituality in Care Giving and Care Receiving," *Holistic Nursing Practice* (January–February 2003); "Spiritual Healing," *Internal Medicine News* (December 15, 2002); "Hypnosis, Relaxation, Imagery, Prayer, and Faith in Healing," *Subconsciously Speaking* (July–August 2002); "Seeing Is Believing? The Form and Substance of French Medical Debates Over Lourdes," *Bulletin of the History of Medicine* (Summer 2002); "The Power of Words: Healing Narratives Among Lubavitcher Hasidim," *Medical Anthropology Quarterly* (March 2002); "The Doctor as God's Mechanic? Beliefs in the Southeastern United States," *Social Science & Medicine* (February 2002); "Spiritual Matters, Earthly Benefits," *Tufts University Health & Nutrition Letter* (August 2001); "Prayer Makes a Difference: I'd Bet My Life on It," *Commonweal* (April 21, 2000); "Can Prayer Heal?" *Health* (March 1998); "Debate on Spirituality," *Ardell Wellness Report* (Winter 1998); "The Greatest Story Never Told," *Utne Reader* (March/April 1997); "Commentary: Into the Heart of Healing," *Making the Rounds in Health, Faith and Ethics* (May 20, 1996); and "Faith and Healing," *Time* (June 24, 1996).

On the Internet . . .

American Cancer Society

The American Cancer Society (ACS) is a nationwide, community-based voluntary health organization. This site offers accurate and credible information about breast cancer.

http://www.cancer.org/docroot/home/index.asp

National Right to Life

This National Right to Life Web site offers comprehensive information on the pro-life movement. Right-to-life issues, including abortion, euthanasia, and infanticide are addressed. Tracking pro-life legislation is also included.

http://www.nrlc.org

NARAL Online

This is the home page of the National Abortion and Reproductive Rights Action League (NARAL), an organization that works to promote reproductive freedom and dignity for women and their families.

http://www.naral.org

The Men's Issues Page

The Men's Issues Page has an alphabetical subject index of men's issues, including fatherhood, physical health, and related topics. This site addresses a variety of men's health, social, and psychological concerns.

http://www.menweb.org/throop/index.html

FDA Office of Women's Health

This site offers information about the U.S. Food and Drug Administration Office of Women's Health, including regulatory guidance, scientific projects, press releases, and publications on a variety of women's health topics.

http://www.fda.gov/womens/default/htm

PART 4

Sexuality and Gender Issues

*F*ew issues could be of greater controversy than those concerning gender and sexuality. Recent generations of Americans have rejected "traditional" sexual roles and values, which has resulted in a significant increase in babies born out of wedlock, the spread of sexually transmitted diseases, and a rise in legal abortions. Discuss in this part is whether or not there is a link between abortion and breast cancer. Despite the fact that women live longer than men, there is a perception among some women that the health care system short-changes them in both clinical care and research. This part debates the alleged gender gap in health care.

- Does Abortion Increase the Risk of Breast Cancer?

- Does Health Care Delivery and Research Benefit Men at the Expense of Women?

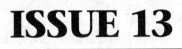

ISSUE 13

Does Abortion Increase the Risk of Breast Cancer?

YES: American Association of ProLife Obstetricians and Gynecologists, from "AAPLOG Statement on Induced Abortion and the Subsequent Risk of Breast Cancer," *Issues in Law and Medicine* (2002)

NO: Joyce Arthur, from "Abortion and Breast Cancer: A Forged Link," *The Humanist* (March/April 2002)

ISSUE SUMMARY

YES: The American Association of ProLife Obstetricians and Gynecologists state that for any woman already pregnant, choosing abortion will leave her with a greater long-term risk of breast cancer than she would have if she were to complete her pregnancy.

NO: Joyce Arthur, editor of the Canadian newsletter *Pro-Choice Press* and abortion rights activist, contends that the assertion that having an abortion significantly increases a woman's risk of breast cancer is deceptive and false.

Few issues have created as much controversy and resulted in as much opposition as abortion, and few diseases evoke as much fear in women as breast cancer. Several scientific studies have shown a correlation between abortion and an increased risk for breast cancer. Pro-life organizations believe that this information should be available to all women contemplating an abortion, while pro-choice organizations believe that the data linking the two are weak.

Those involved in the abortion debate not only have firm beliefs, but each side has a self-designated label—pro-choice and pro-life—that clearly reflects what they believe. The supporters of a woman's right to choose an abortion view individual choice as central to the debate. They maintain that if a woman cannot choose to end an unwanted pregnancy, she has lost one of her most basic human rights. The pro-choice supporters assert that although the fetus is a potential human being, its life cannot be placed on the same level with that of a woman. The supporters of the pro-life movement counter that the fetus *is* a human being and that it has the same right to life as the mother. They contend that abortion is not only immoral; it is murder.

Although abortion appears to be a modern issue, it has a very long history. In the past, women in both urbanized and tribal societies used a variety of dangerous methods to end unwanted pregnancies. Women consumed toxic chemicals, or various objects were inserted into the uterus in hopes of expelling its contents. Modern technology has simplified the abortion procedure and has made it considerably safer. Before abortion was legalized in the United States, approximately 20 percent of all deaths from childbirth or pregnancy were caused by botched illegal abortions.

In 1973 the U.S Supreme Court's decision of *Roe v. Wade* determined that an abortion in the first three months of pregnancy (first trimester) is a decision between a woman and her physician and is protected by a right to privacy. The Court ruled that during the second trimester an abortion can be performed on the basis of health risks. During the final trimester an abortion can be performed only to preserve the mother's life.

The right-to-life movement has recently focused on several studies that link abortion with breast cancer. They believe that if the public were more aware of this connection, fewer women would choose abortion, fearing that it would increase their odds of developing breast cancer. The pro-choice movement disagrees with the findings of these studies, stating that the research is flawed and that abortion either does not increase the risk of breast cancer or increases it very slightly. In the following selections, the editors of the American Association of ProLife Obstetricians and Gynecologists maintain that the data linking abortion to breast cancer is valid and condemn efforts to suppress the data. Joyce Arthur counters that these studies are seriously flawed and that the link between abortion and breast cancer is extremely weak.

American Association of ProLife
Obstetricians and Gynecologists

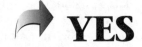 **YES**

AAPLOG Statement on Induced Abortion and the Subsequent Risk of Breast Cancer

There is very strong evidence in the world's scientific medical literature that induced abortion constitutes a significant risk factor for future breast cancer. Is it a real risk that every woman considering elective abortion should be apprised of? Or is it simply an unproven threat thrown into the abortion arena to frighten pregnant women from making "the choice"? These are absolutely vital questions for any abortion inclined pregnant woman. The threat of breast cancer, surgery, radiation, chemotherapy, disfigurement, even death, hang on the correct answers. We depend on "evidence based medicine" to guide us to valid conclusions on such issues. Here is the evidence:

There are two pregnancy related independent risk factors for breast cancer established in the medical literature. The first is the protective effect of an early first full term pregnancy. The landmark study establishing this protective effect by MacMahon et al. is widely accepted in the medical world.[1] MacMahon and group reanalyzed their 1970 data finding that each one year delay in the first full term pregnancy increased relative breast cancer risk by 3.5% (compounded). Obviously, aborting a first pregnancy eliminates the protective effect against breast cancer.[2]

The second independent risk factor for breast cancer is induced abortion. As of March, 2002, there have been published in the world-wide medical literature thirty-seven studies reporting data on the risk of breast cancer among women with a history of induced abortion. Twenty-eight of these studies report increased risk. In the United States, there have been fifteen such studies, thirteen of which reported increased risk, eight with statistical significance (at least 95% probability that the result is not due to chance) irrespective of age at first full-term pregnancy. The relative risk increase of the thirty-seven studies combined is thirty percent.[3]

Consider the implications of the study specifically funded by the United States National Cancer Institute to investigate the abortion/breast cancer [ABC] link.[4] Janet Daling's group found an overall fifty percent breast cancer risk by age forty-five for women who have had an induced abortion. American women today have an approximately 12% lifetime chance of developing breast cancer. But the risk increases even more than fifty percent for certain subgroups. For example, among women with a family history of breast cancer (mother, grandmother, sister, or aunt), the increase in risk was 80%. If the woman had her abortion before she was eighteen, the increase in risk was more than one hundred percent! If the woman had both risk factors (family history, and abortion before age eighteen), the risk was incalculably high, i.e., there were twelve such women out of 1800 in the study, and all twelve developed breast cancer by age forty-five. This subgroup is too small to be statistically significant, but surely it is significant if you are an abortion-minded seventeen year old pregnant teenage with a family history of breast cancer—or if you are a doctor counseling this teen about abortion risks—or if you are the parent or boyfriend concerned for her ultimate welfare.

The only study yet published on American women which relied solely on data from medical records entered at the time of the abortion (and therefore immune to inaccurate interview material) reported a statistically significant ninety percent increase in breast cancer risk with induced abortion.[5]

Authoritative figures in the National Cancer Institute and in the American College of Obstetricians and Gynecologists generally will cite "recall bias" as the scientific reason that they trivialize or outright deny the scientific literature on the subject. They look upon these studies as flawed due to recall bias, and apparently not worthy of serious consideration.

What is "recall bias," also known as "reporting bias" or "response bias," that it is so powerful that it negates twenty-eight of thirty-seven worldwide studies? It is a theory that presumes that women who have breast cancer will be more honest when asked if they have ever had an abortion, whereas healthy women will be less honest if asked the same question. Thus, the theory goes, in interview based studies, the incidence of breast cancer will be statistically (and falsely) higher in the women with previous abortions. A Swedish study published to demonstrate "recall bias" was published in the AJE in 1991. This Swedish team published the only paper we know of which claims to show statistically significant evidence of "recall bias." But this finding was dependent upon the astounding assumption of "over-reporting," i.e., that eight breast cancer patients had imagined (and reported) an abortion of which the computer had no record. (Apparently these women had their abortions in a neighboring country, thus were not on the Swedish computer record.) Importantly, the Swedish team retracted the idea of over-reporting in the March, 1998 issue of the JECH. That rendered their recall bias finding as not statistically significant. We are aware of no studies that substantiate with statistical significance the theory of recall bias. But the assumption of "recall bias," once birthed, has taken on a life of its own, and it has become the rallying cry for those who wish to discredit the world's literature on the subject.

How does induced abortion influence the development, in some women, of breast cancer?[6] We do not know for sure. However, there may be an endocrinological basis. Consider the following facts:

The world's scientific literature on the subject, twenty-eight of thirty-seven world-wide studies, and thirteen of fifteen American studies, sends a very strong message. Why, then, is there deafening silence on the issue by America's medical authorities? There is outright denial of the evidence: The ACOG's 2002 *Compendium of Selected Publications* states: "Long term risks sometimes attributed to surgical abortion include potential effects on reproductive function, cancer incidence, and psychological sequelae. However, the medical literature, when carefully evaluated, clearly demonstrates no significant negative impact on any of these factors with surgical abortion."[7] In the March 2002 issue of *Obstetrics and Gynecology Clinics of North America,* there is a ten page review article entitled "Risk factors for breast cancer." In this article, only the following sentence mentions abortion: "Much has been written regarding the risk of breast cancer and induced abortion; however, an analysis of current data reveals no relationship of induced abortion to breast cancer risk." The National Cancer Institute's March 6, 2002 web page, under "Cancer Facts," section on "Abortion and Breast Cancer" basically denies the abortion/breast cancer link. All of this information is obviously contrary to the great majority of published evidence. On this vital issue, organized medicine, for reasons of its own, is apparently willing to ignore or deny the evidence. This is unacceptable. Women's health, even their lives, may be at risk.

Ultimately, evidence based medicine (and truth) will prevail—but too late for many women who are submitting to their elective abortions without any informed consent regarding breast cancer risk, and with the assurance of many of the leaders in women's health care (and the silence of other leaders) that they need not worry about such risk. If the twenty-eight of thirty-seven world-wide studies, including thirteen of fifteen American studies, are correct, the physicians who have denied the abortion/breast cancer link, and also those who have conveniently ignored it, will stand guilty of an immense disservice to the women they purport to serve—especially to some of those who subsequently develop breast cancer.

Counselor or doctors dealing with pregnant women considering abortion can confidently inform them that:

1. Interruption of her first pregnancy will remove the protective effect of the first full term pregnancy, and subject her to a small but real increased risk of developing breast cancer in the future.

2. According to the only study yet published which was specifically funded by the United States National Cancer Institute to investigate the ABC link, the Daling study, if a woman has a mother, sister, aunt or grandmother with breast cancer she will increase her chance of getting breast cancer by eighty percent; if she is under eighteen she will double her chance of getting breast cancer; and if both conditions pertain her risk is much higher (twelve of twelve in the Daling study). And all these cancers were diagnosed by age forty-five. This is a frightening fact.

3. Seventy-five percent of the world's scientific literature on this subject, and eighty percent of the American scientific literature on the subject, agree with the conclusion that elective abortion results in a significant increase in the risk of developing breast cancer in later life.

Notes

1. MacMahon et al., 43 Bull. WHO 209–221 (1970).

2. D. Trichopolous et al., *Age at Any Birth and Breast Cancer Risk,* 31 Int'l J. Cancer 701–04 (1983).

3. Note: this means that among aborted women there would be a 30% increase in breast cancer cases over what would normally be expected. In the current American abortion experience, this would result in approximately 5,000 additional cases of breast cancer per year in the U.S. There are about 190,000 new cases of breast cancer diagnosed in the U.S. each year.

4. Janet R. Daling et al., *Risk of Breast Cancer Among Young Women: Relationship to Induced Abortion,* 86 J. Nat'l Cancer Inst. 1584–92 (1994).

5. Howe et al., 18 J. Epidemiology 300–04 (1989).

6. Miscarriage—also known as "spontaneous abortion"—has no demonstrated breast cancer link.

7. American College of Obstetrics and Gynecology, Compendium of Selected Publications 392 (2002).

Joyce Arthur

NO

Abortion and Breast Cancer: A Forged Link

A major weapon of the anti-abortion movement is its scare-mongering claim that having an abortion significantly increases a woman's risk of breast cancer—the "ABC link." This allegation is grossly deceptive and just plain false. A substantial weight of evidence counters the ABC link, and a recent international scientific consensus has rejected it.

Unfortunately, this doesn't stop anti-abortionists from presenting the ABC link as an undisputed fact, even manufacturing the lie that half of all abortion patients will go on to develop breast cancer. This is what anxious women were advised in 1996 when they called the toll-free number on east coast subway advertisements that featured the dire warning: "Women Who Choose Abortion Suffer More and Deadlier Breast Cancer!" In spite of new research that largely refutes the ABC link, almost all anti-abortion websites still trumpet the claim without reservation, and scientific-sounding ads hyping the ABC link have appeared in newspapers.

The latest tactic is lawsuits aimed at forcing abortion providers to inform patients of the bogus link. It's all part of the neverending anti-abortion war, and although anti-abortionists want us to believe they're fighting the battle to save women, what they're really doing is turning women into frightened pawns in a strategic campaign against abortion.

Anti-abortionists promote the alleged ABC link because seventeen out of thirty-seven scientific studies that have examined the link showed a small overall increase in breast cancer risk for women who have abortions. These studies had serious flaws, however. In particular, most were older *case control* studies that suffered from a major bias: they relied on women self-reporting their abortion history. Women with breast cancer are more likely to tell the truth about past abortions because people with serious illnesses are motivated to report their medical history accurately to facilitate their treatment and recovery. But control groups of healthy people have less incentive to report honestly and, in fact, many women keep quiet about past abortions since it's a private and sensitive issue.

It's well established that in medical case control studies, patients tend to disclose their histories more fully than healthy control groups (a phenomenon called *recall bias*), and a recent study has confirmed abortion underreporting by healthy women. According to Radha Jagannatha in the November 2001 *American Journal of Public Health,* within a randomly selected group of Medicaid recipients in New Jersey, only 29 percent of those who had a Medicaid billing for an abortion actually admitted to the abortion in a reproductive health survey. Other studies on underreporting have found that only 35 percent to 60 percent of actual abortions are reported in surveys. What this means is that the detection of an ABC link by self-report studies is untrustworthy. Women with breast cancer only *appear* to have had more abortions than healthy women.

The best studies of the alleged link are called *historical cohort studies* because they rely on complete medical records for entire populations of women, over decades. This means researchers have accurate statistics from a large sample from which to calculate exactly how many women suffered breast cancer, how many had abortions, and which ones had either or both. *No cohort study has shown evidence of an ABC link,* at least for abortions performed in the first trimester.

The definitive cohort study on the ABC link was conducted by the Danish Epidemiology Science Center at Statens Serum Institute in Copenhagen and reported in the January 9, 1997, *New England Journal of Medicine.* Researchers M. Melbye, M. Wohlfahrt, J. H. Olsen, M. Frisch, T. Westergaard, K. Helweg-Larsen, and P. K. Andersen used data from detailed government medical registries of 1.5 million Danish women, which recorded all cases of breast cancer or legally induced abortion since 1973. The researchers found *zero* increased risk of breast cancer for women who have abortions by the fourteenth week of pregnancy. (The study left open the question of whether a risk may be present for late abortions performed after eighteen weeks, but the rarity of these abortions would render any such risk statistically less problematic.)

Attempts by the anti-abortion movement to refute the Danish study have failed. Anti-abortionist Joel Brind accused the study authors of making gross errors in their research design. In response the authors said, "We find [Brind's] argument self-contradictory and based on fundamental misconceptions about the cohort design." Although they corrected Brind's specific misunderstandings, their rebuke failed to modify Brind's position; he continues to propagate the same criticisms to his exclusive audience, the anti-abortion movement.

Brind, a professor of biology and endocrinology at New York City's Baruch College, is a tireless proponent of the ABC link. He has devoted an entire website—www.abortioncancer.com—to the issue. The website states that Brim "has written and lectured extensively" on this topic since 1992, but his lecturing is confined essentially to the anti-abortion speaker circuit, and he has published only one peer-reviewed research paper on the supposed connection between induced abortion and breast cancer. This 1996 paper, "Induced Abortion As an Independent Risk Factor for Breast Cancer: A Comprehensive Review and Meta-Analysis" (*Journal of Epidemiology and Community Health,* October), has been heavily criticized. Brind pooled the data from twenty-three studies on the ABC link and came up with a 30 percent increase in risk. However, most of the studies he included were those flawed by reporting bias, so it was a classic case of "garbage in, garbage out." Brind's work has been supplanted by a December

2001 review of twenty-eight studies of the ABC link by British researcher Tim Davidson, who concluded in the *Lancet Oncology* there was "insufficient data to justify warning women of future breast-cancer risk when counseling them about abortion."

There simply is no known mechanism that would cause the alleged ABC link.

Brind speculates that abortion suddenly interrupts the estrogen surge, leaving rapidly growing breast cells in an undifferentiated state and more vulnerable to carcinogens. However, this hypothesis has no empirical support. Besides, how would one then explain the fact that studies show no link between miscarriage and breast cancer, as anti-abortionists acknowledge? Brind claims the "raging-hormones-cut-short" problem doesn't affect miscarriage, since most miscarriages are caused by a lack of pregnancy hormones. Not so—the majority of miscarriages are actually caused by genetic defects in the egg/embryo, and other causes; only an estimated 10 percent or so of miscarriages are caused by hormonal deficiencies. This means there is probably no significant difference between the effects of miscarriage and abortion—so if miscarriage doesn't lead to an increased risk of breast cancer, then, of course, neither would abortion.

For the sake of argument, let's suppose that Brind's ABC link is real. What would it really mean? He claims that abortion may boost the risk of breast cancer by 30 percent, but this increase is not really that significant. For example, the risk is 200 percent to 300 percent higher for a woman whose mother or sister had breast cancer after age fifty. Even this well-established risk factor is considered moderate by scientists. In comparison, the alleged ABC link barely qualifies; even if it's real, the risk is close to negligible. To put it another way, the National Cancer Institute estimates the current risk of breast cancer to be one in 2,525 for a woman in her thirties; if that risk were increased by 30 percent, it would mean one in 1,942 women would get breast cancer.

Second, correlation doesn't equal causation, which means some other factor could be responsible for any increased breast cancer risk, thus confounding the study results. For example, women with a first full-term pregnancy after age thirty face a breast cancer risk two to three times higher than women with a full-term pregnancy before age twenty. If a study included many women who had aborted their first pregnancy when they were young, effectively postponing motherhood, we might find a correlation between abortion and breast cancer, but delayed childbearing would be the more probable cause of the increased risk.

Anti-abortion "researchers" are notorious for confusing correlation with causation, which is showcased by a new study, privately funded by a British anti-abortion group. The "study"—published by lone author Patrick Carroll and not peer reviewed—blames thirty years of legalized abortion for rising rates of breast cancer in some countries. Dismissed or ignored are many other probable causes that have also proliferated in the last thirty years—including delayed childbearing, smaller family size, better cancer-screening methods, environmental contaminants, obesity in mid-life, and the use of oral contraceptives and hormone replacement therapy.

Many reputable organizations have released position statements or articles discounting the ABC link, and citing the Danish cohort study and other reliable studies in support. Such groups include the American Cancer Society, the National Cancer Institute, the National Breast Cancer Coalition, the World Health Organization, the Center for Reproductive Law and Policy, the Alan Guttmacher Institute, the Planned Parenthood Federation of America, and others. On its website (cis.nci.nih.gov/fact/3_53.htm), the National Cancer Institute says: "Although it has been the subject of extensive research, there is no convincing evidence of a direct relationship between breast cancer and either induced or spontaneous abortion." After reviewing the research on the ABC link, the World Health Organization's online article (www.who.int/inf-fs-/en/fact240.html) concludes: "Therefore, results from epidemiological studies are reassuring in that they show no consistent effect of first trimester induced abortion upon a woman's risk of breast cancer later in life." Impervious to reality, however, Brind and other anti-abortionists make the preposterous claim that these groups are conspiring in a "pro-abortion cover-up" of the ABC link.

Anti-abortionists are now taking their crusade to legislatures and courtrooms. Laws have been sponsored in about two dozen states to force abortion providers to inform patients of the supposed breast cancer risk, and so far two states—Montana and Mississippi—have passed them. In 1999, anti-abortionists launched a "false advertising" lawsuit against a North Dakota abortion clinic for distributing a pamphlet saying the ABC link is unsupported by medical research. The case is currently before the courts, and a new suit has recently been filed by three California women against Planned Parenthood for "misleading" women about the ABC link.

Raising the stakes even higher, a dubious lawsuit was settled in Australia in September 2001, in which the plaintiff had sued her abortion provider for not informing her of the alleged risk of "psychiatric damage" from abortion (there's actually little or no risk). Tacked onto the lawsuit was the additional "failure" to warn of an increased risk of breast cancer. Settled confidentially out of court, the case highlights the disconnect between law and science. Anti-abortionists are naively touting the settlement as "proof" of the ABC link, but lawsuit settlements are the crafty negotiations of lawyers, have nothing to do with science, and are incapable of establishing scientific facts. Defendants are often pressured to settle out of court for expediency's sake, not because they're in the wrong.

More lawsuits like the Australia case are on the way. Behind them lies the enduring modus operandi of the anti-abortion movement—demonizing abortion providers and intimidating women out of abortions. But given the current evidence against the ABC link, it would be irresponsible for health professionals to advise abortion patients of any alleged risk. Anti-abortionists' fear-mongering promotion of the ABC link is reprehensible as well as fanatical. Although aware that their evidence is highly disputed, anti-abortionists continue to advise women, without qualification, that having an abortion puts them at great danger of breast cancer. For a pregnant woman faced with the traumatic, life-changing decision of whether or not to have a baby, such hypocritical posturing to advance a political anti-abortion agenda is callous in the extreme.

POSTSCRIPT

Does Abortion Increase the Risk of Breast Cancer?

The abortion issue continues to be complex and polarizing. With pressure and support from pro-life groups throughout the country, *Roe v. Wade* may continue to come before the Supreme Court for reconsideration. Pro-life groups have been successful in keeping the abortion issue in the media and in the political arena.

The literature on abortion and its relationship to breast cancer is prolific. In "Abortion, Breast Cancer, and Consent," *Issues in Law & Medicine* (Spring 2000) attorney John Kindley argues that the current level of scientific evidence linking induced abortion with increased breast cancer risk is sufficient enough to support an ethical and legal duty to disclose fully the risk to women who are considering abortion. Studies that have found a relationship between abortion and the subsequent development of breast cancer include "Women's Health After Abortion," *The Human Life Review* (Fall 2002); "It's Simple as ABC—Deny, Deny, Deny," *The Report Newsmagazine* (February 4, 2002); "Abortion and Breast Cancer," *National Right to Life News* (February 2002); "Past Study Indicates Abortion Increases Risk of Breast Cancer," *Nutrition Health Review* (Winter 2001); and "Another Study Finds Abortion and Cancer Link," *Cancer Weekly Plus* (December 16, 1996). An article in the *American Family Physician* (April 1997) found that full-term pregnancy increases a woman's risk of breast cancer in the short-term but decreases the long-term risk. Other studies of the association between induced abortion and the risk of breast cancer have been inconsistent. The authors concluded that induced abortion appears to have no overall effect on the incidence of breast cancer, although the small number of women with a history of second-trimester abortion had a statistically significant increase in breast cancer risk. A three-percent increase in the risk of breast cancer was associated with each one-week increase in the gestational age of the fetus at the time of the abortion.

Selections that dispute the abortion/breast cancer relationship include "Abortion-Cancer Link Is Rejected," *Science News* (March 15, 2003); "An Enduring Debate: Cancer and Abortion," *The Los Angeles Times* (March 10, 2003); "Risk Is Significantly Reduced by Both Induced and Spontaneous Abortions," *Cancer Weekly* (March 11, 2003); "Review Rules Out Abortion-Cancer Link," *Science* (March 7, 2003); "Abortion and Breast Cancer: A Struggle to Link Them," *Catholic Insight* (January–February 2003); "Abortion and Breast Cancer: A Case-Control Record Linkage Study," *Journal of Epidemiology & Community Health* (May 2001); "Abortion Does Not Raise Breast Cancer Risk in Massive Danish Study," *Biotechnology Newswatch* (January 20, 1997); and "Induced Abortion and the Risk of Breast Cancer," *The New England Journal of Medicine* (January 9, 1997).

Articles about groups and organizations using the breast cancer/abortion relationship for political purposes include "Bearer of Bad News; An Alberta Woman Crashes a World Conference With Her Message: Abortion Causes Breast Cancer," *The Report Newsmagazine* (July 8, 2002); "Abortion & Breast Cancer: National Cancer Institute's Disinformation Halted," *National Right to Life News* (July 2002); "Abortion, Breast Cancer, and Ideology," *First Things: A Monthly Journal of Religion and Public Life* (May 1997); and "The Politics of Cancer Research," *The Wall Street Journal* (February 28, 1997).

ISSUE 14

Does Health Care Delivery and Research Benefit Men at the Expense of Women?

YES: Gayle Feldman, from "Women *Are* Different," *Self* (July 1997)

NO: Sally L. Satel, from "Sick Sisters: How Feminist Politics Is Warping Medicine," *The American Enterprise* (April/May 2001)

ISSUE SUMMARY

YES: Health and medical reporter Gayle Feldman contends that most disease research is done almost exclusively on men, yet the results of these studies have been extrapolated to draw conclusions concerning women and disease.

NO: Psychiatrist Sally L. Satel argues that the feminist political agenda has inaccurately asserted that women are second-class subjects in the world of medicine.

According to many researchers, women appear to respond differently from men to a varied array of medications and diseases. For instance, although heart disease is the leading killer of both men and women, women are less likely to survive heart attacks and heart surgery. Since the most influential studies of heart disease have studied only men, scientists and researchers are unable to explain the gender differences. Women activists state that medical research has focused on men for too long and that it is now time to change this pattern.

Heart disease, the leading killer of both men and women, has long been considered a male condition by both physicians and the public. This is probably because men develop the affliction at an earlier age than women do. But women catch up after menopause. By age 65 about one-third of women have some form of heart disease, high blood pressure, or stroke.

As a result of this perception, doctors tended to ignore womens' complaints of chest pains and other symptoms of heart disease or considered them to be psychosomatic. When women *were* treated for heart disease, they were often treated less aggressively than men with similar symptoms.

In 1989 Harvard University reported that taking an aspirin tablet every other day could prevent heart disease based on a study involving 22,000 male physicians. The findings were generalized to include both men and women, and the final reports maintained that aspirin, which helps prevent blood clotting, would be useful to all adults. Dr. Suzanne Oparil, president of the American Heart Association, however, believes that aspirin might not be beneficial to women because they have generally faster rates of blood clotting than men.

Why were women excluded in the Harvard aspirin study or in other research that might help prevent their premature deaths or disabilities? The answer goes back to 1975, when the National Commission for the Protection of Human Subjects of Biomedical and Behavioral Research issued guidelines limiting research on pregnant women. This ban on using women stemmed from fears following the thalidomide crisis in the late 1950s.

In 1985 the National Institutes of Health (NIH) issued a statement urging researchers to include women in their studies. In 1990 it was reported, however, that women were still excluded in major federally funded clinical studies and that the NIH was not enforcing its policy of including women.

Things began to change, beginning with the 1991 launching of the *Women's Health Initiative,* a 14-year study of women's health. And in 1993 the FDA lifted its ban on using women in drug trials.

A relatively recent concern pertains to AIDS and HIV-related conditions. In particular, AIDS research has a proportionately higher number of men participating in drug and other scientific trials. What is known about HIV and AIDS seems to have been acquired from research on men only.

Despite concerns that health care and research in the United States benefit men at the expense of women, there is ample evidence to the contrary: Department of Health and Human Services studies show that women see their physicians more frequently, have more surgery, and are admitted to hospitals more often than men. Currently, two out of three medical dollars are spent by women.

Women have benefited from medical research involving high-tech procedures. Laparoscopic surgery and ultrasound are two advanced techniques that were first developed for use on women's bodies (these procedures were later adapted for men). Women's diseases have also been the recipient of research dollars. Breast cancer, the second leading cancer killer of women, has received more funding than any other tumor research. In 1993 the National Cancer Institute spent over $213 million dollars on breast cancer and $51 million dollars on prostate cancer. Although one-third more women die of breast cancer than men of prostate cancer, research into breast cancer received more than four times the funding of prostate cancer research.

In the following selections, Gayle Feldman argues that women have been shortchanged with regard to health care and medical research. Sally L. Satel disagrees, stating that although it is often believed that women do not get the same consideration in medical care and research as men, the truth appears to be exactly the opposite.

Gayle Feldman

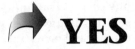 **YES**

Women *Are* Different

Linda is 36 years old, on the go all day, and can hardly spare the time for her annual physical. She knows what the doctor will tell her: Lose weight, quit smoking, work out. Fat chance, given her schedule. In fact, she would like to put off the physical, but she's been feeling so tired and short of breath lately. On top of that, the past couple of weeks she's been sick to her stomach. She can't figure out why—she hasn't changed her diet or routine, and she's on the Pill, for goodness' sake, so she can't be pregnant. She'd better get the physical over with and find out what's going on.

What's going on, the doctor tells her, is that Linda has heart disease; in fact, she's already had a mild heart attack. It's a complete shock. Like most women, Linda thinks heart disease is something that happens to men. Her image of a heart attack is a man clutching his chest or doubling over in life-stopping pain. The truth is, heart disease is the number-one killer of women, too; it kills more women than all cancers, AIDS, domestic violence and osteoporosis combined.

Most women are like Linda, not only completely unaware that heart disease could happen to them, but also that its symptoms and risk factors are often very different in women and in men. Their ignorance isn't surprising since heart disease—along with almost every other disease or condition outside the reproductive area—was until recently studied almost exclusively in men, and the results extrapolated, undifferentiated, to women.

But ignorance is not bliss; it's dangerous. Women are not simply pint-size men with different sexual plumbing. Now a new medical frontier is opening up, one that researchers are calling gender-based medicine. It is not only saying vive la différence but is aggressively setting out to learn from that difference and to make up for the years of neglect. It's looking at the biological specifics in areas that range from heart disease to pain management to how our bodies metabolize drugs.

Government and business are paying attention. Procter & Gamble is investing more than $2.5 million over the next few years to help establish the Partnership for Women's Health at Columbia University, located at Columbia–Presbyterian Medical Center in New York City, precisely to study gender-based medicine. Drug industry surveys show that more products are being developed specifically for women. And the Women's Health Initiative (WHI), the largest-ever prevention study funded by the U.S. government, is, among other things, researching how female hormones and lifestyles affect the development over time of heart disease, osteoporosis and other conditions in women.

Researchers know that women are far more prone to certain diseases or conditions than men. For example, we are:

- Twice as likely to suffer from major depression, anxiety disorders and phobias.
- Fifteen times more likely to have autoimmune or thyroid diseases.
- Three times more prone to rheumatoid arthritis and irritable bowel syndrome.
- Far more likely to suffer from migraine headaches.

The challenge that gender-based medicine has set for itself is to find out what causes the disproportion in women, and how treatment options might eventually be tailored more specifically—and more successfully—to help them.

Think about Linda's situation: A doctor grounded in gender-based medicine would recognize that her fatigue, shortness of breath and nausea were common heart disease symptoms in women. This doctor would know the best tests for coronary disease in women and would recognize that Linda is putting herself at risk for major heart problems by the very fact that she smokes while taking birth-control pills, which can cause the development of life-threatening blood clots. Smoking while on the Pill is something no woman over age 35 should ever do. A gender-based approach would recognize the heart benefits of hormone-replacement therapy after menopause for a woman like Linda.

Unfortunately, though, many primary-care physicians aren't yet looking at patients through a gender-specific lens. Astonishingly, a 1995 Gallup survey for the American Medical Women's Association (AMWA) found that one out of three of the 300 primary-care doctors surveyed didn't know that heart disease is the number-one cause of death in American women; two out of three didn't know risk factors for women are different; and nine out of 10 thought that male and female symptoms were the same. All the more reason for women to be educated participants in their own care.

One of the easiest ways to begin to appreciate what gender-based medicine is about is to look more closely into the female heart. Women's hearts are smaller, they weight 50 to 100 grams less, and they beat more often and more quickly than men's. Our arteries also tend to be smaller, so it takes less fatty plaque to block them. When these arteries do become blocked and bypass operations, balloon angioplasty or other procedures are necessary to open or circumvent them, it can be trickier and riskier for heart surgeons to use on their female patients the standard instruments that have been designed to go into bigger male arteries. Sometimes they have to use surgical instruments that were designed for use on children; on other occasions, they just can't operate on certain arteries.

WHAT WE'LL LEARN IN THE YEAR 2006

Ten years from now we will have answers to some of our gender-based women's health questions, courtesy of the Women's Health Initiative (WHI), an unprecedented 15-year, 40-site, $628 million study of 164,500 postmenopausal women from 50 to 79 years old that was begun in 1991.

The largest part of this study is "observational," with 100,000 women participating. They will have periodic physical exams and respond to annual surveys about their health, focusing on heart disease, cancer and osteoporosis. Lifestyle, attitude, diet and medications will be taken into account.

The other 64,500 women will each be in one or more of three clinical trials:

- 27,500 will be involved in a randomized HRT [hormone replacement therapy] trial. No previous randomized trials of estrogen have gone on longer than three years, so up till now doctors have essentially been dispensing HRT in the dark. This study should finally tell us about its real benefits and risks.
- 48,000 will be studied to see if a low-fat, high-fiber, high-fruit-and-vegetable diet lowers breast and colon cancer rates.
- 45,000 women from the two previous groups will also be tracked to see the effects of calcium and vitamin D supplements on osteoporosis and colon cancer risk.

In 1995, another project, the $25 million, five-year Study of Women's Health Across the Nation (SWAN), involving women ages 42 to 52, was begun. It is studying 3,200 women for alterations in body composition, bone density and cardiovascular function; risk factors for cardiovascular disease and arthritis; the endocrine system; and sexuality. Lifestyle and psychological factors will also be taken into account, and a special feature of the study is that it was designed to include a large proportion of African Americans, Hispanics and Asian Americans.

We'll have to wait for an equivalent study of younger women.—*G.F.*

Statistically, our 36-year-old friend Linda was unlucky, since most premenopausal women are—to a large degree—protected against heart disease by their own estrogen. Once a woman enters menopause, heart problems can mushroom. One in nine women ages 45 to 64 has some cardiovascular disease, and the statistics skyrocket to one in three after age 65. Of course, until modern medical advancements like antibiotics extended women's life spans from an average of 48 years in 1900 to 79 years today, chronic illnesses such as heart disease, stroke and late-onset diabetes were hardly a problem at all: Women tended to die of infectious diseases or during childbirth; many never reached menopause. That is one of the reasons why the study of these diseases in women has lagged.

SHAKING UP THE MEDICAL ESTABLISHMENT

Throughout history, a woman's unique ability to bear children has largely determined society's attitude toward her, and medicine was no exception. Inspired by feminism, groups such as the Boston Women's Health Collective—authors of the pathbreaking book *Our Bodies, Ourselves*—began in the 1970s to look at women's health in a new way. Only during the past decade have the medical and political establishments started to catch up.

Pressure to shift the focus to gender-specific aspects of women's health has been coming from grassroots advocacy and the efforts of female scientists who have worked to change the agenda. One of them, gynecologist Florence Haseltine, Ph.D., M.D., arrived at the National Institutes of Health to direct the Center for Population Research in 1985. Once there, she became angry about the unfairness of excluding women from government-funded clinical trials.

From 1977 to 1993, women were officially barred from early drug trials overseen by the FDA, partly in response to the tragic birth defects of children whose pregnant mothers had taken thalidomide and DES. The FDA feared the possible side effects of experimental drugs on fetuses or on future pregnancies, as well as legal liability issues. Women were also excluded to ensure a "homogeneous" testing population, and because of the extra "complications" in cost, timing and "unreliability" of dealing with people who have menstrual cycles.

So, for example, during the 1980s, when 25,000 men were studied to see if aspirin worked as a preventive measure for heart disease, not one woman was included. Even earlier, estrogen was tested to see if it helped prevent heart disease—in men only. Dr. Haseltine also discovered that in the NIH there were fewer gynecologists than veterinarians. So in 1988, with psychiatrist Susan J. Blumenthal, M.D. (now deputy assistant secretary for women's health at the Department of Health and Human Services, or HHS), she co-founded the Society for the Advancement of Women's Health Research.

To be fair, the government hadn't been completely unaware of the need for change. A Public Health Service report in 1985 clearly stated that "biomedical and behavioral research should be expanded to ensure an emphasis on conditions and diseases unique to, or more prevalent in, women," and in 1986 the NIH issued a policy statement advising that women be included in clinical trials. But those good intentions had not been carried out. So Haseltine, Dr. Blumenthal and others turned to the Congressional Caucus for Women's Issues for help.

The caucus requested that the Government Accounting Office (GAO) determine the extent to which women had been left out of federally funded research. The GAO findings, issued in a June 1990 report, were scathing.

The reaction was swift. Within two months, the NIH instructed its staff that beginning the following February, no grant applications for studies would be accepted unless women were adequately represented; soon thereafter, the organization established the Office for Research on Women's Health. In fall 1990, Bernadine Healy, M.D., became the first female head of the NIH. That September, the NIH conference in Hunt Valley, Maryland, issued the watershed "Hunt Valley report," setting its priorities for women's health research. Finally, in 1993, it was mandated that women be included in clinical trials. A year later, President Clinton named Blumenthal to the first senior level post at HHS exclusively devoted to women's health.—*G.F.*

Although we know that estrogen protects the cardiovascular system, we still don't completely understand how. Traditionally, doctors thought that the hormone's beneficial effect was to help maintain a high level of high-density lipoproteins (HDLs, or "good cholesterol") and a low level of low-density lipoproteins (LDLs, or "bad cholesterol"). Now, it has become clear that LDL levels are a better predictor of heart disease risk for men; HDL and triglyceride levels (triglycerides are another kind of fat, not found in cholesterol) are a better predictor for women, according to Debra R. Judelson, M.D., the Beverly Hills cardiologist who is the current president of AMWA. Linda's HDL level was found to be low and her triglyceride level was very high.

A unique benefit of estrogen that we do know is that it preserves the normal dilating response of blood vessels during stress. "You preserve the dilating response even in damaged blood vessels, an effect that is totally different between men and women," Dr. Judelson says.

Women often have very distinctive cardiovascular disease symptoms. According to Elizabeth Ross, M.D., author of *Healing the Female Heart*, the pain that a man with heart disease in danger of a heart attack feels tends to be severe and sudden. A woman may feel that, too, or, like Linda, may only feel nausea, pain in the arm or shoulder or jaw, extreme fatigue or shortness of breath. Or, she might only suffer from swelling in the ankles or lower legs.

Thanks to her estrogen, a woman tends to get heart disease, on average, 10 years later than a man, and yet she is twice as likely to die after a heart attack. How can that be? First, many women are so completely unaware of their risk that they don't realize their bodies are giving them warning signs. Second, many primary-care physicians are unaware of women's more subtle symptoms. Third, Dr. Ross emphasizes, the traditional gold-standard exercise stress test "is not as accurate in women as it is in men, because women's physiology of response to exercise may be different." Some doctors still don't realize that heart disease can be diagnosed more accurately in women by two other tests (a nuclear stress test or a stress echocardiogram). So by the time many women are diagnosed, they are far sicker than men.

Knowing already that heart disease was a factor in her life, Linda's physician wasn't surprised to find some evidence of mild diabetes when her blood test results came back from the lab. Diabetes is a stronger cardiovascular risk factor in women than in men, and as our population ages, its prevalence is greatly increasing, even more so in the African American population. Obesity and a sedentary lifestyle are the two biggest predictors of diabetes risk. Ross reminds us that "one third of American women past the age of 30 are obese, and too many subscribe to the concept that dieting makes you healthy. But unless you also begin to exercise regularly, dieting will accomplish nothing useful in the long term."

Then, of course, there's smoking. Quite simply, it cancels out the beneficial effects of estrogen. According to Judelson, "smoking makes a man get a heart attack seven years earlier than usual, but a woman 19 years earlier than usual."

In fact, one of the major goals of gender-specific medicine is to determine how much lifestyle factors (regular exercise, eating a low-fat diet and not smoking, for example) can affect a woman's health. Researchers already know that how a woman treats her body when she's young affects what happens after menopause. Yet findings also show that too many young women are ignorant about that relationship or feel immune to it.

A 1993 survey by the Commonwealth Fund's Commission on Women's Health found that nearly one out of three women never exercised, and one out of four smoked. In addition, tobacco seems to slow lung function and growth in adolescent girls more than in boys. Since cigarette manufacturers recognized the profits to be made in targeting advertising to women decades ago, preventive medicine has lot of catching up to do to tailor antismoking campaigns specifically to young girls.

And, of course, the whole debate over whether women should take hormone replacement therapy (HRT) after they have reached menopause is connected to their risk of cardiovascular disease. The higher their risk, the more they should consider HRT. Hormone replacement also looms large in any discussion of osteoporosis.

The next time you're in a crowd, notice all the senior citizens whose shoulders and backs are stooped and bent. Most of them are women, not men. That's because older women are the main victims of the disintegrating bone disease osteoporosis. In fact, two out of five women now alive will have had an osteoporosis-related fracture by the age of 70, according to Marianne J. Legato, M.D., the Columbia University professor who is directing the Partnership for Women's Health. The loss of estrogen after menopause is the most obvious factor in female osteoporosis, so why should younger women pay attention to a disease of middle and old age? Simple: because how we treat our bodies when we're young affects development of the disease after menopause. The osteoporosis that younger women should be concerned about is Type 1, which affects women six times more often than men and is associated with estrogen decline. (Type 2 affects women twice as often as men, but isn't really a factor until after age 70.)

Osteoporosis is the loss of bone mass or density, which leads to fragility and unexpected fractures. Throughout our lives, our bones are constantly being rebuilt, with new bone matter replacing the bone mass we lose. But around age 30, bone loss begins very subtly to exceed bone formation in both men and women. Once a woman reaches menopause—and for eight to 10 years immediately afterward—the hormonal changes cause increased breakdown of bone. During that decade, as much as 5 percent of bone mass can be lost in a single year.

Building Better Bones

So it's essential to build maximum bone mass when young and lead a lifestyle that will help maintain as much of it as possible later on. But women's bones are at a disadvantage from a very early age. Since most women have smaller frames and are less physically active as teenagers, they have less bone density than men do. If a teenager does not eat well or diets a lot, she will have a calcium deficiency and never build optimum mass. Similarly, if a woman is an exercise fanatic and begins to have irregular periods (or none at all), her body isn't producing enough estrogen. She'll pay the price later on.

Obviously, estrogen deficiency is not the only factor in the disease, since not every postmenopausal woman has osteoporosis. All women require a certain amount of calcium, but many don't get it through their diet. Although researchers agree that calcium supplements can be a beneficial preventive measure, according to the Commonwealth Fund survey, four out of five women ages 18 to 44 (and three out of five women 45 and older) do not take them.

Smoking, caffeine, too much alcohol and lack of weight-bearing physical exercise throughout adulthood make a woman susceptible to the disease. So, too, does the abuse of thyroid medications, which some women misguidedly use to speed up their metabolisms to lose weight.

Thyroid disorders predispose women to osteoporosis, and they are much more a woman's problem than a man's. One in eight women develops some thyroid problem during her lifetime; one in 20 does so after having a baby. That's why during the past few years some doctors have started to advocate the TSH (thyroid stimulating hormone) test as part of a regular physical exam.

Drugs for Women Only?

The drugs men and women take may affect them differently solely because of gender, and the instructions that come with them may one day contain dosage variations for sex, weight, age and other factors. Freda Lewis-Hall, M.D., who heads the Lilly Center for Women's Health in Indianapolis, says that drug companies will have to address two major questions when developing new medications: first, whether there are differences in their effectiveness or in adverse side effects in men and women; and, second, whether the effectiveness of the medicine varies during a woman's menstrual cycle.

Think of the changes the menstrual cycle imposes on women's bodies; indeed, consider the multiplicity of hormonal changes through a woman's life and the effects they can have. Judelson describes a scenario that is all too familiar to every woman: "When I'm premenstrual, my GI tract slows down, my stomach takes forever to empty, and my belly bloats—doesn't that affect medication absorption?"

Remember, standard dosages of most medications until very recently were designed for and tested on men. According to a 1993 research report by the Food and Drug Administration's Working Group on Women in Clinical Trials, the popular painkillers acetaminophen, aspirin and lidocaine take longer to be eliminated from a woman's body. Does that mean women need different dosages or need to time them differently for optimum effect? We don't know. Seventy percent of psychotropic drugs are prescribed to women, yet basic studies of them were done primarily on male rats.

We have only limited knowledge about how oral contraceptives lessen some of the gender differential effects for drug metabolism and heighten others; we know even less about how HRT enters into the equation. The tranquilizer Valium, for example, takes longer to clear a woman's body than a man's, but only until menopause. What happens if a menopausal woman is on both Valium and HRT? As yet, nobody knows.

Then, too, consider not only the variations of the monthly cycle, but also the fact that women's circadian rhythms are different from men's. There may be certain times of day when a woman's body would do a quicker, better job of absorbing a drug and circulating it throughout her system, and it may be very different from the timing that works best in a man. We need to find out.

One thing we do know is that our higher body-fat content and lower body-water volume contribute to higher blood-alcohol concentrations. Women produce less of a liver enzyme—alcohol dehydrogenase—that breaks down alcohol. This is why a woman who drinks a smaller amount of an alcoholic beverage than does a man of the same size will nevertheless get more intoxicated.

Then there are drugs that have been tested and abandoned in men-only clinical trials, but if given a chance might work beautifully in women. Take, for example, the recent discovery by a team of researchers at the University of California San Francisco regarding a group of painkilling drugs called kappa-opioids. These drugs do not have the significant side effects of the more familiar mu-opioids—morphine, codeine, etc.—and had originally been developed as an alternative to them. In men-only tests, their effectiveness had been disappointing.

The team at San Francisco decided to try them out again, this time on a group of 48 young men and women who were having impacted wisdom teeth removed. The kappa-opioids worked very well for the women in the group—so well that the leader of this National Institutes of Health (NIH)−funded project, Jon D. Levine, M.D., Ph.D., recommended that their use for women with moderate to severe pain be reevaluated. Further, Dr. Levine stated, "our studies provide evidence that biologically, women and men do not obtain pain relief in the same way. It may be that the brain circuitry regulating pain relief differs between the sexes."

There's much to find out about gender differentiation in brain function. Some experts, like Dr. Legato, speculate that it may reveal the most fascinating gender specificity of all. Sex differences have already been recognized in cognition as well as in epilepsy, Alzheimer's disease and sleep disorders.

While research is crucial, it must be accompanied by new attitudes in the medical profession. AMWA believes doctors must fundamentally change the way they think about women. The organization has developed an education program for practicing physicians, the Advanced Curriculum in Women's Health, to help them do so. "Instead of grouping information by organ systems, it's much more suitable to look at life phases and consider how to prevent illness and maintain health in each phase," says Lila Wallis, M.D., clinical professor of medicine at

Cornell University Medical College, head of the team that designed the course. The five life phases are adolescence (12 to 20 years old); young adulthood (from 20 to 45); perimenopause (45 to 60); postmenopausal, "mature" (60 to 85); and "advanced" (85-plus).

Changes also must be made in the way future doctors are trained. In 1994, doctors at Philadelphia's Allegheny University of the Health Sciences joined with AMWA to create *Women's Health in the Curriculum,* a resource guide for medical school professors and health care educators. But experts say that curriculum shifts will only occur if gender-specific questions become part of the licensing exams that every aspiring physician must take. Florence Haseltine, Ph.D., M.D., director of the Center for Population Research at the NIH, doesn't see "real changes happening for another 10 years."

The research establishment needs to rethink the way it conducts medical studies and reports results. Experts like Vivian W. Pinn, M.D., director of the Office of Research on Women's Health at the NIH, are concerned that medical journal articles don't routinely address gender differences in studies. Hormonal variations are not typically taken into account; rarely does a study report whether the subjects were pre- or postmenopausal, or taking HRT.

Dr. Haseltine believes medical students will be the agents of change, actively seeking out gender-specific information in their courses, as will the pharmaceutical industry, which sees the profit potential in new, differentiated products for the two sexes. In the end, gender-specific women's health also implies gender-specific men's health. Learning more about the special characteristics of women will inevitably produce corresponding action for men. That can only be good for both.

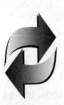

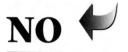

Sally L. Satel

Sick Sisters: How Feminist Politics Is Warping Medicine

We are now on the threshold of politically correct medicine. P.C. health care is powered by the idea that injustice produces disease, and that political empowerment is the cure. It is a false promise.

Though the activists behind politically correct medicine appear to be fighting for better health, their actions do not prevent disease, alleviate symptoms, or perfect treatments. At best, they create distractions and waste money; at worst, they interfere with effective diagnosis and doctoring. Although the agitators themselves may end up feeling better for having taken part in a "social justice" movement, they undermine the Hippocratic ideal of putting patients first. Instead, P.C. medicine puts ideology first.

⋘◉⋙

According to Patricia Ireland, president of the National Organization for Women, the toxicity of women's breasts will be one of the major political issues of the new millennium. "There are hundreds of synthetic chemicals in breast milk," Ireland pronounced recently on Capitol Hill. "We are poisoning the earth, and women are dying because of it." About 60 women's and health advocacy organizations joined with Ireland to demand more federal funding for diseases that are supposedly killing more and more women. "The evidence—and our bodies—continue to pile up," claim the advocates. A male-dominated medical system, they say, systematically slights America's females. "Women are invisible in the health care system beyond their reproductive systems. The medical model using male science, male body, male culture is still the norm. Women die unnecessarily due to this male perspective," asserts the Foundation for Women's Health.

The foundation's goal is to create a specialty in "women's health" similar to surgery or pediatrics. The American College of Women's Health Physicians is lobbying for the same thing. "Those of us who were exposed to Women's

Studies in college find Women's Health a very natural transition and progression," writes Kelley Phillips, president of the college.

It may seem odd that women would need their own specialty. For most doctors (except urologists and orthopedists), treating women patients is the norm, since women make greater use of health care services than men do. Women are especially overrepresented in the age groups that rely most heavily on medical services—the elderly. Indeed, apart from the urological problems that beset old men, geriatrics could reasonably be said to be a woman's specialty, because there are more than two women for every man over age 85.

Nonetheless, the Office of Women's Health at the Department of Health and Human Services (HHS) has been promoting a separate medical school curriculum in women's health. "Curricula in women's health should begin to erase the misconceptions caused by a generation of training physicians in the male model of disease," explains HHS official Elena V. Rios.

These calls for special treatment are rooted in the belief that women are second-class citizens in medicine. Hillary Rodham Clinton complained while First Lady about the "appalling degree to which women were routinely excluded from major clinical trials of most illnesses." During his presidential campaign Al Gore told an audience: "Throughout my career, I have fought for more research funds for those diseases so recently considered less important because they befell only women, such as breast cancer. I pledge to you: Women's health will always be at the top of my agenda."

It is hard to imagine what more Gore could do. Women represented 62 percent of the more than six million participants in ongoing National Institutes of Health-funded research in the latest year. Breast cancer research has received more money than any other type of cancer research each year since 1985, when the National Cancer Institute began keeping track of disease-specific funding. It has always received many times the funding of prostate cancer—about five times the amount in 1997, and triple the expenditure in 1999—even though the incidence of breast cancer in women is less than the incidence of prostate cancer in men. In the latest year's data, 115 women per 100,000 received a diagnosis of invasive breast cancer, compared to 147 men per 100,000 for prostate cancer. Overall death rates are almost identical (though breast cancer victims tend to be younger).

Breast cancer also receives considerable funding compared to other diseases. A 1999 analysis in the *New England Journal of Medicine* calculated that according to the number of years of healthy life lost to a disease, breast cancer was among the five conditions most "generously" funded (the other four were heart disease, dementia, AIDS, and diabetes).

The enormous focus on breast cancer by women's health groups has skewed American women's health fears. Activists have popularized the idea that "one out of every nine" women will get breast cancer. Actually, a 40-year-old woman with no special risk factors has less than a 1-in-200 chance of getting breast cancer, and an even smaller likelihood of dying from it.

Only one in four women recognize that lung cancer is the leading cancer killer among females today. In 1997, about 70,000 women died from lung cancer; fewer than 42,000 died from breast cancer. And the biggest killer of all among women is not cancer at all, but rather heart disease—annual deaths from heart disease exceed deaths from all cancers *combined*. Less than 4 percent of women will die of breast cancer, while about one-third will die of heart disease.

Elaine Ratner, author of *The Feisty Woman's Breast Cancer Book*, is worried that the "fear of breast cancer has reached epidemic proportions, because breast cancer has moved into the spotlight." Having been treated for cancer herself, Ratner says she feels lucky that it was in her breast. "No other body part is as expendable," she writes. But she suspects that many women forgo mammography because their inflated idea of breast cancer's lethality scares them away.

•

Women's health has recently been a favorite cause in Congress. Dozens of women's health bills were introduced just in the last two years. Free pap smears and mammograms have been made available; minimum hospital stay lengths have been dictated by law; postmastectomy reconstructive surgery has been mandated; the Women's Health and Cancer Rights Act ensures coverage for second opinions and other assurances.

In its 1999 report to Congress and the President, the U.S. Commission on Civil Rights expressed concern about "gender bias" in our health care system. The commission accused medical schools of steering female medical students "toward the more 'accepted' specialties such as pediatrics and general practice," while men are "more likely to enter the richly rewarding surgical subspecialties." The commission presented no evidence whatever for this claim, however, and a fuller picture shows that many women doctors who want to have a family are attracted to specialties with the shortest residencies (family practice, internal medicine, pediatrics, and psychiatry). Surgical subspecialty training after medical school can take up to seven years at a time of life when women are in their prime childbearing years. The culture of surgery, with its brutal hours and strict hierarchy, may not appeal to many women, but those who burn to be surgeons will make it through. And female surgeons are highly sought after by both employers and patients, especially those with breast disease.

The Commission on Civil Rights also leveled a charge of sexism in medical research funding. Noting that women received 22 percent of all research project funding from the National Institutes of Health between 1981 and 1992, and that their grants were, on average, $30,000 lower than grants given to male scientists, the commissioners called this "a blatant civil rights violation." The federal government "must mandate that female scientists are awarded grants at the same ratio as men," they concluded.

Remarkably, these accusers possessed no evidence that quality proposals from women were being rejected at a greater rate than comparable proposals from men. The commission was simply advocating, in effect, that grants be distributed according to the applicant's sex rather than the merit of the proposed research. Ironically, the most recent data show that the percentage of female applicants winning grants (18.3 percent) is actually higher than the percentage of male applicants who succeed (17.1 percent).

The Commission on Civil Rights also alleges that women have been systematically excluded from clinical trials for new medicines and therapies. Many other women's health activists have pushed this same claim, and they've had political effects. "It was my female colleagues and I who led the charge to put an end to clinical trials conducted entirely on men—even for breast cancer," Senator Olympia Snowe (R-Maine) proudly states.

The topic makes great media fodder. "Government-funded Studies Deny Women Key Health Data" was the headline on a May 2000 *USA Today* editorial. "The habit of overlooking women in medical research is deeply ingrained and hard to shake," it pontificated. "For decades, women have been alternatively ignored or overprotected. And the research hierarchy is still largely dominated by the interests and concerns of white males."

In reality, this whole contention is a myth. As Andrew Kadar, an anesthesiologist at the UCLA School of Medicine, points out, those studies that have looked more at one sex than another usually focused on *women* rather than men. That is certainly the case with antidepressants. One of the largest and earliest studies I could find involved 215 subjects—*most* of whom were women (or "housewives," as the 1950s authors called them). Nevertheless, women's health advocates routinely claim, without evidence, that the hormonal fluctuations brought on by women's menstrual cycles led researchers to bar them from antidepressant research.

Have women ever been systematically omitted from clinical trials? Yes, starting in 1977, the Food and Drug Administration excluded pregnant and fertile women from participating in the toxicity testing of pharmaceuticals. The policy, withdrawn in 1993, evolved in the wake of the birth defect tragedies associated with thalidomide and diethylstilbestrol (DES). Women were excluded from the safety-testing phases of pharmaceutical trials to protect fetuses and, to some extent, avoid liability. Though the policy deserved its label of paternalistic, the point was to protect women and babies, not to favor men at their expense. Indeed, men themselves have not been rushing to volunteer for toxicity tests; why else would so many of the subjects who sign up be men from military bases and prisons?

Overall, government surveys have found that "both sexes had substantial representation in clinical trials, in proportions that usually reflected the prevalence of the disease in the sex and age groups included in the trials." Conditions such as depression, osteoporosis, and arthritis have always been *more* thoroughly studied among women—which should come as no surprise, since researchers tend to study the group most at risk. The Office of Research on Women's Health at NIH, created to respond to just these concerns, found that research subjects for NIH clinical trials funded in 1997 were 69 percent women and 31 percent men.

Still, as late as 1999 advocates like Phyllis Greenberger of the Society for Women's Health Research continued to make remarks like, "It's going to take some time before it's generally accepted that women and men have to be in clinical trials." In the spring of 2000 I received a promotional letter from the *Harvard Women's Health Watch* newsletter telling readers that "nearly all drug testing has been done on men." What will it take to convince these activists of the truth?

⟨⦿⟩

Advocates also claim that certain specific medical procedures are evidence of the devaluation of women's health. For instance, the treatment of breast cancer with mastectomy. In her 1999 book *A Darker Ribbon*, Ellen Leopold, a member of the Women's Community Cancer Project in Cambridge, Massachusetts, opines,

> The surgical removal of the breast has to be seen as a violent act. The apparent barbarity of the procedure raises the question of male intent. It is not much of a stretch to view surgery as yet another opportunity to punish a woman for the ambivalent feelings she provokes. The aura surrounding breast surgery reinforced the worst gender stereotypes, attributing all power to the male hero.

Today we know that radical mastectomy is not necessary for most women. But before the late 1970s and early 1980s it was the accepted lifesaving procedure. A surgeon who did not perform it would have been considered derelict. In hindsight, we can see that many women underwent needlessly aggressive surgery, but there wasn't a gender bias: Men too have been subject to the radical nature of cancer surgery. Thousands of men with positive blood tests as their only sign of possible prostate cancer have undergone needless radical prostatectomies, sometimes involving the removal of pelvic nerves, which destroys the ability to perform sexually. Then, if metastases appeared, men were castrated, since testosterone seemed to promote cancer growth.

In a response to Leopold's feminist interpretation of breast cancer, Jerome Groopman, an oncologist and professor of medicine at Harvard, asks, "Does this mean that urological surgeons were, consciously or subconsciously, acting out as alpha males to dominate and abase the vulnerable men of the tribe?" The development of more conservative operations for both women and men is a continuing priority for physicians, but surgical practice must not be taken out of its historical context.

⟨⦿⟩

Contrary to what ideologues ranging from Clinton administration Secretary of Health and Human Services Donna Shalala on down have maintained, there is no women's health crisis today. Women's health research is first-rate. Women are well represented in the ranks of health care administrators. Female consumers have enormous influence in the medical marketplace. In 1999 at least 3,600 programs across the country called themselves women's health centers. There are few comparable centers for men.

To say that mainstream medicine caters to men is ludicrous. Women visit doctors much more often than men. Pharmaceutical companies are advertising vigorously to women. In many specialties women physicians are in high de-mand. And at the end of the century, 44 percent of the entering class in our medical schools were women.

But some will always portray women as deprived no matter what. Except for the tiny Office of Research on Women's Health, "the whole rest of the Na-tional Institutes of Health is the men's office," claims Marianne Legato, who di-rects the Partnership for Women's Health.

Apparently, such partisans count only the portion of the NIH budget ear-marked for diseases specific to women as beneficial to females. But by that barometer, less than 7 percent of medical funding goes to male diseases. So at least 93 percent goes to diseases that affect either women only or both sexes. Pit-ting the well-being of women against men in this way is not only petty but—considering that women outlive men by six years—rather absurd.

Women are hurt by the half-truths disseminated by the women's health movement and by the righteous indignation it seeks to provoke. People worry needlessly. Patients clamor for procedures that ultimately do them more harm than good. Medical relationships are contaminated with distrust. "When I give lectures on the doctor-patient relationship to physicians, many of the over-worked doctors—male *and* female—comment on how frustrating it is to deal with women who come into their office with an attitude of 'Prove that you're not going to take advantage of me,'" says Edward Bartlett, associate adjunct pro-fessor at the George Washington University School of Public Health.

Assuredly, there is more to know about the treatment of diseases in women. But it is wrongheaded to confuse the need to know more—an impera-tive that will always be with us—with the unwarranted and poisonous notion that women are somehow second-class subjects in the world of medicine.

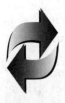

POSTSCRIPT

Does Health Care Delivery and Research Benefit Men at the Expense of Women?

Many articles, in both the popular press and the scientific literature, maintain that there is a gender bias in medicine. These include "Biology or Bias: Practice Patterns and Long-Term Outcomes for Men and Women With Acute Myocardial Infarction," *The Journal of the American Medical Association* (September 11, 2002); "Gender Bias in the Diagnosis of COPD," *The Journal of the American Medical Association* (August 15, 2001); and "Do Women With Hearth Attacks Get Fewer Heart Procedures Than Men?" *Annals of Internal Medicine* (September 17, 2002). There are researchers who have found the opposite—that gender is not a significant issue. See "Age, Not Gender, Determines Treatment, Survival After Heart Attack," *Health & Medicine Week* (July 15, 2002) and "False Diagnosis: When it Comes to Gender, Doctors Don't Play Favorites," *Reason* (May 2001). In "Men With Osteoporosis Often Fall Through the Cracks of Detection," *Family Practice News* (April 15, 2003) and "Men and Osteoporosis: Red Flags That Are Often Overlooked," *Tufts University Health & Nutrition Letter* (September 2001), it was found that men with "women's" diseases often do not get the diagnoses and treatment they need.

For an overview on women's health, see *Encyclopedia of Women's Health Issues* (Oryx Press, 2002), which addresses such topics as hormone therapy debates, whether or not women's health should be a separate medical specialty, breast cancer, hysterectomies, and leading causes of death for men and women. See also "Disparities in Women's Health and Health Care Experiences in the United States and Israel: Findings From 1998 National Women's Health Surveys," *Women & Health* (January 2003); "The Cost of Being a Woman," *The New England Journal of Medicine* (June 4, 1998); and "Women in the New World Order: Where Old Values Command New Respect," *Journal of the American Dietetics Association* (May 1997). Two reports on gender issues in women's health are *Report of the Advisory Committee on Research on Women's Health: Office of Research on Women's Health and NIH Support for Research on Women's Health Issues* by the United States Advisory Committee on Research on Women's Health, U.S. Department of Health and Human Services, Public Health Service, National Institutes of Health (2001) and *Improving Women's Health: Why Contraceptive Insurance Coverage Matters: Hearing Before the Committee on Health, Education, Labor, and Pensions, United States Senate, One Hundred Seventh Congress, First Session on S. 104 to Require Equitable Coverage of Prescription Contraceptive Drugs and Devices, and Contraceptive Services Under Health Plans* by the United States Congress, Senate, Committee on Health, Education, Labor, and Pensions. Washington: U.S. G.P.O. (2002).

On the Internet . . .

National Rifle Association

This National Rifle Association Web site contains multiple links. This site addresses the issue of gun control and the Second Amendment.

http://www.nra.org

Global Vaccine Awareness League

The Global Vaccine Awareness League Web site is dedicated to the education of parents and concerned citizens regarding vaccination. This site includes a live, interactive message board and a list of related links and articles that reflect both pro-vaccine and pro-choice opinions.

http://www.gval.com

National Institute on Drug Abuse: Anabolic Steriod Abuse

This site by the U.S. National Institute on Drug Abuse contains news articles, medical examinations, and links related to anabolic steriod abuse.

http://www.steroidabuse.org

National Clearinghouse for Alcohol and Drug Information

Affiliated with the U.S. Department of Health and Human Services, this National Clearinghouse for Alcohol and Drug Information site offers information aimed at preventing alcohol and drug abuse. It includes a "Prevention Primer," which is a reference for prevention practitioners and contains a variety of studies about drug use.

http://www.health.org

PART 5

Public Health Issues

There are many health issues that concern the public. This part addresses a number of these, including the issue of gun control. This issue questions if gun control really is a public health issue or more a matter of social policy. Many are concerned with the potential risks of childhood immunization. Does parental refusal to immunize their children risk potential disease outbreaks? Instead, does immunization depress the immune system, thereby increasing one's risk of disease? The increasing threat of biological terrorism only adds to this controversy. This part also examines the topic of anabolic steriod abuse among athletes. Also discussed is whether marijuana is dangerous and addictive. Is it potentially beneficial to those with some terminal illnesses or is it a gateway to more dangerous drugs?

- Is Gun Control a Public Health Issue?

- Should Parents Be Allowed to Opt Out of Vaccinating Their Children?

- Does Anabolic Steroid Use Cause Serious Health Problems for Athletes?

- Is Marijuana Dangerous and Addictive?

ISSUE 15

Is Gun Control a Public Health Issue?

YES: Josh Sugarmann, from "Reverse Fire," *Mother Jones* (January/February 1994)

NO: Don B. Kates, Henry E. Schaffer, and William C. Waters IV, from "Public Health Pot Shots: How the CDC Succumbed to the Gun 'Epidemic,'" *Reason* (April 1997)

ISSUE SUMMARY

YES: Josh Sugarmann, executive director of the Violence Policy Center, an education foundation that researches firearm violence and advocates gun control, argues that guns increase the costs of hospitalization, rehabilitation, and lost wages, making them a serious public health issue.

NO: Attorney Don B. Kates, professor of genetics Henry E. Schaffer, and William C. Waters IV, a physician, counter that most gun-related violence is caused by aberrants, not ordinary gun owners.

More and more people in the United States are buying guns to protect themselves and their families in response to increasing crime rates. There are currently over 216 million firearms—close to 900,000 assault weapons—in private hands in the United States, more than double the number in 1970. Also, each year more than 24,000 Americans are killed with handguns in homicides, suicides, and accidents (an average of 65 people each day). Firearms are used in 70 percent of all murders committed in the United States. These statistics raise important questions: Does gun ownership afford protection against crime or increase the risk of gun-related death? And are gun control and gun ownership public health concerns? Gun owners and opponents of gun control state that weapons kept at home will prevent crime. Proponents of gun control maintain that weapons kept at home are involved in too many fights that lead to injury or death, accidental shootings, and suicides.

To attempt to resolve these issues, Arthur Kellermann, an emergency room physician at the University of Tennessee, and his associates conducted a study, "Gun Ownership as a Risk Factor for Homicide in the Home," *The New England Journal of Medicine* (October 7, 1993). Kellermann's study concluded that people who keep guns in their homes are much more likely to kill or injure another family member than use the gun in self-defense against a criminal. Kellermann believes that a gun almost automatically makes any fight potentially more dangerous and that the risks of having a gun outweigh the benefits. Many supporters of gun control say that the study confirmed their warnings about the basic dangers of owning guns and keeping them in the home.

The contention that gun ownership is more dangerous than beneficial is not without its critics. The Kellermann et al. study, for instance, only measured *risks* associated with gun ownership. They did not study cases in which guns actually deterred crime. Kellermann et al. also did not discuss the possibility that the guns may not have caused the violence; the violence may have caused the use of guns. For instance, in areas of high crime, citizens are more likely to arm themselves for self-protection.

Although it is unclear whether guns deter crime or cause it, gun control in one form or another has been around since the early part of the twentieth century. The first major gun control act strengthening restrictions on handguns followed the assassinations of John F. Kennedy, Dr. Martin Luther King, Jr., and Robert Kennedy in the 1960s. Other laws banning the sale of handguns and the manufacture and sale of certain types of assault weapons followed. In 1993 President Bill Clinton signed the Brady Bill, which imposed a five-day waiting period for handgun purchases. (The bill was named for James Brady, aide to former president Ronald Reagan. Both Brady and Reagan were shot during an assassination attempt in the early 1980s). Unfortunately for gun control advocates, in June 1997 the Supreme Court ruled that the Brady gun control law violated "the very principle of separate state sovereignty" by requiring state officials to conduct background checks of prospective handgun buyers. In a five-to-four decision, the Court invalidated the background check of the 1993 law. This decision did not address, however, a separate portion of the Brady Bill that imposes a five-day waiting period before a gun sale can be completed.

Gun control is a controversial issue in the United States. Its opponents assert that it infringes on the constitutional rights of Americans to bear arms as granted by the Second Amendment. The gun lobby also pictures America under stricter gun controls as a country where honest citizens would be helpless against well-armed criminals. Many advocates of gun control, however, regard the deaths and injuries related to guns as a public health problem that can be treated only by getting rid of guns themselves.

In the following selections, Josh Sugarmann asserts that guns are definitely a public health issue and supports stricter gun control. He states that guns offer no protective benefit even in homicide cases that follow forced entry. Don B. Kates, Henry E. Schaffer, and William C. Waters IV argue that violence is not a matter of honest citizens killing simply because a gun is nearby but of criminals committing violent acts. The authors also maintain that health organizations, such as the Centers for Disease Control, should focus on true public health issues and not veer off into social policy.

Josh Sugarmann

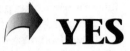 **YES**

Reverse Fire

For seven years gun-control advocates have lobbied for the Brady Bill, which mandates a national waiting period for buying handguns. But ironically, the bill's passage may actually benefit the gun industry. Oversold by its supporters, the Brady Bill has become synonymous in American minds with gun control itself. If violence continues once a national waiting period goes into effect (as it likely will), the gun lobby will offer the Brady Bill as proof that gun control doesn't work.

A Lack of Regulation

With its passage in 1993, gun-control advocates find themselves at a crossroads. We can continue to push legislation of dubious effectiveness. Or we can acknowledge that gun violence is a public-health crisis fueled by an inherently dangerous consumer product. To end the crisis, we have to regulate—or, in the case of handguns and assault weapons, completely ban—the product.

The romantic myths attached to gun ownership stop many people from thinking of them as a consumer product. As a result, the standard risk analysis applied to other potentially dangerous products—pesticides, prescription drugs, or toasters—has never been applied to firearms.

Yet guns are manufactured by corporations—with boards of directors, marketing plans, employees, and a bottom line—just like companies that manufacture toasters. What separates the gun industry from other manufacturers is lack of regulation.

For example, when a glut in the market caused handgun production to plummet from 2.6 million in 1982 to 1.4 million in 1986, the industry retooled its product line. To stimulate sales, manufacturers added firepower, technology, and capacity to their new models. The result: assault weapons, a switch from six-shot revolvers to high-capacity pistols, and increased use of plastics and high-tech additions like integral laser sights.

The industry was free to make these changes (most of which made the guns more dangerous) because guns that are 50 caliber or less and not fully automatic can be manufactured with virtually no restrictions. The Bureau of Alcohol, Tobacco, and Firearms (ATF) lacks even the common regulatory powers—including safety-standard setting and recall—granted government agencies such as the Consumer Product Safety Commission, the Food and Drug Administration, and the Environmental Protection Agency.

A Deadly Product

Yet guns are the second most deadly consumer product (after cars) on the market. In Texas and Louisiana the firearms-related death rate already exceeds that for motor vehicles, and by the year 2000 firearms will likely supplant automobiles as the leading cause of product-related death throughout the United States.

But since Americans view firearm suicides, murders, and fatal accidents as separate problems, the enormity of America's gun crisis goes unrecognized. In 1990, American guns claimed an estimated 37,000 lives. Federal Bureau of Investigation data shows that gun murders that year reached an all-time high of 15,377; a record 12,489 involved handguns.

The Human Toll

In 1990 (the most recent year for which statistics are available), 18,885 Americans took their own lives with firearms, and an estimated 13,030 of those deaths involved handguns. Unlike pills, gas, or razor blades—which are of limited effectiveness—guns are rarely forgiving. For example, self-inflicted cutting wounds account for 15 percent of all suicide attempts but only 1 percent of all successful suicides. Poisons and drugs account for 70 percent of suicide attempts but less than 12 percent of all suicides. Conversely, nonfatal, self-inflicted gunshot wounds are rare—yet three-fifths of all U.S. suicides involve firearms.

In addition to the human toll, the economic costs of not regulating guns are staggering. The Centers for Disease Control (CDC) estimated that the lifetime economic cost—hospitalization, rehabilitation, and lost wages—of firearms violence was $14.4 billion in 1985, making it the third most expensive injury category. The average lifetime cost per person for each firearms fatality—$373,520—was the highest of any injury.

Such human and economic costs are not tolerated for any other product. Many consumer products from lawn darts to the Dalkon Shield have been banned in the United States, even though they claimed only a fraction of the lives guns do in a day. The firearms industry is long overdue for the simple, regulatory oversight applied to other consumer products. For public safety, the ATF must be given authority to control the design, manufacture, distribution, and sale of firearms and ammunition.

Under such a plan, the ATF would subject each category of firearm and ammunition to an unreasonable-risk analysis to weed out products whose potential for harm outweighs any possible benefit. This would result in an immediate ban on the future production and sale of handguns and assault weapons because of their high risk and low utility.

Because they are easily concealed and accessed, handguns hold the dubious honor of being our number-one murder and suicide tool. Assault weapons—high-capacity, semiautomatic firearms designed primarily for the military and police—pose a public-safety risk as the result of their firepower. A 1989 study of ATF data conducted by Cox Newspapers found that assault firearms were twenty times more likely to turn up in crime traces than conventional firearms.

In addition, a regulatory approach to firearms would exert far greater control over the industry and its distribution network. It would not, however, affect the availability of standard sporting rifles and shotguns, which would continue to be sold because of their usefulness and relatively low risk.

A Public-Health Issue

Such an approach is the industry's worst nightmare—conjuring images of an all-powerful "gun czar." And in a sense, gun manufacturers would be right: the ATF would become a gun czar in the same way that the EPA is a pesticide czar, the FDA is a prescription-drug-and-medical-device czar, and the Consumer Product Safety Commission is a toaster czar. Yet it is just such a regulatory approach that has dramatically reduced motor-vehicle deaths and injuries over the past twenty years.

Gun-control advocates cannot afford to spend another seven years battling over piecemeal measures that have little more to offer than good intentions. We are far past the point where registration, licensing, safety training, background checks, or waiting periods will have much effect on firearms violence. Tired of being shot and threatened, Americans are showing a deeper understanding of gun violence as a public-health issue, and are becoming aware of the need to restrict specific categories of weapons.

As America's health-care debate continues, discussion of the role of guns—from the human price paid in mortality to the dollars-and-cents cost of uninsured gunshot victims—can only help clarify that gun violence is not a crime issue but a public-health issue. This shift in attitude is apparent in the firearms component of Bill Clinton's domestic violence prevention group, which is co-chaired not only by a representative from the Justice Department—as expected—but also by a CDC official.

Even if the only legacy of this current wave of revulsion is that gun violence will now be viewed as a public-health issue, America will still have taken a very large first step toward gun sanity.

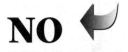

NO

Don B. Kates, Henry E. Schaffer, and William C. Waters IV

Public Health Pot Shots: How the CDC Succumbed to the Gun "Epidemic"

Last year Congress tried to take away $2.6 million from the U.S. Centers for Disease Control and Prevention. In budgetary terms, it was a pittance: 0.1 percent of the CDC's $2.2 billion allocation. Symbolically, however, it was important: $2.6 million was the amount the CDC's National Center for Injury Prevention and Control had spent in 1995 on studies of firearm injuries. Congressional critics, who charged that the center's research program was driven by an anti-gun prejudice, had previously sought to eliminate the NCIPC completely. "This research is designed to, and is used to, promote a campaign to reduce lawful firearms ownership in America," wrote 10 senators, including then–Majority Leader Bob Dole and current Majority Leader Trent Lott. "Funding redundant research initiatives, particularly those which are driven by a social-policy agenda, simply does not make sense."

After the NCIPC survived the 1995 budget process, opponents narrowed their focus, seeking to pull the plug on the gun research specifically, or at least to punish the CDC for continuing to fund it. At a May 1996 hearing, Rep. Jay Dickey (R-Ark.), co-sponsor of the amendment cutting the CDC's budget, chastised NCIPC Director Mark Rosenberg for treating guns as a "public health menace," suggesting that he was "working toward changing society's attitudes so that it becomes socially unacceptable to own handguns." In June the House Appropriations Committee adopted Dickey's amendment, which included a prohibition on the use of CDC funds "to advocate or promote gun control," and in July the full House rejected an attempt to restore the money.

Although the CDC ultimately got the $2.6 million back as part of a budget deal with the White House, the persistent assault on the agency's gun research created quite a stir. *New England Journal of Medicine* Editor Jerome Kassirer, who has published several of the CDC-funded gun studies, called it "an attack that strikes at the very heart of scientific research." Writing in *The Washington Post*, CDC Director David Satcher said criticism of the firearm research did not bode well for the country's future: "If we question the honesty of scientists who give every evidence of long deliberation on the issues before them, what are our expectations of anyone else? What hope is there for us as a society?" Frederick P. Rivara, a pediatrician who has received CDC money to do gun research, told *The Chronicle of Higher Education* that critics of the program were trying "to block scientific discovery because they don't like the results. This is a frightening trend for academic researchers. It's the equivalent of book burning."

That view was echoed by columnists and editorial writers throughout the country. In a *New York Times* column entitled "More N.R.A. Mischief," Bob Herbert defended the CDC's "rigorous, unbiased, scientific studies," suggesting that critics could not refute the results of the research and therefore had decided "to pull the plug on the funding and stop the effort altogether." Editorials offering the same interpretation appeared in *The Washington Post* ("NRA: Afraid of Facts"), *USA Today* ("Gun Lobby Keeps Rolling"), the *Los Angeles Times* ("NRA Aims at the Messenger"), *The Atlanta Journal* ("GOP Tries to Shoot the Messenger"), the *Sacramento Bee* ("Shooting the Messenger"), and the *Pittsburgh Post-Gazette* ("The Gun Epidemic").

Contrary to this picture of dispassionate scientists under assault by the Neanderthal NRA and its know-nothing allies in Congress, serious scholars have been criticizing the CDC's "public health" approach to gun research for years. In a presentation at the American Society of Criminology's 1994 meeting, for example, University of Illinois sociologist David Bordua and epidemiologist David Cowan called the public health literature on guns "advocacy based on political beliefs rather than scientific fact." Bordua and Cowan noted that *The New England Journal of Medicine* and the *Journal of the American Medical Association*, the main outlets for CDC-funded studies of firearms, are consistent supporters of strict gun control. They found that "reports with findings not supporting the position of the journal are rarely cited," "little is cited from the criminological or sociological field," and the articles that are cited "are almost always by medical or public health researchers."

Further, Bordua and Cowan said, "assumptions are presented as fact: that there is a causal association between gun ownership and the risk of violence, that this association is consistent across all demographic categories, and that additional legislation will reduce the prevalence of firearms and consequently reduce the incidence of violence." They concluded that "[i]ncestuous and selective literature citations may be acceptable for political tracts, but they introduce an artificial bias into scientific publications. Stating as fact associations which may be demonstrably false is not just unscientific, it is unprincipled." In a 1994 presentation to the Western Economics Association, State University of New York at Buffalo criminologist Lawrence Southwick compared public health firearm studies to popular articles produced by the gun lobby: "Generally the level of analysis done on each side is of a low quality. . . . The papers published in the medical literature (which are uniformly anti-gun) are particularly poor science."

◦✤◦

As Bordua, Cowan, and Southwick observed, a prejudice against gun ownership pervades the public health field. Deborah Prothrow-Stith, dean of the Harvard

School of Public Health, nicely summarizes the typical attitude of her colleagues in a recent book. "My own view on gun control is simple," she writes. "I hate guns and cannot imagine why anybody would want to own one. If I had my way, guns for sport would be registered, and all other guns would be banned." Opposition to gun ownership is also the official position of the U.S. Public Health Service, the CDC's parent agency. Since 1979, its goal has been "to reduce the number of handguns in private ownership," starting with a 25 percent reduction by the turn of the century.

Since 1985 the CDC has funded scores of firearm studies, all reaching conclusions that favor stricter gun control. But CDC officials insist they are not pursuing an anti-gun agenda. In a 1996 interview with the *Times-Picayune*, CDC spokeswoman Mary Fenley adamantly denied that the agency is "trying to eliminate guns." In a 1991 letter to CDC critic Dr. David Stolinsky, the NCIPC's Mark Rosenberg said "our scientific understanding of the role that firearms play in violent events is rudimentary." He added in a subsequent letter, "There is a strong need for further scientific investigations of the relationships among firearms ownership, firearms regulations and the risk of firearm-related injury. This is an area that has not been given adequate scrutiny. Hopefully, by addressing these important and appropriate scientific issues we will eventually arrive at conclusions which support effective, preventive actions."

Yet four years *earlier,* in a 1987 CDC report, Rosenberg thought the area adequately scrutinized, and his understanding sufficient, to urge confiscation of all firearms from "the general population," claiming "8,600 homicides and 5,370 suicides could be avoided" each year. In 1993 *Rolling Stone* reported that Rosenberg "envisions a long term campaign, similar to [those concerning] tobacco use and auto safety, to convince Americans that guns are, first and foremost, a public health menace." In 1994 he told *The Washington Post,* "We need to revolutionize the way we look at guns, like what we did with cigarettes. Now it *[sic]* is dirty, deadly, and banned."

As Bordua and Cowan noted, one hallmark of the public health literature on guns is a tendency to ignore contrary scholarship. Among criminologists, Gary Kleck's encyclopedic *Point Blank: Guns and Violence in America* (1991) is universally recognized as the starting point for further research. Kleck, a professor of criminology at Florida State University, was initially a strong believer that gun ownership increased the incidence of homicide, but his research made him a skeptic. His book assembles strong evidence against the notion that reducing gun ownership is a good way to reduce violence. That may be why *Point Blank* is never cited in the CDC's own firearm publications or in articles reporting the results of CDC-funded gun studies.

Three Kleck studies, the first published in 1987, have found that guns are used in self-defense up to three times as often as they are used to commit crimes. These studies are so convincing that the doyen of American criminologists, Marvin Wolfgang, conceded in the Fall 1995 issue of *The Journal of Criminal Law and Criminology* that they pose a serious challenge to his own anti-gun views. "I am as strong a gun-control advocate as can be found among the criminologists in this country . . . What troubles me is the article by Gary Kleck and

Mark Gertz. The reason I am troubled is that they have provided an almost clear-cut case of methodologically sound research in support of something I have theoretically opposed for years, namely, the use of a gun against a criminal perpetrator."

Yet Rosenberg and his CDC colleague James Mercy, writing in *Health Affairs* in 1993, present the question "How frequently are guns used to successfully ward off potentially violent attacks?" as not just open but completely unresearched. They cite neither Kleck nor the various works on which he drew.

When CDC sources do cite adverse studies, they often get them wrong. In 1987 the National Institute of Justice hired two sociologists, James D. Wright and Peter H. Rossi, to assess the scholarly literature and produce an agenda for gun control. Wright and Rossi found the literature so biased and shoddy that it provided no basis for concluding anything positive about gun laws. Like Kleck, they were forced to give up their own prior faith in gun control as they researched the issue.

But that's not the story told by Dr. Arthur Kellermann, director of Emory University's Center for Injury Control and the CDC's favorite gun researcher. In a 1988 *New England Journal of Medicine* article, Kellermann and his co-authors cite Wright and Rossi's book *Under the Gun* to support the notion that "restricting access to handguns could substantially reduce our annual rate of homicide." What they actually said was: "There is no persuasive evidence that supports this view." In a 1992 *New England Journal of Medicine* article, Kellermann cites an *American Journal of Psychiatry* study to back up the claim "that limiting access to firearms could prevent many suicides." But the study actually found just the opposite—i.e., that people who don't have guns find other ways to kill themselves.

At the same time that he misuses other people's work, Kellermann refuses to provide the full data for any of his studies so that scholars can evaluate his findings. His critics therefore can judge his results only from the partial data he chooses to publish. Consider a 1993 *New England Journal of Medicine* study that, according to press reports, "showed that keeping a gun in the home nearly triples the likelihood that someone in the household will be slain there." This claim cannot be verified because Kellerman will not release the data. Relying on independent sources to fill gaps in the published data, SUNY-Buffalo's Lawrence Southwick has speculated that Kellermann's full data set would actually vindicate defensive gun ownership. Such issues cannot be resolved without Kellermann's cooperation, but the CDC has refused to require its researchers to part with their data as a condition for taxpayer funding.

Even without access to secret data, it's clear that many of Kellermann's inferences are not justified. In a 1995 *JAMA* study that was funded by the CDC, he and his colleagues examined 198 incidents in which burglars entered occupied homes in Atlanta. They found that "only three individuals (1.5%) employed a firearm in self-defense"—from which they concluded that guns are rarely used for self-defense. On closer examination, however, Kellermann et al.'s data do not support that conclusion. In 42 percent of the incidents, there was no confrontation between victim and offender because "the offender(s) either left silently or fled when detected." When the burglar left silently, the victim was not even aware of the crime, so he did not have the opportunity to use a gun in self-defense (or to call the police, for that matter). The intruders who "fled when detected" show how defensive gun ownership can protect all victims, armed and unarmed alike, since the possibility of confronting an armed resident encourages burglars to flee.

These 83 no-confrontation incidents should be dropped from Kellermann et al.'s original list of 198 burglaries. Similarly, about 50 percent of U.S. homes do not contain guns, and in 70 percent of the homes that do, the guns are kept unloaded. After eliminating the burglaries where armed self-defense was simply not feasible, Kellermann's 198 incidents shrink to 17, and his 1.5 percent figure for defensive use rises to 17 percent. More important, this study covers only burglaries reported to the police. Since police catch only about 10 percent of home burglars, the only *good* reason to report a burglary is that police documentation is required to file an insurance claim. But if no property was lost because the burglar fled when the householder brandished a gun, why report the incident? And, aside from the inconvenience, there are strong reasons *not* to report: The gun may not be registered, or the householder may not be certain that guns can legally be used to repel unarmed burglars. Thus, for all Kellermann knows, successful gun use far exceeds the three incidents reported to police in his Atlanta study.

Similar sins of omission invalidate the conclusion of a 1986 *New England Journal of Medicine* study that Kellermann coauthored with University of Washington pathologist Donald T. Reay, another gun researcher who has enjoyed the CDC's support. (This particular study was funded by the Robert Wood Johnson Foundation.) Examining gunshot deaths in King County, Washington, from 1978 to 1983, Kellermann and Reay found that, of 398 people killed in a home where a gun was kept, only two were intruders shot while trying to get in. "We noted 43 suicides, criminal homicides, or accidental gunshot deaths involving a gun kept in the home for every case of homicide for self-protection," they wrote, concluding that "the advisability of keeping firearms in the home for protection must be questioned."

❧❀❧

But since Kellermann and Reay considered only cases resulting in death, which Gary Kleck's research indicates are a tiny percentage of defensive gun uses, this conclusion does not follow. As the researchers themselves conceded, "Mortality studies such as ours do not include cases in which burglars or intruders are wounded or frightened away by the use or display of a firearm. Cases in which would-be intruders may have purposely avoided a house known to be armed are also not identified." By leaving out such cases, Kellermann and Reay excluded almost all of the lives saved, injuries avoided, and property protected by keeping a gun in the home. Yet advocates of gun control continue to use this study as the basis for claims such as, "A gun in the home is 43 times as likely to kill a family member as to be used in self-defense."

Another popular factoid—"having a gun in the home increases the risk of suicide by almost five times"—is also based on a Kellermann study, this one funded by the CDC and published by *The New England Journal of Medicine* in 1992. Kellermann and his colleagues matched each of 438 suicides to a "control" of the same race, sex, approximate age, and neighborhood. After controlling for arrests, drug abuse, living alone, and use of psychotropic medication (all of which were more common among the suicides), they found that a household with one or more guns was 4.8 times as likely to be the site of a suicide.

Although press reports about gun research commonly treat correlation and causation as one and the same, this association does not prove that having a gun in the house raises the risk of suicide. We can imagine alternative explanations: Perhaps gun ownership in this sample was associated with personality traits that were, in turn, related to suicide, or perhaps people who had contemplated suicide bought a gun for that reason. To put the association in perspective, it's worth noting that living alone and using illicit drugs were both better predictors of suicide than gun ownership was. That does not necessarily mean that living alone or using illegal drugs leads to suicide.

Furthermore, Kellermann and his colleagues selected their sample with an eye toward increasing the apparent role of gun ownership in suicide. They started by looking at all suicides that occurred during a 32-month period in King County, Washington, and Shelby County, Tennessee, but they excluded cases that occurred outside the home—nearly a third of the original sample. "Our study was restricted to suicides occurring in the victim's home," they explained with admirable frankness, "because a previous study has indicated that most suicides committed with guns occur there."

⋯◈⋯

Kellermann also participated in CDC-funded research that simplistically compared homicide rates in Seattle and Vancouver, attributing the difference to Canada's stricter gun laws. This study, published in *The New England Journal of Medicine* in 1988, ignored important demographic differences between the two cities that help explain the much higher incidence of violence in Seattle. Furthermore, the researchers were aware of nationwide research that came to strikingly different conclusions about Canadian gun control, but they failed to inform their readers about that evidence.

Two years later in the same journal, the same research team compared suicide rates in Seattle and Vancouver. Unfazed by the fact that Seattle had a *lower* suicide rate, they emphasized that the rate was higher for one subgroup, adolescents and young men—a difference they attributed to lax American gun laws. Gary Mauser, a criminologist at Simon Fraser University, called the Seattle/Vancouver comparisons "a particularly egregious example" of "an abuse of scholarship, inventing, selecting, or misinterpreting data in order to validate *a priori* conclusions."

These and other studies funded by the CDC focus on the presence or absence of guns, rather than the characteristics of the people who use them. Indeed, the CDC's Rosenberg claims in the journal *Educational Horizons* that murderers are "ourselves—ordinary citizens, professionals, even health care workers": people who kill only because a gun happens to be available. Yet if there is one fact that has been incontestably established by homicide studies, it's that murderers are not ordinary gun owners but extreme aberrants whose life histories include drug abuse, serious accidents, felonies, and irrational violence. Unlike "ourselves," roughly 90 percent of adult murderers have significant criminal records, averaging an adult criminal career of six or more years with four major felonies.

Access to juvenile records would almost certainly show that the criminal careers of murderers stretch back into their adolescence. In *Murder in America* (1994), the criminologists Ronald W. Holmes and Stephen T. Holmes report that murderers generally "have histories of committing personal violence in childhood, against other children, siblings, and small animals." Murderers who don't have criminal records usually have histories of psychiatric treatment or domestic violence that did not lead to arrest.

Contrary to the impression fostered by Rosenberg and other opponents of gun ownership, the term "acquaintance homicide" does not mean killings that stem from ordinary family or neighborhood arguments. Typical acquaintance homicides include: an abusive man eventually killing a woman he has repeatedly assaulted; a drug user killing a dealer (or vice versa) in a robbery attempt; and gang members, drug dealers, and other criminals killing each other for reasons of economic rivalry or personal pique. According to a 1993 article in the *Journal of Trauma,* 80 percent of murders in Washington, D.C., are related to the drug trade, while "84% of [Philadelphia murder] victims in 1990 had antemortem drug use or criminal history." A 1994 article in *The New England Journal of Medicine* reported that 71 percent of Los Angeles children and adolescents injured in drive-by shootings "were documented members of violent street gangs." And University of North Carolina-Charlotte criminal justice scholars Richard Lumb and Paul C. Friday report that 71 percent of adult gunshot wound victims in Charlotte have criminal records.

As the English gun control analyst Colin Greenwood has noted, in any society there are always enough guns available, legally or illegally, to arm the violent. The true determinant of violence is the number of violent people, not the availability of a particular weapon. Guns contribute to murder in the trivial sense that they help violent people kill. But owning guns does not turn responsible, law-abiding people into killers. If the general availability of guns were as important a factor in violence as the CDC implies, the vast increase in firearm ownership during the past two decades should have led to a vast increase in homicide. The CDC suggested just that in a 1989 report to Congress, where it asserted that "[s]ince the early 1970s the year-to-year fluctuations in firearm availability has [sic] paralleled the numbers of homicides."

But this correlation was a fabrication: While the number of handguns rose 69 percent from 1974 to 1988, handgun murders actually dropped by 27 percent. Moreover, as U.S. handgun ownership more than doubled from the early 1970s through the 1990s, homicides held constant or declined for every major population group except young urban black men. The CDC can blame the homicide surge in this group on guns only by ignoring a crucial point: Gun ownership is far less common among urban blacks than among whites or rural blacks.

The CDC's reports and studies never give long-term trend data linking gun sales to murder rates, citing only carefully selected partial or short-term correlations. If murder went down in the first and second years, then back up in the third and fourth years, only the rise is mentioned. CDC publications focus on fluctuations and other unrepresentative phenomena to exaggerate the incidence of gun deaths and to conceal declines. Thus, in its *Advance Data from Vital and Health Statistics* (1994), the CDC melodramatically announces that gun deaths now "rival" driving fatalities, as if gun murders were increasing. But this trend simply reflects the fact that driving fatalities are declining more rapidly than murders.

While the CDC shows a selective interest in homicide trends, it tends to ignore trends in accidental gun deaths—with good reason. In the 25 years from 1968 to 1992, American gun ownership increased almost 135 percent (from 97 million to 222 million), with handgun ownership rising more than 300 percent. These huge increases coincided with a two-thirds *decline* in accidental gun fatalities. The CDC and the researchers it funds do not like to talk about this dramatic development, since it flies in the face of the assumption that more guns mean more deaths. They are especially reluctant to acknowledge the drop in accidental gun deaths because of the two most plausible explanations for it: the replacement of rifles and shotguns with the much safer handgun as the main weapon kept loaded for self-defense, and the NRA's impressive efforts in gun safety training.

⋅◦❀◦⋅

The question is, why hasn't it been studied? The answer illustrates how the CDC's political agenda undermines its professed concern for saving lives. In the absence of an anti-gun animus, a two-thirds decrease in accidental gun deaths would surely have been a magnet for studies, especially since it coincided with a big increase in handgun ownership. But the CDC wants to reduce gun deaths only by banning guns, not by promoting solutions that are consistent with more guns. So the absence of studies is an excuse to dismiss gun safety training rather than an incentive for research.

Taken by itself, any one of these flaws—omission of relevant evidence, misrepresentation of studies, questionable methodology, overreaching conclusions—could be addressed by a determination to do better in the future. But the consistent tendency to twist research in favor of an anti-gun agenda suggests that there is something inherently wrong with the CDC's approach in this area. Implicit in the decision to treat gun deaths as a "public health" problem is the notion that violence is a communicable disease that can be controlled by attacking the relevant pathogen.

Dr. Katherine Christoffel, head of the Handgun Epidemic Lowering Plan, a group that has received CDC support, stated this assumption plainly in a 1994 interview with *American Medical News:* "Guns are a virus that must be eradicated. . . . They are causing an epidemic of death by gunshot, which should be treated like any epidemic—you get rid of the virus. . . . Get rid of the guns, get rid of the bullets, and you get rid of the deaths."

In the same article, the CDC's Rosenberg said approvingly, "Kathy Christoffel is saying about firearms injuries what has been said for years about AIDS: that we can no longer be silent. That silence equals death and she's not willing to be silent anymore. She's asking for help." Similarly, in a 1993 *Atlanta Medicine* article on the public health approach to violence, Arthur Kellermann subtitled part of his discussion "The Bullet as Pathogen."

It is hardly surprising that research based on this paradigm would tend to indict gun ownership as a cause of death. The inadequacy of the disease metaphor, which some public health specialists seem to take quite literally, is readily apparent when we consider Koch's postulates, the criteria by which suspected pathogens are supposed to be judged: 1) The microorganism must be observed in all cases of the disease; 2) the microorganism must be isolated and grown in a pure culture medium; 3) microorganisms from the pure culture must reproduce the disease when inoculated in a test animal; and 4) the same kind of microorganism must be recovered from the experimentally diseased animal. A strict application of these criteria is clearly impossible in this case. But applying the postulates as an analogy, we can ask about the consistency of the relationship between guns and violence. Gun ownership usually does not result in violence, and violence frequently occurs in the absence of guns. Given these basic facts, depicting violence as a disease caused by the gun virus can only cloud our thinking.

It may also discredit the legitimate functions of public health. "The CDC has got to be careful that we don't get into social issues," Dr. C.J. Peters, head of the CDC's Special Pathogens Branch, told the *Pittsburgh Post-Gazette* last year, in the midst of the controversy over taxpayer-funded gun research. "If we're going to do that, we ought to start a center for social change. We should stay with medical issues."

If treating gun violence as a public health issue invites confusion and controversy, why is this approach so popular? The main function of the disease metaphor is to lend a patina of scientific credibility to the belief that guns cause violence—a belief that is hard to justify on empirical grounds. "We're trying to depoliticize the subject," Rosenberg told *USA Today* in 1995. "We're trying to transform it from politics to science." What they are actually trying to do is disguise politics as science.

POSTSCRIPT

Is Gun Control a Public Health Issue?

Between 1960 and 1970 both the murder rate in the United States and the rate of handgun ownership doubled. Was it coincidence that violence and gun ownership grew at nearly the same pace? Can it be assumed from this fact that more guns cause more violence? The conventional wisdom is that guns and violence are related in the same sense that owning a gun increases the risk that the *gun owner,* rather than the criminal, will be hurt.

In several major studies, Dr. Arthur Kellermann attempted to prove just that. In 1986 he published "Protection or Peril? An Analysis of Firearm-Related Deaths in the Home," *The New England Journal of Medicine* (vol. 314). His other publications on guns as a public health issue include "Validating Survey Responses to Questions About Gun Ownership Among Owners of Registered Handguns," *American Journal of Epidemiology* (vol. 131, 1990); "Men, Women, and Murder: Gender-Specific Differences in Rates of Fatal Violence and Victimization," *Journal of Trauma* (vol. 33, 1992); "Suicide in the Home in Relation to Gun Ownership," *The New England Journal of Medicine* (vol. 327, 1992); and "Gun Ownership as a Risk Factor for Homicide in the Home," *The New England Journal of Medicine* (vol. 329, 1993). Kellermann, quoted in "Should You Own a Gun?" *U.S. News and World Report* (August 15, 1994), says, "Most gun homicides occur in altercations among family members, friends or acquaintances. In a heated dispute, few carefully weigh the legal consequences of their actions. They are too busy reaching for a weapon. If it's a gun, death is more likely to result." Kellermann and his colleagues are not the only physicians who consider homicide and gun ownership public health issues. In *Mother Jones* (May/June 1993), Mark Rosenberg, an epidemiologist at the Centers for Disease Control, maintains that violence is a public health issue and that violence prevention should be pushed to the top of the public health agenda. A similar study found comparable results. See "Association Between Handgun Purchase and Mortality From Firearm Injury," *Injury Prevention* (March 2003).

Is violence really a *health* issue? Each year, more than 500,000 Americans, including children, are brought to hospital emergency rooms for treatment of a violent injury. These injuries, including shootings and assaults, add over $5 billion dollars in direct medical costs to current health care expenditures. Lifetime costs of violent injuries, which include medical care and loss of productivity, is over $45 billion. And since many gunshot victims are uninsured, the public at large pays the bill. Gunshot wounds can also strain the health care system by diverting resources away from other illnesses and injuries.

Articles on the relationship between guns and public health include "Gun Availability and Violent Death," *American Journal of Public Health* (June 1997);

"Private Arsenals and Public Peril," *The New England Journal of Medicine* (May 7, 1998); and "Confronting the Small Arms Pandemic: Unrestricted Access Should Be Viewed as a Public Health Disaster," *British Medical Journal* (April 27, 2002).

Doctors who treat gunshot victims may feel that controlling gun ownership will reduce the number of shootings, but there is opposition to controlling the sale or possession of guns in the United States. Despite this opposition, a majority of gun owners and the general public favor stricter gun controls, including safety classes for gun owners. Only 39 percent of the American public backs a total ban on handguns, according to an article in *USA Today* (December 17, 1993). And although gun control may save some lives, the availability of guns can never be truly stemmed. In "The False Promise of Gun Control," *The Atlantic Monthly* (March 1994), law professor Daniel Polsby argues that gun control also diverts attention away from the roots of the crime problem in America: lack of job opportunities, inadequate education, and the breakdown of families. Polsby compares gun control with Prohibition. Jacob Sullum, senior editor of *Reason,* presents evidence that crime rates increase in countries that do not recognize a right to carry a weapon in "Gun Shy," *Reason* (April 1998). However, an article in *Health Letter on the CDC* (May 4, 1998) reports on the results of the Centers for Disease Control's study on firearm death rates among 36 nations. This study shows that the highest rate of gun-related death occurs in the United States.

Overviews of the gun control issue include "Struggling Against Common Sense: The Pluses and Minuses of Gun Control," *The World & I* (February 1997); "Still Under the Gun," *Time* (July 6, 1998); "Congressional Voting Behavior on Firearm Control Legislation: 1993–2000," *Journal of Community Health* (December 2002); "Guns in the World: Old News and New News; The Worldwide Small Arms Epidemic Must Be Controlled," *Injury Prevention* (September 2002); "The Art of Self-Defense: Gun Control on Trial," *Reason* (March 2003); and Big Band: The Loud Debate Over Gun Control," *School Library Journal* (March 2003).

ISSUE 16

Should Parents Be Allowed to Opt Out of Vaccinating Their Children?

YES: Barbara Loe Fisher, from "Should Parents Be Allowed to Opt Out of Vaccinating Their Kids? Yes," *Insight on the News* (April 24, 2000)

NO: Steven P. Shelov, from "Should Parents Be Allowed to Opt Out of Vaccinating Their Kids? No," *Insight on the News* (April 24, 2000)

ISSUE SUMMARY

YES: Barbara Loe Fisher, cofounder and president of the National Vaccine Information Center, states that parents should have the right to make informed, voluntary decisions about vaccination and that the government should not have the right to force the issue.

NO: Pediatrician Steven P. Shelov maintains that it would be poor public health philosophy and practice to consider not immunizing children against infectious diseases.

A number of infectious diseases are almost completely preventable through childhood immunization. These diseases include diphtheria, meningitis, pertussis (whooping cough), tetanus, polio, measles, mumps, and rubella (German measles). Largely as a result of widespread vaccination, these once-common diseases have become relatively rare. Before the introduction of the polio vaccine in 1955, polio epidemics occurred each year. In 1952 a record 20,000 cases were diagnosed, as compared to the last outbreak in 1979, when only 10 cases were identified.

The incidence of measles, which can cause serious complications or death, has also declined considerably since the measles vaccine became available. In 1962 there were close to 500,000 cases in the United States, as compared to 138 confirmed cases in 1997. However, in some parts of the United States, particularly urban areas, measles epidemics occur among nonimmunized children.

Many diseases that were thought to be nearly eradicated are making a comeback. In 1983 an outbreak of whooping cough in Oklahoma affected over 300 people. By 1988 nearly 3,000 cases nationwide had been diagnosed.

Whooping cough is a serious and sometimes fatal disease, especially among infants. Although the risks of whooping cough and other childhood diseases are serious, many children have not been vaccinated. Currently, between 37 percent and 56 percent of preschool children in the United States have not received immunization. Some parents either cannot afford vaccination or are unaware of the dangers of childhood diseases. Others believe that the risks of vaccination outweigh the benefits—the last of these reasons is the basis for this debate.

The whooping cough vaccine has been the subject of more concern than any other immunization. Although almost all of the 18 million doses administered each year cause little or no reaction, approximately 50 to 75 children who receive the vaccine suffer serious neurological injury. In a few cases the vaccine has been fatal. Some consider this risk to be too high, but before the vaccine was available, nearly 8,000 children died annually from whooping cough. Still, many parents who are concerned about the dangers of the vaccine have chosen not to immunize their children, and an antivaccine movement has grown in the United States and other developed countries. This movement may prove to be dangerous, as indicated in "Impact of Anti-Vaccine Movements on Pertussis Control: The Untold Story," *The Lancet* (January 31, 1998). This study reports that whooping cough is 10–100 times less prevalent in countries with high vaccination rates compared to countries with low vaccination rates due to antivaccine movements.

In the following articles, Steven P. Shelov states that the growing antivaccine movement is dangerous and may trigger disease outbreaks. Barbara Loe Fisher disagrees and maintains that vaccines can cause serious injury and that parents should have the option of not immunizing their children.

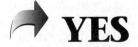

Children at Risk for Adverse Reactions Should Be Given a Pass Without Penalty

P arents do not want their children to be injured or die from a disease or a vaccination. As guardians of their children until those children are old enough to make life-and-death decisions for themselves, parents take very seriously the responsibility of making informed vaccination decisions for the children they love. That responsibility includes becoming educated about the relative risks of diseases when compared to vaccines aimed at preventing them.

Like every encounter with a viral or bacterial infection, every vaccine containing lab-altered viruses or bacteria has an inherent ability to cause injury or even death. Vaccination either can produce immunity without incident or can result in mild to severe brain and immune-system damage, depending upon the vaccine or combination of vaccines given, the health of the person at the time of vaccination and whether the individual is genetically or otherwise biologically at risk for developing complications.

The fact that vaccines can cause injury and death officially was acknowledged in the United States in 1986 when Congress passed the National Childhood Vaccine Injury Act, creating a no-fault federal compensation system for vaccine-injured children to protect the vaccine manufacturers and doctors from personal-injury lawsuits. Since then, the system has paid out more than $1 billion to 1,000 families, whose loved ones have died or been harmed by vaccines, even though three out of four applicants are turned away.

Since 1990, between 12,000 and 14,000 reports of hospitalizations, injuries and deaths following vaccination are made to the federal Vaccine Adverse Event Reporting System, or VAERS, annually, but it is estimated that only between 1 and 10 percent of all doctors make reports to VAERS. Therefore, the number of vaccine-related health problems occurring in the United States every year may be more than 1 million.

In the late 1980s, the Institute of Medicine, or IOM, and the National Academy of Sciences convened committees of physicians to study existing medical knowledge about vaccines and, in 1991 and 1994, IOM issued historic reports confirming vaccines can cause death, as well as a wide spectrum of brain

From Barbara Loe Fisher, "Should Parents Be Allowed to Opt Out of Vaccinating Their Kids? Yes," *Insight on the News* (April 24, 2000). Copyright © 2000 by News World Communications, Inc. Reprinted by permission of *Insight*.

and immune-system damage. But the most important conclusion, which deserves greater public attention and congressional action, was: "The lack of adequate data regarding many of the [vaccine] adverse events under study was of major concern to the committee. [T]he committee encountered many gaps and limitations in knowledge bearing directly or indirectly on the safety of vaccines."

Because so little medical research has been conducted on vaccine side effects, no tests have been developed to identify and screen out vulnerable children. As a result, public-health officials have taken a "one-size-fits-all" approach and have aggressively implemented mandatory vaccination laws while dismissing children who are injured or die after vaccination as unfortunate but necessary sacrifices "for the greater good." This utilitarian rationale is of little comfort to the growing number of mothers and fathers who watch their once-healthy, bright children get vaccinated and then suddenly descend into mental retardation, epilepsy, learning and behavior disorders, autism, diabetes, arthritis and asthma. Some adverse reactions are fatal.

As vaccination rates have approached 98 percent for children entering kindergarten in many states, there is no question that mass vaccination in the last quarter-century has suppressed infectious diseases in childhood, eradicating polio in the Western hemisphere and lowering the number of cases of measles from a high of more than 400,000 cases in 1965 to only 100 in 1999. Yet, even as infectious-disease rates have fallen, rates of chronic disease and disability among children and young adults have risen dramatically.

A University of California study published by the U.S. Department of Education in 1996 found that "the proportion of the U.S. population with disabilities has risen markedly during the last quarter-century. [T]his recent change seems to be due not to demographics, but to greater numbers of children and young adults reported as having disabilities." The study concluded the change was due to "increases in the prevalence of asthma, mental disorders (including attention-deficit disorder), mental retardation and learning disabilities that have been noted among children in recent years."

Instead of epidemics of measles and polio, we have epidemics of chronic autoimmune and neurological disease: In the last 20 years rates of asthma and attention-deficit disorder have doubled, diabetes and learning disabilities have triple, chronic arthritis now affects nearly one in five Americans and autism has increased by 300 percent or more in many states. The larger unanswered question is: To what extent has the administration of multiple doses of multiple vaccines in early childhood—when the body's brain and immune system is developing at its most rapid rate—been a cofactor in epidemics of chronic disease? The assumption mass-vaccination policies have played no role is as unscientific and dangerous as the assumption that an individual child's health problems following vaccination are only coincidentally related to the vaccination.

Questions about vaccination only can be answered by scientific research into the biological mechanism of vaccine injury and death so that pathological profiles can be developed to distinguish between vaccine-induced health problems and those that are not. Whether the gaps in scientific knowledge about vaccines will be filled in this decade or remain unanswered in the next depends upon the funding and research priorities set by Congress, the National Institutes of Health and industry.

With the understanding that medical science and the doctors who practice it are not infallible, today's better-educated health-care consumer is demanding more information, more choices and a more equal decision-making partnership with doctors. Young mothers, who are told that their children must be injected with 33 doses of 10 different vaccines before the age of 5, are asking questions such as: "Why does my 12-hour-old newborn infant have to be injected with hepatitis B vaccine when I am not infected with hepatitis B and my infant is not an IV-drug user or engaging in sex with multiple partners—the two highest risk groups for hepatitis B infection?" And: "Why does my 12-month-old have to get chicken-pox vaccine when chicken pox is a mild disease and once my child gets it he or she will be immune for life?"

Informed parents know that hepatitis B is not like polio and that chicken pox is not like smallpox. They know the difference between taking a risk with a vaccine for an adult disease that is hard to catch, such as the blood-transmitted hepatitis B, and using a vaccine to prevent a devastating, highly contagious childhood disease such as polio.

All diseases and all vaccines are not the same and neither are children. Parents understand the qualitative difference between options freely taken and punishing dictates. They are calling for enlightened, humane implementation of state vaccination laws, including insertion of informed-consent protections that strengthen exemptions for sincerely held religious or conscientious beliefs. This is especially critical for parents with reason to believe that their child may be at high risk for dying or being injured by one or more vaccines but cannot find a doctor to write an exemption.

Informed consent has been the gold standard in the ethical practice of medicine since World War II, acknowledging the human right for individuals or their guardians to make fully informed, voluntary decisions about whether to undergo a medical procedure that could result in harm or death. To the extent that vaccination has been exempted from informed-consent protections and vaccine makers and doctors have been exempted from liability for vaccine injuries and deaths, the notion that a minority of individuals are expendable in service to the majority has prevented a real commitment of will and resources to develop ways to screen out vulnerable children and spare their lives. It is not difficult to understand why some parents resist offering up their children as sacrifices for a government policy that lacks scientific and moral integrity.

But even as educated health-care consumers are asking for more information and choices, mechanisms are being set up to restrict those choices. Government-operated, electronic vaccine-tracking systems already are in place in most states, using health-care identifier numbers to tag and track children without the parent's informed consent in order to enforce use of all government-recommended vaccines now and in the future. Health-maintenance organizations are turning down children for health insurance and federal entitlement programs are economically punishing parents who cannot show proof their child got every state-recommended vaccine. Even children who have suffered severe vaccine reactions are being pressured to get revaccinated or be barred from getting an education.

Drug companies and federal agencies are developing more than 200 new vaccines, including ones for gonorrhea and herpes that will target 12-year-olds. On March 2, President Clinton joined with the international pharmaceutical industry, multinational banks and the Bill and Melinda Gates Foundation to launch the Millennium Vaccine Initiative with several billion dollars committed to vaccinating all children in the world with existing and future vaccines, including those in accelerated development for AIDS, tuberculosis and malaria.

With so many unanswered questions about the safety and necessity of giving so many vaccines to children, the right to informed consent to vaccination takes on even greater legal and ethical significance as we head into the 21st century. In a broader sense, the concept of informed consent transcends medicine and addresses the constitutional concept of individual freedom and the moral concept of individual inviolability. If the state can tag, track down and force individuals into being injected with biological agents of unknown toxicity today, will there be any limit on what individual freedoms the state can take away in the name of the greater good tomorrow?

Parents, who know and love their children better than anyone else, have the right to make informed, voluntary vaccination decisions for their children without facing state-sanctioned punishment. Whether a child is hurt by a vaccine or a disease, it is the mother and father—not the pediatrician, vaccine maker or public-health official—who will bear the lifelong grief and burden of what happens to that child.

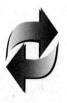

Steven P. Shelov 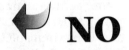 **NO**

That Would Open the Door for Epidemics of Some Deadly Childhood Diseases

Some parents today are in a quandary regarding the need for immunizing their children. They need not be.

True, recent media stories about an increase in childhood autism associated with immunizations and other illnesses have led some to question the need to give their children the full range of vaccinations required by most school districts in the country. In addition, numerous others have had unfortunate experiences with their own children or relatives with respect to a bad reaction to an immunization. Yet, it is important to keep all these issues and incidents in perspective and not to erode public confidence in immunizing our children. In fact, if the U.S. population or any population regards immunizing children as optional, we risk having large numbers of children becoming vulnerable to the most deadly diseases known to man. As a practicing pediatrician, I am passionately opposed to that. The following are a few questions some skeptical parents are asking about the vaccination issue:

What would happen if I did not have my child immunized?

Without immunizations there would be a significant possibility that your child would contract some of the diseases that are now waiting to come back. These include: whooping cough (pertussis), tetanus, polio, measles, mumps, German measles (rubella), bacterial meningitis and diphtheria.

These illnesses all may injure children severely, leaving them deaf, blind, paralyzed or they even may cause death. For example, in 1960 there were more than 1.5 million cases of measles and more than 400 deaths associated with this disease. As a result of our active immunization process in 1998 the United States had only 89 cases of measles and there were no deaths.

Why should I accept any risk of immunization for my child when other children already are immunized? Won't that protect my child?

It is important to understand the concept of herd immunity and public health vs. individual risk. Individual risk is always a possibility with any procedure, medication, new activity or vaccine. The key to any program or new intervention is to minimize the risk. There is no question that vaccines are the safest, most risk-free type of medication ever developed. Nevertheless, occasionally—very occasionally—children have been known to experience a bad, or adverse, reaction to a vaccine. In some cases—polio vaccine, for example—one in 1 million doses appears to have been associated with vaccine-related mild polio disease. The reactions to other vaccines also have been very, very small, though nevertheless significant for the child or family who have experienced one.

It is not, however, good public policy to give those few at-risk situations priority over the goal of protecting the population as a whole from those diseases. If the pool of unimmunized children becomes large enough, then the disease itself may reemerge in those unimmunized children, possibly in epidemic proportions. This has occurred in countries where immunizations have been allowed to decrease; most recently pertussis (whooping cough) resurfaced in Europe. Failure to immunize a child not only puts that child at risk of illness but also increases the potential for harm to other children who are not able to be vaccinated because they are too young or too ill or to those who in rare cases are vaccinated but the vaccination fails to provide the expected protection.

Are immunizations safe? Don't they hurt?

Reactions to vaccines may occur, but they usually are mild. Serious reactions are very, very rare but also may occur. Remember, the risks from these potentially dangerous childhood illnesses are far greater than any risk of serious reaction from immunization. Even though immunizations may hurt a little when they are given, and your baby may cry for a few minutes, and there might be some swelling, protecting your child's health is worth a few tears and a little temporary discomfort.

Isn't it better that children get a disease such as chicken pox to give them a permanent immunity?

If a child gets the disease, the danger is that the child may develop serious complications from the disease. The immunity conferred following the recommended immunization schedule will give excellent immunity and not place the child at risk.

Is it true that hepatitis B vaccine can cause autism or juvenile diabetes, sudden infant death syndrome, or SIDS, multiple sclerosis or asthma?

There have been occasional reports in the media associating this vaccine with all of the above illnesses. Scientific research has not found any evidence linking the hepatitis B vaccine to autism, SIDS, multiple sclerosis, juvenile diabetes or asthma. In fact, SIDS rates have declined during the same time period that the hepatitis B vaccine has been recommended for routine immunization. Although some media have circulated reports that health authorities in France have stopped giving the hepatitis vaccine to children, that is not true. French health officials did not stop giving the hepatitis vaccine but decided not to administer the vaccine in the schools and recommended that the vaccine be given in medical settings.

Is there a link between measles vaccine and autism?

No. There is no scientifically proven link between measles vaccine and autism. Autism is a chronic developmental disorder often first identified in toddlers ages 18 months to 30 months. The MMR (mumps, measles, rubella vaccine) is administered just before the peakage of autism that has caused some parents to assume a causal relationship, but a recent study in a British journal showed there was no association between the MMR vaccine and autism.

It is assumed that there has been an increase in the diagnosis of autism because the definition for who would fall under that category has changed. In addition, parents and medical professionals are more aware of this condition and are more likely to pursue that diagnosis. Though there may be an increase in the number of children who have autism, there have been many studies completed that show that the MMR does not cause autism.

Aren't measles, mumps and rubella relatively harmless illnesses?

Measles is a highly contagious respiratory disease. It causes a rash, high fever, cough and runny nose. In addition, it can cause encephalitis, which leads to convulsions, deafness or mental retardation in one to two children of every 2,000 who get it. Of every 1,000 people who get measles, one to two will die. MMR can prevent this disease. Mumps is less serious than measles but may cause fever, headache and swelling of one or both sides of the jaw. Four to 6 percent of those who get mumps will get meningitis, which puts the child at risk for significant disability and potential retardation. In addition, inflammation of the testicles occurs in four of every 10 adult males who get mumps, and mumps may result in hearing loss that usually is permanent. The effects of rubella are mild in children and adults—causing only a minor rash—but the major reason to prevent rubella in the community is to prevent exposure of pregnant women to children who have rubella. When contracted by a pregnant woman, rubella may infect her unborn baby, leading to a significant potential for mental retardation and a host of serious defects. This devastating disease, known as congenital rubella syndrome, essentially has been eliminated with the use of rubella vaccine.

Given that measles, rubella and mumps essentially have disappeared from the United States and therefore are uncommon, why should we continue to immunize?

The measles virus continues to be present in other countries outside the United States. Given the large number of immigrants to this country, the potential for exposure to measles remains a real potential. Just [recently] several young children who recently emigrated from the United Kingdom came into one of our pediatrician's offices. Due to the decrease in immunization vigilance in the United Kingdom against measles, these young children were infected with measles, and they put at risk the other infants and children in the waiting room of this busy pediatrician's office. If those other children contract measles, they will be at risk for developing serious sequela of the disease. And, should they develop the disease, they potentially will expose others as well. A mini-epidemic could have been caused by these infected children with measles.

Should parents be able to choose not to vaccinate their child without being barred from enrolling that child in school? Immunizing children is a public-health issue. Public-health laws in all 50 states require immunization of children as a condition of school enrollment. This is as it should be, since public health must take precedence. Immunizations have a clear community benefit and, therefore, individual preferences should not be permitted to expose the public to the hazards of infectious diseases.

In summary, it is clear that the risk of exposing children to infectious disease should there be a decline in immunizations is a risk to which the population of the United States should not be exposed. It always is regrettable when an individual case of an adverse event occurs no matter what might have taken place. These adverse events clearly affect the child and obviously the family as well, and there indeed is always an outcry when this does occur. However, as with all safe, proven interventions, an exception could always occur given a normal risk ratio.

It would be actual malpractice and poor public-health philosophy and practice to consider not immunizing our children against the potentially deadly infectious diseases. We should be thankful to our research scientists, epidemiologists, and medical and pharmaceutical industry for the skill and care with which these important vaccines have been developed and the care with which the vaccine policies have been developed and monitored. There is no question in my mind that immunizations are one of the most important ways parents can protect their children against serious diseases. Without immunizations the children of the United States would be exposed to deadly diseases that continue to occur throughout the world.

POSTSCRIPT

Should Parents Be Allowed to Opt Out of Vaccinating Their Children?

The possibility of biologic warfare, particularly the release of the smallpox virus, has recently become a serious issue. Vaccination against smallpox has already begun despite the small risk of serious reaction. The risk of an attack of the deadly and often fatal virus could potentially involve over 120 million Americans who were born after the mass vaccination was ended in 1972. In addition, the immunity of the approximately 155 million U.S. residents who were immunized prior to 1972 may be waning or gone. While the disease can be disfiguring and/or fatal, the vaccination also has risks. Approximately one or two persons per million does die from vaccine complications. Should the government once again force all children to be vaccinated against smallpox in case of a terrorist attack? Information on the smallpox issue may be found in "Smallpox Vaccination: The Call to Arms," *The New England Journal of Medicine* (January 30, 2003) and "Smallpox Vaccination Policy: The Need for Dialogue," *The New England Journal of Medicine* (April 25, 2002).

Currently, all 50 states require children to be vaccinated, though not for smallpox, before enrolling in school. Exemptions apply for children whose parents' religious beliefs prohibit vaccinations. Some children are exempt for medical reasons, which must be certified by their doctors. Almost all children are vaccinated by the time they enter school. However, the safety of various vaccines, particularly the diphtheria, pertussis, and tetanus (DPT) vaccine, continues to be the subject of debate. Although both the American Academy of Pediatrics and the U.S. Public Health Service continue to endorse the DPT vaccine, many parents and health providers believe that the risks associated with it are too high.

Widespread publicity about the genuine but extremely rare adverse effects of the pertussis vaccine is causing concern among drug manufacturers. Fewer companies are willing to produce vaccines due to expensive lawsuits brought by parents of injured children. This will lead to vaccine shortages and higher costs (which will be passed on to the consumer). The following articles discuss cost factors in relation to the low rates of immunizations: "Persistent Low Immunization Coverage Among Inner City Children," *Pediatrics* (April 1998) and "Shots in the Dark," *Reason* (November 1994).

Vaccines other than the DPT vaccine are also thought to be harmful. "Changing Concepts of Epstein-Barr Syndrome: An Immunization Reaction?" *Medical Hypothesis* (January 1988) reports a study of 200 patients who contracted Epstein-Barr syndrome when vaccinated with a live rubella (German measles) virus. Other articles discussing the risks of vaccination include "Juvenile Diabetes and Vaccination: New Evidence for a Connection," *The Vaccine Reaction* (February 1998); "Experts Forum," *Mothering* (Summer 1996); and "Immunizations: Do You Know the Risks?" *Second Opinion* (May 1994).

The medical community's endorsement of vaccination is evident in "U.S. Measles Cases at Record Low," *Health Letter on the CDC* (May 4, 1998); "Safety of Vaccinations," *Journal of the American Medical Association* (December 18, 1996); and "The War We Thought We Had Won," *Medical Update* (April 1996). For a comprehensive update on vaccine safety, see "Update: Vaccine Side Effects, Adverse Reactions, Contraindications, and Precautions," *Morbidity and Mortality Weekly Report* (September 6, 1996).

ISSUE 17

Does Anabolic Steroid Use Cause Serious Health Problems for Athletes?

YES: Steven Ungerleider, from "Steroids: Youth at Risk," *The Harvard Mental Health Letter* (May 2001)

NO: Dayn Perry, from "Pumped-Up Hysteria," *Reason* (January 2003)

ISSUE SUMMARY

YES: Clinical psychologist Steven Ungerleider asserts that anabolic steroids are dangerous to the health of athletes and should not be used.

NO: Freelance writer Dayn Perry states that the health risks of anabolic steroids are greatly exaggerated and that they pose limited harm to athletes.

Anabolic steroids are synthetic derivatives of the male hormone testosterone. These derivatives promote the growth of skeletal muscle and increase lean body tissue. Both athletes and nonathletes use steroids to enhance athletic performance and to change physical appearance. The drugs are injected or taken orally in cycles of weeks or months and in patterns. This is a practice known as *cycling*. Cycling involves taking multiple doses of anabolic steroids over a specified period, stopping, and then restarting. Some users combine several different types of steroids to increase their effectiveness while attempting to reduce the negative side effects. This is a practice known as *stacking*.

While anabolic steroids produce increased strength, lean muscle mass, and the ability to train harder and longer, their long-term health effects may be risky. Former NFL defensive end Lyle Alzado, who died in 1992 at the age of 43, used steroids for much of his career and believed that the drugs were responsible for the brain cancer that ultimately killed him. Researchers, however, do not have conclusive proof that long-term steroid use is linked to cancer. Many, but not all, of the risks associated with *short* term use are reversible. Side effects of the drug include liver disease, fluid retention, high blood pressure, acne, and trembling. Other noted effects in male users are reduced sperm count, breast enlargement, and shrinking of the testicles. Among female users, cessation of the menstrual cycle, deepening of the voice, and growth of facial hair have been observed. For both males and females, steroid use can lead to serious muscle and tendon injuries as players overuse and overextend their bodies while on the drug. In addition to physical side effects, there are concerns that anabolic steroids improve athletic performance by increasing aggression. Uncontrollable aggression, or "roid rage," has been used in criminal cases as a legal defense.

Despite the health concerns, the number of athletes who use or have used anabolic may be as high as three million. This includes up to 11 percent of male high school students, one-third of whom are nonathletes. Although most professional and collegiate sports organizations ban the use of steroids, their use among professional athletes, especially baseball players and professional body builders, is widespread. Use by nonprofessional body builders is increasing. Major league baseball has agreed to start testing in the 2003 season because of claims that steroids are heavily used by players. However, many athletes consider the benefit of an enhanced performance due to steroid use outweighs the risks. Many wonder how much emphasis should be placed on the risks. Are the assertions concerning the health problems due to steroid use overblown or are they not taken seriously enough?

In the following selections, Steven Ungerleider argues that steroids cause both physical and mental health risks and should be avoided. Dayn Perry contends that the health risks associated with steroid use among athletes is grossly exaggerated and that the political response to the drugs has been driven more by the illegality of steroids more than the actual danger.

Steven Ungerleider

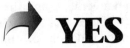 **YES**

Steroids: Youth at Risk

Several years ago, in a well-known research project, elite athletes were asked whether they would take a pill that guaranteed an Olympic gold medal if they knew it would kill them within a year. More than half of the athletes said they would take the pill.

The need to win at all costs has permeated many areas of our lives. In sports, one of the forms it takes is the use of anabolic-androgenic steroids (AAS). "Anabolic" refers to constructive metabolism or muscle-building, and "androgenic" means masculinizing. All AAS are derived from the hormone testosterone, which is found primarily in men, although women also produce it in smaller concentrations. There are at least thirty AAS, some natural and some synthetic.

Use of these substances has been pervasive for years among collegiate, Olympic, and professional competitors. Experiments with steroids began in Germany in the thirties, and their use by East German Olympic athletes is well known. More than 10,000 East German athletes in 22 events were given these synthetic hormones over 30 years. In August 2000, after a long battle in the criminal courts, more than 400 doctors, coaches, and trainers from the former East Germany were convicted of giving steroids to minors without their informed consent. But despite these revelations and convictions, scandals persist. Recently the chief of sports medicine for the United States Olympic Committee resigned in protest, saying that "some of our greatest Olympians have been using performance-enhancing drugs for years, and we have not been honest about our drug testing protocols."

Now anabolic steroids are becoming available to middle school and high school children as well. Concerns about body image and athletic performance lead adolescents to use the substances despite their serious side effects. Young athletes are responding to encouragement, social pressure, and their own desire to excel, as well as admonitions from coaches to put on muscle and build strength and resilience.

A recent survey by the National Institute on Drug Abuse indicates that steroid use by eighth- and tenth-graders is increasing, and twelfth-graders are increasingly likely to underestimate their risks. Some 2.7% of eighth- and tenth-graders and 2.9% of twelfth-graders admitted they had taken steroids at least once—a significant increase since 1991, the first year that full data were available. Other studies suggest that as many as 6% of high school students have used steroids. The numbers are especially alarming because many students will not admit that they take drugs. Sixth-graders report that these drugs are available in schoolyards, and they are increasingly used by nonathletes as well to impress their peers and attract the opposite sex.

Anabolic-androgenic steroids fall into three classes: C-17 alkyl derivatives of testosterone; esters or derivatives of 19-nortestosterone; and esters of testosterone.

C-17 alkyl derivatives are soluble in water and can be taken orally. Among them are Anavar, Anadrol, Dianabol (a favorite among Olympians), and the most famous, Winstrol, also known as stanozolol. Stanozolol was taken in large doses by the Canadian sprint champion Ben Johnson, who was stripped of a gold medal in the 1988 Olympics. These steroids are often favored by athletes trying to avoid drug screens because they clear the body quickly (within a month).

The 19-nortestosterone derivatives are oil-based; they are usually injected and absorbed into fat deposits, where long-term energy is stored. The most popular steroid in this group is nandrolone (Deca-Durabolin). It has recently made headlines because it is found in food supplements and other preparations that can be bought without a prescription. Many athletes who test positive for nandrolone say they had no idea what was in the vitamin supplements they took. Because nandrolone is stored in fatty tissue and released over a long period of time, it may take 8–10 months to clear the body.

Esters of testosterone, the third class, are especially dangerous. Among them are testosterone propionate, Testex, and cypionate. Active both orally and by injection, they closely mimic the effects of natural testosterone and are therefore difficult to detect on drug screens. The International Olympic Committee determines their presence by measuring the ratio of testosterone to the related substance epitestosterone in an athlete's urine; if the ratio exceeds 6:1, the athlete is suspected of cheating.

How do anabolic steroids work? The scientific literature demonstrates their effects, but it is not clear how they enhance the synthesis of proteins and the growth of muscles. They apparently increase endurance, allowing longer periods of exercise, and improve the results of strength training by increasing both the size (mass) of muscles and the number of muscle fibers.

Especially when taken in high doses, AAS can induce irritability and aggression. When Hitler's SS troops took steroids to build strength and stave off fatigue, they found that the hormones also made them more fearless and willing to fight. Among young athletic warriors today, steroids not only permit harder training and faster recovery from long workouts but may also induce a sense of invincibility and promote excessively macho behavior—and occasionally, attacks of rage or psychosis.

These drugs have a great many other risks as well. Men may develop reduced sperm production, shrunken testicles, impotence, and irreversible breast enlargement. Women may develop deep voices and excessive body hair. In either sex, baldness and acne are risks. The ratio of good to bad lipids may change, increasing the danger of heart attacks, strokes, and liver cancer. In adolescents bone growth may stop prematurely. (See Table 1 for details on side effects). Injecting steroids with contaminated needles creates a risk of HIV and other blood-borne infections.

Mental health professionals must consider how to address this problem in our schools. The National Institute on Drug Abuse and its nongovernmental partners have established Web sites to educate youth about the dangers of steroids. These sites may be found at *steroidabuse.org, archpediatrics.com,* and *drugabuse.gov.* A useful site for professionals interested in intervention and prevention is *tpronline.org.* Researchers at the Oregon Health Sciences University have devised an effective program known as Adolescents Training and Learning to Avoid Steroids (ATLAS). It is a team-centered and gender-specific approach that educates athletes about the dangers of steroids and other drugs while providing alternatives including nutritional advice and strength training. A three-year study demonstrated the benefits of the program for 3,000 football players in 31 Oregon high schools. ATLAS reduced not only anabolic steroid use but also alcohol and illicit drug use and drunk driving. Still more research is needed both to address the potentially deadly consequences of youthful steroid use and to discover ways of preventing it.

SIDE EFFECTS OF ANABOLIC-ANDROGENIC STEROIDS

In men:
- Gynecomastia (breast development), usually permanent
- Testicular or scrotal pain
- Testicular atrophy and decreased sperm production
- Premature baldness, even in adolescents
- Enlargement of the prostate gland, causing difficult urination

In women:
- Enlargement of the clitoris, usually irreversible
- Disruption of the menstrual cycle
- Permanent deepening of the voice
- Excessive facial and body hair

In both sexes:
- Nervous tension
- Aggressiveness and antisocial behavior
- Paranoia and psychotic states
- Acne, often serious enough to leave permanent scars on the face and body
- Burning and pain during urination
- Gastrointestinal and leg muscle cramps
- Headaches
- Dizziness
- High blood pressure
- Heart, kidney, and liver damage
- In adolescents, premature end to the growth of long bones, leading to shortened stature

NO ↰

Dayn Perry

Pumped-Up Hysteria

Had Ken Caminiti been a less famous ballplayer, or had he merely confessed his own sins, then it would have been a transient controversy. But it wasn't. Last May [2002], Caminiti, in a cathartic sit-down with Tom Verducci of *Sports Illustrated,* became the first major league baseball player, current or retired, to admit to using anabolic steroids during his playing days. Specifically, he said he used them during the 1996 season, when he was named the National League's Most Valuable Player. And his truth session didn't stop there.

"It's no secret what's going on in baseball. At least half the guys are using [steroids]," Caminiti told *SI.* "They talk about it. They joke about it with each other. . . . I don't want to hurt fellow teammates or fellow friends. But I've got nothing to hide."

The suggestion that steroids are a systemic problem in professional athletics is hardly shocking, but such candor from players—particularly baseball players, who until recently weren't subject to league-mandated drug testing—was virtually unheard of. Before the Caminiti flap had time to grow stale, Jose Canseco, another high-profile ex-ballplayer, upped the ante, declaring that a whopping 85 percent of current major league players were "juicing."

The estimates were unfounded, the sources unreliable, and the implications unclear. But a media orgy had begun. The questions that are being asked of the players—Do you think it's worth it? How many are using? Why did the players union wait so long to adopt random testing? Why won't you take a test *right now?*—are mostly of the "Have you stopped beating your wife?" variety. The accusation is ensconced in the question.

This approach may be satisfying to the self-appointed guardians of baseball's virtue, but it leaves important questions unexplored. Indeed, before the sport can solve its steroid problem, it must determine whether it even has one.

From those sounding the clarion call for everything from stricter league policies to federal intervention, you'll hear the same two-pronged concern repeated time and again: Ballplayers are endangering their health and tarnishing baseball's competitive integrity. These are defensible, if dogmatic, positions, but the sporting media's fealty to them obscures the fact that both points are dubious.

From Dayn Perry, "Pumped-Up Hysteria," *Reason* (January 2003). Copyright © 2003 by The Reason Foundation, 3415 S. Sepulveda Boulevard, Suite 400, Los Angeles, CA 90034. www.reason.com. Reprinted by permission.

A more objective survey of steroids' role in sports shows that their health risks, while real, have been grossly exaggerated; that the political response to steroids has been driven more by a moral panic over drug use than by the actual effects of the chemicals; and that the worst problems associated with steroids result from their black-market status rather than their inherent qualities. As for baseball's competitive integrity, steroids pose no greater threat than did other historically contingent "enhancements," ranging from batting helmets to the color line. It is possible, in fact, that many players who use steroids are not noticeably improving their performance as a result.

There are more than 600 different types of steroids, but it's testosterone, the male sex hormone, that's most relevant to athletics. Testosterone has an androgenic, or masculinizing, function and an anabolic, or tissue-building, function. It's the second set of effects that attracts athletes, who take testosterone to increase their muscle mass and strength and decrease their body fat. When testosterone is combined with a rigorous weight-training regimen, spectacular gains in size and power can result. The allure is obvious, but there are risks as well.

Health Effects

Anecdotal accounts of harrowing side effects are not hard to find—everything from "'roid rage" to sketchy rumors of a female East German swimmer forced to undergo a sex change operation because of the irreversible effects of excess testosterone. But there are problems with the research that undergirds many of these claims. The media give the impression that there's something inevitably Faustian about taking anabolics—that gains in the present will undoubtedly exact a price in the future. Christopher Caldwell, writing recently in *The Wall Street Journal*, proclaimed, "*Doctors are unanimous that [anabolic steroids] increase the risk of heart disease, and of liver, kidney, prostate and testicular cancer.*"

This is false. "We know steroids can be used with a reasonable measure of safety," says Charles Yesalis, a Penn State epidemiologist, steroid researcher for more than 25 years, and author of the 1998 book *The Steroids Game*. "We know this because they're used in medicine all the time, just not to enhance body image or improve athletic performance." Yesalis notes that steroids were first used for medical purposes in the 1930s, some three decades before the current exacting standards of the Food and Drug Administration (FDA) were in place.

Even so, anabolic steroids or their derivatives are commonly used to treat breast cancer and androgen deficiencies and to promote red blood cell production. They are also used in emerging anti-aging therapies and to treat surgical or cancer patients with damaged muscle tissue.

Caldwell cites one of the most common fears: that anabolics cause liver cancer. There is dubious evidence linking oral anabolics to liver tumors, but athletes rarely take steroids in liquid suspension form. Users almost uniformly opt for the injectable or topical alternatives, which have chemical structures that aren't noxious to the liver. And as Yesalis observes, even oral steroids aren't causally linked to cancer; instead, some evidence associates them with benign liver tumors.

More specifically, it's C-17 alkylated oral steroids that are perhaps detrimental to liver function. But the evidence is equivocal at best. A 1990 computer-assisted study of all existing medical literature found but three cases of steroid-associated liver tumors. Of those three cases, one subject had been taking outrageously large doses of C-17 oral anabolics without cessation for five years, and a second case was more indicative of classic liver malignancy. It's also C-17 orals, and not other forms of steroids, that are associated with decreased levels of HDL, or "good" cholesterol. But, again, C-17s are almost never used for athletic or cosmetic purposes.

Another commonly held belief is that steroid use causes aggressive or enraged behavior. Consider the case of San Francisco Giants outfielder Barry Bonds, whose impressive late-career home run hitting and built-up physique have long raised observers' eyebrows. Last season, Bonds, long known for being irascible, had a dugout shoving match with teammate Jeff Kent. A few columnists, including Bill Lankhof of *The Toronto Sun* and Jacob Longan of the *Stillwater News-Press,* obliquely diagnosed "'roid rage" from afar. "There's very inconsistent data on whether 'roid rage even exists," says Yesalis. "I'm more open to the possibility than I used to be, but its incidence is rare, and the studies that concluded it does exist largely haven't accounted for underlying factors or the placebo effect."

Scientists are nearly unanimous that excessive testosterone causes aggression in animals, but this association begins to wither as you move up the evolutionary ladder. Diagnosing such behavior in athletes is especially tricky. "There's a certain degree of aggression that's not only acceptable but necessary in competitive sports," Yesalis says. "What's perhaps just the intensity that's common to many athletes gets perceived as steroid-linked outbursts."

Fears about steroid use also include other cancers, heart enlargement, increased blood pressure, elevated cholesterol levels, and musculoskeletal injuries. Upon closer examination, these too turn out to be overblown. Reports associating heart enlargement, or cardiomegaly, with steroid use often ignore the role of natural, nonthreatening enlargement brought on by prolonged physical exertion, not to mention the effects of alcohol abuse. The relationship is unclear at best. Evidence supporting a link between steroids and ligament and tendon damage is weak, since steroid-related injuries are virtually indistinguishable from those occurring normally. And blood pressure problems, according to Yesalis, have been exaggerated. There is some associative evidence that steroid use can increase the risk of prostate cancer, but this link has yet to be borne out in a laboratory setting. No studies of any kind link the use of anabolics to testicular cancer.

Addiction is a legitimate concern, and Yesalis says a quarter to a half of those who use steroids solely to improve their body image exhibit signs of psychological dependence. "But in all my years of research," Yesalis continues, "I've only known three professional athletes who were clinically addicted to steroids." The distinction, he explains, is that professional athletes see steroids as little more than a tool to help them do their job—the way "an office worker views his computer." Once their playing days are over, almost all the athletes within Yesalis' purview "terminate their use of the drug."

One reason the health effects of steroids are so uncertain is a dearth of research. In the almost 65 years that anabolic steroids have been in our midst, there has not been a single epidemiological study of the effects of long-term use. Instead, Yesalis explains, concerns about extended usage are extrapolated from what's known about short-term effects. The problem is that those short-term research projects are often case studies, which Yesalis calls the "lowest life form of scientific studies." Case studies often draw conclusions from a single test subject and are especially prone to correlative errors.

"We've had thousands upon thousands [of long-term studies] done on tobacco, cocaine, you name it," Yesalis complains. "But for as much as you see and hear about anabolic steroids, they haven't even taken that step."

What about the research that has been done? At least some of it seems to yield engineered results. "The studies linking steroid use to cancer were performed by and large on geriatric patients," notes Rick Collins, attorney, former bodybuilder, and author of the book *Legal Muscle,* which offers an exhaustive look at anabolic steroid use under U.S. law. The hazard of such research is that side effects observed in an older patient could be the result of any number of physiological problems unrelated to steroid intake. Moreover, the elderly body is probably more susceptible to adverse reactions than the body of a competitive athlete.

Collins believes that some studies were performed with a conclusion in mind at the outset. "Their hearts were in the right place," says Collins. "Curtailing nonessential steroid use is a good and noble goal, but they undermined their efforts by exaggerating the dangers." Call it the cry-wolf effect.

For instance, it's long been dogma that use of anabolic steroids interferes with proper hepatic (liver) function and causes thickening of the heart muscle. However, a 1999 study at the University of North Texas found that it's not steroid use that causes these medical phenomena; rather, it's intense resistance training. Weight-lifting causes tissue damage, and, at high extremes, can elevate liver counts and thicken the left ventricular wall of the heart. Both disorders were observed in high-intensity weightlifters irrespective of steroid use. The researchers concluded that previous studies had "misled the medical community" into embellishing the side effects of use.

Testosterone-Fueled Panic

The cry-wolf effect may have as much to do with the boom in steroid use as anything else. Athletes were inclined to be skeptical of warnings about steroids because their own experience contradicted what critics were saying. When use of Dianabol and other anabolics began to surge in the 1960s and '70s, opponents decried them as ineffective. The message was: *They don't work, so don't take the risk.* But steroids did work, and users knew it. Once weightlifters, bodybuilders, and other athletes realized they were being lied to about the efficacy of steroids, they were less likely to believe warnings about health hazards, especially when the evidence backing them up was vague or anecdotal.

One of the chief drumbeaters for the steroids-don't-work movement was Bob Goldman, author of the hysterical anti-steroids polemic *Death in the Locker Room*. Goldman, a former competitive power-lifter turned physician and sports medicine specialist, was an early, and shrill, critic of performance pharmacology. In his 1984 exposé, Goldman attributes steroids' tissue-building qualities almost entirely to the placebo effect. His agenda may have been morally sound, but his conclusions ran counter to the preponderance of scientific evidence at the time. Today, his claims are even less supportable. Goldman is working on a new edition of the book, one that he says will better crystallize current scientific thought on the subject. Of his 1984 edition and its seeming histrionics, Goldman says the book was intended "as an educational tool to warn high school students of the possible hazards of drug use, but then it became something else."

Whatever his intentions at the time, Goldman's views played well in the media, which cast the book as a sobering empirical assault on performance-enhancing drugs. Its warnings soon gained traction with lawmakers. Although the Anti-Drug Abuse Act of 1988 had already made it illegal to dispense steroids for nonmedical reasons, Congress, ostensibly out of concern over reports of increasing steroid use among high school athletes, revisited the matter in 1989.

Congressional hearings convened to determine whether steroids should become the first hormone placed on Schedule III of the Controlled Substances Act, reserved for drugs with substantial abuse potential. Such legislation, if passed, would make possession of anabolic steroids without a prescription a federal offense punishable by up to a year in prison. Distributing steroids for use, already prohibited by the 1988 law, would be a felony punishable by up to five years in prison. What's usually forgotten about these hearings, or perhaps simply ignored, is the zeal with which many regulatory agencies, research organizations, and professional groups objected to the proposed changes. The American Medical Association (AMA), the FDA, the National Institute on Drug Abuse, and even the Drug Enforcement Administration all opposed the reclassification. Particularly adamant was the AMA, whose spokespersons argued that steroid users did not exhibit the physical or psychological dependence necessary to justify a change in policy.

Nevertheless, Congress voted into law the 1990 Anabolic Steroids Control Act, which reclassified steroids as Schedule III controlled substances, placing them on legal par with barbiturates and narcotic painkillers such as Vicodin, just one step down from amphetamines, cocaine, and morphine. Now even first-time steroid users faced possible jail time.

Black-Market 'Roids

Prohibition naturally produced a black market, and unintended consequences followed. Besides creating yet another economic niche for the criminal underworld, the legislation scuttled any hope of using steroids as a legitimate and professionally administered performance enhancer.

Criminalization of steroids created dangers more serious than any that had prompted the ban. Once steroids became contraband, many athletes bought black-market anabolics that, unbeknownst to them, were spiked or cut with other drugs or intended solely for veterinary use. Physicians were forbidden to prescribe steroids for promoting muscle growth and thus were not able to provide steroid users with responsible, professionally informed oversight. New league policies even ban the use of steroids for recovery from injuries.

Combine the lack of medical supervision with the mind-set of the garden-variety steroid user, and you have a potentially perilous situation. "Many of those using anabolic steroids," says Penn State's Yesalis, "have the attitude that if one [dose] works, then five or 10 will work even better. That's dangerous."

Athletes who acquire steroids on the black market are loath to consult with their physician after they begin using regularly. If they do disclose their habit and ask for guidance, the physician, for fear of professional discipline or even criminal charges, may refuse to continue seeing the patient. For professional athletes, another deterrent to proper use is that all responsible doctors keep rigorously accurate records of their dealings with patients. The fear that those records might be leaked or even subpoenaed makes pro athletes even less likely to seek medical guidance.

Since many of the observed side effects of steroids—anecdotal, apocryphal, or otherwise—most likely result from excessive or improper use of the drug, one wonders: Can steroids be used for muscle building with a reasonable degree of safety? "The candid answer is yes, but with caveats," says Collins, the attorney who specializes in steroid law. "It would need to be under the strict direction of a physician and administered only after a thorough physical examination, and it would need to be taken at reasonable and responsible dosages."

It's a statement that even Goldman, once the bellwether scaremonger, says is "something I could probably agree with."

Herbert Haupt, a private orthopedist and sports medicine specialist in St. Louis, is "absolutely, unequivocally, positively opposed" to steroid use as a training or cosmetic tool. But he concedes that properly supervised use of the drug for those purposes can be reasonably safe. "The adverse side effects of steroids typically subside upon cessation of use," says Haupt, "and use over a short span, say a six-week duration, probably carries nominal risk."

Moreover, the official attitude toward steroid use seems anomalous when compared to the treatment of other methods that people use to improve their bodies. "People die from botched liposuctions," Collins notes. "We're also allowed to inject botulism into people's faces [in botox therapy], but no one is allowed to use steroids for similar cosmetic reasons."

Collins is quick to add that adolescents, whose bodies are already steeped in hormones, cannot use steroids safely. But the fact remains that the illegality of steroids makes responsible professional oversight virtually impossible.

Another puzzling distinction is the one made between steroids and other training supplements. Many baseball players have openly used androstenedione, a muscle-building compound that major league baseball hasn't banned even though it's merely a molecular puddle-jump from anabolic steroids. Androstenedione is a chemical precursor that is converted to testosterone by the liver. Creatine monohydrate, another effective supplement, is far more widely used than androstenedione and is virtually free of stigma. Creatine is chemically unrelated to anabolic steroids or androstenedione and also differs in that it does not manipulate hormone levels; rather, creatine allows muscle cells to recover from fatigue more quickly. But all three substances—creatine, androstenedione, and anabolic steroids—increase a naturally occurring substance in the body to promote the building of muscle tissue. Anabolic steroids simply accomplish this end more quickly and dramatically.

The list of "artificial" enhancements doesn't stop there. Indeed, the boundaries of what constitutes a "natural" modern athlete are increasingly arbitrary. Pitchers benefit from computer modeling of their throwing motions. Medical and pharmacological technologies help players to prevent and recover from injuries better than ever before. Even laboratory-engineered protein shakes, nutrition bars, and vitamin C tablets should theoretically violate notions of "natural" training. Yet no one claims these tools are tarnishing the competitive integrity of the game.

Muscle Beach Zombies

Rangers pitcher Kenny Rogers has said, in a bizarre admission, that he doesn't throw as hard as he can because he fears that the line drives hit by today's players, if properly placed, could kill him on the mound. And you need not read the sports pages for long to find someone complaining that today's "juiced" ballplayers are toppling the game's sacrosanct records by the shadiest of means. This sentiment began percolating when Roger Maris' single-season home run record tottered and fell to Mark McGwire in 1998. Since the Caminiti and Canseco stories broke, sportswriters have been resorting to preposterous rhetorical flourishes in dismissing the accomplishments of the modern hitter. Bill Conlin of the *Philadelphia Daily News,* for example, writes: "To all the freaks, geeks and 'roid zombies who have turned major league baseball into a Muscle Beach version of the Medellin Cartel: Take your records and get lost."

Yet baseball statistics have never existed in a vacuum. Babe Ruth became the sport's chief pantheon dweller without ever competing against a dark-skinned ballplayer. Chuck Klein of the Philadelphia Phillies posted some eye-popping numbers in the 1930s, but he did it in an era when runs were scored in bundles, and he took outrageous advantage of the Baker Bowl's right field fence, which was a mere 280 feet from home plate. Detroit pitcher Hal Newhouser won two most valuable player awards and a plaque in Cooperstown in part by dominating competition that had been thinned out by World War II's conscription. Sandy Koufax crafted his run of success in the '60s with the help of a swollen strike zone. Also a boon to Koufax was the helpfully designed Dodger Stadium, which included, according to many, an illegally heightened mound. Gaylord Perry succored his Hall of Fame career by often calling upon an illegal spitball pitch. Take any baseball statistic, and something is either inflating or depressing it to some degree.

Beginning in the mid-'90s in the American League and the late '90s in the National League, home runs reached unseen levels. This fact has encouraged much of the present steroids conjecture. But correlation does not imply causation, as the deductive reasoning platitude goes, and there are more likely explanations for the recent increase in homers.

Home runs are up, in large part, because several hitter-friendly ballparks have opened in recent years. Coors Field, home of the Colorado Rockies since 1995, is the greatest run-scoring environment in major league history. Until the 2000 season, the Houston Astros played in the Astrodome, a cavernous, run-suppressing monstrosity with remarkably poor visuals for hitters. They replaced it with Enron Field (now renamed Minute Maid Park), which is second only to Coors Field in terms of helping hitters and boasts a left field line that's so short it's in violation of major league rules. The Pittsburgh Pirates, Milwaukee Brewers, and Texas Rangers also have recently replaced their old ballparks with stadiums far more accommodating to hitters. The Arizona Diamondbacks came into being in 1998; they too play in a park that significantly inflates offensive statistics. The St. Louis Cardinals, Baltimore Orioles, and Chicago White Sox have all moved in their outfield fences in the last few years. Add to all that the contemporary strike zone, which plainly benefits hitters, and it's little wonder that home runs are at heretofore unimaginable levels.

And then there is Barry Bonds and the momentous season he had in 2001. In the midst of Bonds' siege on McGwire's still freshly minted single-season home run record, Bob Klapisch of the Bergen County, New Jersey, *Record* made a transparent observation-cum-accusation by writing, "No one has directly accused Bonds of cheating—whether it be a corked bat or steroids. . . ."

Bonds is plainly bigger than he was early in his career. That fact, considered in tandem with his almost unimaginable statistical achievements, has led many to doubt the purity of his training habits. But Bonds had bulked up to his current size by the late '90s, and from then until 2001 his home run totals were in line with his previous yearly levels. So there's obviously a disconnect between his body size and his home runs. Last season, bulky as ever, Bonds hit "only" 46 homers, which isn't out of step with his pre-2001 performance. More than likely, Bonds had an aberrant season in 2001—not unlike Roger Maris in 1961.

Steroids vs. the Perfect Swing

This is not to suggest that no ballplayers are taking advantage of modern pharmacology. Rick Collins says he knows some major league ballplayers are using steroids but can't hazard a guess as to how many. And Yesalis believes that at least 30 percent of major league ballplayers are on steroids.

But then there are skeptics like Tony Cooper of the *San Francisco Chronicle*, a longtime sportswriter and 20-year veteran of the weightlifting and body-building culture. During the 2001 season, as Bonds was assailing McGwire's freshly minted home run record, Cooper responded to the groundswell of steroid speculation by writing that he saw no evidence of steroid use in baseball. Cooper had seen plenty of steroid users and plenty of "naked baseball players," and he couldn't name one obvious juicer in the entire sport. As for Bonds, Cooper called the accusations "ludicrous," writing that the Giants' slugger "merely looks like a man who keeps himself in condition."

Canseco, of course, claims 85 percent of players are on steroids. Caminiti initially said half, then backpedaled to 15 percent. Other players have dotted the points in between with guesses of their own. Whatever the actual figure, such widely divergent estimates suggest that not even the ballplayers themselves know the extent of the problem. And if *they* don't know, the pundits assuredly don't either.

A more reasonable (and answerable) question is: If players are on steroids, how much of a difference is it making?

Not much of one, according to Chris Yeager, a human performance specialist, private hitting instructor, and longtime weightlifter. Yeager's argument is not a replay of Bob Goldman's assertion that steroids function merely as placebos. Yeager posits that the engorged arms, chests, and shoulders of today's ballplayers could well be the result of steroid use—but that they aren't helping them hit home runs.

"Upper body strength doesn't increase bat speed," he explains, "and bat speed is vital to hitting home runs. The upper body is used in a ballistic manner. It contributes very little in terms of power generation." Yeager likens the arms, in the context of a hitter's swing, to the bat itself: simply a means to transfer energy. A batter's pectoral muscles, says Yeager, "are even less useful."

Yeager isn't saying steroid use *couldn't* increase a batter's power. He's saying most ballplayers don't train properly." There's a difference between training for strength and training for power," he says, "and most baseball players train for strength." If hitters carefully and specifically trained their legs and hips to deliver sudden blasts of power, then steroids could be useful to them, but by and large that's not what they do. "Mark McGwire hit 49 home runs as a 23-year-old rookie," Yeager says. "And, while I think he probably used steroids at some point in his career, he hit home runs primarily because of his excellent technique, his knowledge of the strike zone, and the length of his arms. Barry Bonds could be on steroids, but his power comes from the fact that he has the closest thing to a perfect swing that I've ever seen."

Much Ado About Nothing

In what at first blush seems counterintuitive, Yeager asserts that steroid use may have *decreased* home run levels in certain instances. Specifically, he points to Canseco. "I'm almost positive Canseco used steroids, and I think it hurt his career," says Yeager. "He became an overmuscled, one-dimensional player who couldn't stay healthy. Without steroids, he might have hit 600, 700 home runs in his career."

In short, steroids are a significant threat to neither the health of the players nor the health of the game. Yet the country has returned to panic mode, with both private and public authorities declaring war on tissue-building drugs.

The chief instrument in that war is random drug testing, which major league baseball adopted in September 2002 with the ratification of the most recent collective bargaining agreement. Players can be tested for drugs at any time, for any reason whatsoever. Leaving aside what this implies for players' privacy, testing is easily skirted by users who know what they're doing.

Sprinter Ben Johnson tested positive for steroids at the 1988 Summer Olympics and forfeited his gold medal, but subsequent investigation revealed that he'd passed 19 drug tests prior to failing the final one at the Seoul games. Yesalis says most professional athletes who use steroids know how to pass a drug test. Whether by using masking agents, undetectable proxies like human growth hormone, or water-based testosterone, they can avoid a positive reading. At the higher levels of sports, Yesalis believes, drug testing is done mostly "for public relations." Image protection is a sensible goal for any business, but no one should be deluded into thinking it eliminates drug use.

Nevertheless, lawmakers are lining up to push the process along. California state Sen. Don Perata (D-East Bay) has introduced a bill that would require all professional athletes playing in his state to submit to random drug testing. Federal legislation could be forthcoming from Sen. Byron Dorgan (D-N.D.). It's unlikely that any bill calling for this level of government intrusion will pass. But the fact that such legislation is even being considered suggests how entrenched the steroid taboo is. Meanwhile, baseball's new collective bargaining agreement has firmly established drug testing in the sport. The Major League Baseball Players Association, contrary to what some expected, agreed to the testing program with little resistance.

The measure won't do much to prevent the use of performance-enhancing drugs in baseball, but it may serve as a palliative for the media. At least until the next cause celebre comes along.

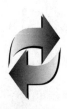

POSTSCRIPT

Does Anabolic Steroid Use Cause Serious Health Problems for Athletes?

Since the death of NFL star Lyle Alzado in 1992 the dangers of anabolic steroids have been promoted by the media. The use of these drugs is banned by the International Olympic Committee, the National Football League, the National Basketball Association, the NCAA, and high schools. Obtaining and using these drugs is illegal except by prescription for purposes deemed as medically necessary. In addition, many within the athletic community believe that the use of steroids is unethical and a form of cheating.

Are people overreacting when it comes to steroid use? Do the risks outweigh the benefits? For further reading see "Anabolic-Androgenic Steroids for Athletes: Adverse Effects," *Alternative Medicine Alert* (January 2003); "A Bulked-Up Body of Knowledge," *Los Angeles Times* (June 10, 2002); "Androgenic-Anabolic Steroid-Induced Body Changes in Strength Athlete," and "Anabolic Steroid Abuse and Cardiac Sudden Death: A Pathologic Study," *Archives of Pathology & Laboratory Medicine* (February 2001); "Performance-Enhancing Drugs: The Truth Behind the Hype," *Current Health* (February 2003); "The Safety and Efficacy of Anabolic Steroid Precursors: What Is the Scientific Evidence?" *Journal of Athletic Training* (July–September 2002); and "Athletes Risk Their Lives by Use of Drugs, Says British Medical Association," *British Medical Journal* (April 13, 2002). Other studies have found a relationship between steroid use and injuries on the field. See "The Injury Toll: Steroid Use May Explain a Sharp Rise in the Time Players Spend on the Disabled List," *Sports Illustrated* (June 3, 2002).

While illicit steroids make headlines, wholly legal, over-the-counter dietary supplements have become a $17.7 billion business, including $1.7 billion in sports-nutrition supplements. Largely outside the FDA's jurisdiction, supplements are not federally approved. They have not been subjected to rigorous clinical trials, and often little is known about their chemical composition, side effects, or efficacy. However, millions of athletes are taking supplements containing everything from ephedra to creatine to andro in any of several forms, including pills, powders, and gums, in hopes of gaining a competitive edge. Further reading includes "Safety of Ephedra, Links to Deaths and Illness Debated," *Knight Ridder/Tribune News Service* (March 24, 2003); "Use of Ephedra Supplements, Steroids Up, NCAA Says," *Food Chemical News* (August 20, 2001); "The Scoop on Ephedra," *Health* (July/August 2001); and "Steroid Suspicions Abound in Major-League Dugouts," *The New York Times* (October 11, 2000).

ISSUE 18

Is Marijuana Dangerous and Addictive?

YES: Eric A. Voth, from "Should Marijuana Be Legalized as a Medicine? No, It's Dangerous and Addictive," *The World & I* (June 1994)

NO: Ethan A. Nadelmann, from "Reefer Madness 1997: The New Bag of Scare Tactics," *Rolling Stone* (February 20, 1997)

ISSUE SUMMARY

YES: Eric A. Voth, medical director of Chemical Dependency Services at St. Francis Hospital in Topeka, Kansas, argues that marijuana produces many adverse effects and that its effectiveness as a medicine is supported only by anecdotes.

NO: Ethan A. Nadelmann, director of the Lindesmith Center, a New York drug policy research institute, asserts that government officials continue to promote the myth that marijuana is harmful and leads to the use of hard drugs. He states that the war on marijuana is being fought for purely political, not health, reasons.

At one time there were no laws in the United States regulating the use or sale of drugs, including marijuana. Rather than by legislation, their use was regulated by religious teaching and social custom. As society grew more complex and more heterogeneous, the need for more formal regulation of drug sales, production, and use developed.

Attempts at regulating patent medications through legislation began in the early 1900s. In 1920 Congress, under pressure from temperance organizations, passed an amendment prohibiting the manufacture and sale of all alcoholic beverages. From 1920 until 1933, the demand for alcohol was met by organized crime, who either manufactured it illicitly or smuggled it into the United States. The government's inability to enforce the law, as well as increasing violence, finally led to the repeal of Prohibition in 1933.

Many years later, in the 1960s, drug usage again began to worry many Americans. Heroin abuse had become epidemic in urban areas, and many middle-class young adults had begun to experiment with marijuana and LSD by the end of the decade. Cocaine also became popular first among the middle class and later among inner-city residents. Today, crack houses, babies born with drug addictions, and drug-related crimes and shootings are the images of a new epidemic of drug abuse.

Many of those who believe illicit drugs are a major problem in America, however, are usually referring to hard drugs, such as cocaine and heroin. Soft drugs like marijuana, though not legal, are not often perceived as a major threat to the safety and well-being of citizens. Millions of Americans have tried marijuana and did not become addicted. The drug has also been used illegally by those suffering from AIDS, glaucoma, and cancer to alleviate their symptoms and to stimulate their appetites. Should marijuana be legalized as a medicine, or is it too addictive and dangerous? In California, Proposition 215 passed in the November 1996 ballot. A similar measure passed in Arizona. These initiatives convinced voters to relax current laws against marijuana use for medical and humane reasons.

Opponents of these recent measures argue that marijuana use has been steadily rising among teenagers and that this may lead to experimentation with hard drugs. There is concern that if marijuana is legal via a doctor's prescription, the drug will be more readily available. There is also concern that the health benefits of smoking marijuana are overrated. For instance, among glaucoma sufferers, in order to achieve benefits from the drug, patients would literally have to be stoned all the time. Unfortunately, the efficacy of marijuana is unclear because, as an illicit drug, studies to adequately test it have been thwarted by drug control agencies.

Although marijuana's effectiveness in treating the symptoms of disease is unclear, is it actually dangerous and addictive? Scientists contend that the drug can negatively affect cognition and motor function. It can also have an impact on short-term memory and can interfere with perception and learning. Physical health effects include lung damage. Until recently, scientists had little evidence that marijuana was actually addictive. Whereas heavy users did not seem to experience actual withdrawal symptoms, studies with laboratory animals given large doses of THC, the active ingredient in marijuana, suffered withdrawal symptoms similar to those of rodents withdrawing from opiates.

Not all researchers agree, however, that marijuana is dangerous and addictive. The absence of well-designed, long-term studies on the effects of marijuana use further complicates the issue, as does the current potency of the drug. Growers have become more skilled about developing strains of marijuana with high concentrations of THC. Today's varieties may be three to five times more potent than the pot used in the 1960s. Much of the data are unclear, but what is known is that young users of the drug are likely to have problems learning. In addition, some users are at risk for developing dependence.

In the following selections, Eric A. Voth argues that marijuana causes many physical and psychological effects, including potential addiction. Ethan A. Nadelmann states that there are no proven studies to support the view that marijuana is more dangerous than previously thought or that it is a gateway to more dangerous drugs.

Eric A. Voth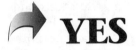

Should Marijuana Be Legalized as a Medicine? No, It's Dangerous and Addictive

To best understand the problems associated with legalizing marijuana, it is useful to examine drug legalization in general and then to discuss the specific pitfalls of legal marijuana.

Advocates generally argue that crime would decrease under legalization, that dealers would be driven out of the market by lower prices, that legalization works in other countries, that government would benefit from the sales tax on drugs, that Prohibition did not work, and that the "war on drugs" has failed.

Examining currently legal drugs provides an insight as to the possible effect of legalizing other drugs. First, alcohol is responsible for approximately 100,000 deaths every year and 11 million cases of alcoholism. Virtually every bodily system is adversely affected by alcoholism. While Prohibition was an unfortunately violent time, many of the hardships of that era were really the result of the Depression. Prohibition did decrease the rate of alcohol consumption; alcohol-related deaths climbed steadily after Prohibition was repealed.

Tobacco use is responsible for 400,000 premature deaths per year. It causes emphysema, chronic bronchitis, heart disease, lung cancer, head and neck cancers, vascular disease, and hypertension, to name a few disorders. The taxes on tobacco come nowhere close to paying for the health problems caused by the drug.

The argument that legalization would decrease crime exemplifies a great lack of understanding of drug abuse. Most drug-associated crime is committed to acquire drugs or under the influence of drugs. The Netherlands has often been heralded by the drug culture as a country where decriminalization has worked. In fact, drug-related holdups and shootings have increased 60 percent and 40 percent, respectively, since decriminalization. This has caused the government to start enforcing the drug laws more strictly.

Because of its powerful drug lobby, the Netherlands has never been able to mount a taxation campaign against its legal drugs. We suffer a similar phenomenon in the United States in that the tobacco lobby has successfully defeated most taxation initiatives against tobacco.

The argument that drug dealers would be driven out of the market by lower prices ignores the fact that legalization will probably result in as many as 250,000 to over two million new addicts. Broader markets, even with lower prices, certainly will not drive dealers out of the market. Our overburdened medical system will not be able to handle the drastic increase in the number of addicts.

Medical Marijuana

Richard Cowan, national director of the National Organization for the Reform of Marijuana Laws (NORML), has stated that acceptance of medicinal uses of marijuana is pivotal for its legalization.

In 1972, the drug culture petitioned the Drug Enforcement Administration (DEA) to reschedule marijuana from a Schedule I drug (unable to be prescribed, high potential for abuse, not currently accepted for medicinal use, unsafe) to a Schedule II drug (high potential for abuse, currently accepted for medical use, potential for abuse, but prescribable).

This rescheduling petition was initiated by NORML, the Alliance for Cannabis Therapeutics (ACT), and the Cannabis Corporation of America. Of note is the fact that none of these drug-culture organizations has a recognized medical or scientific background, nor do they represent any accredited medical entity.

After substantial legal maneuvering by the drug culture, the DEA carefully documented the case against the rescheduling of marijuana and denied the petition. To examine the potential for therapeutic uses of marijuana, the DEA turned to testimony from nationally recognized experts who rejected the medical use of marijuana (published in the *Federal Register,* December 29, 1989, and March 26, 1992).

In the face of this expert testimony, the drug lobby could only produce anecdotes and the testimony of a handful of physicians with limited or absent clinical experience with marijuana. (Marijuana has not been accepted as a medicine by the AMA, the National Multiple Sclerosis Society, the American Glaucoma Society, the American Academy of Ophthalmology, and the American Cancer Society.)

The drug culture organizations appealed the DEA's decision. Recently, the U.S. Court of Appeals for the District of Columbia denied their petition to reschedule marijuana. This important decision also sets forth the new guideline that only rigorous scientific standards can satisfy the requirement of "currently accepted medical use." These preconditions are:

1. The drug has a known and reproducible chemistry;
2. Adequate safety studies;
3. Adequate and well-controlled studies proving efficacy; and
4. Qualified experts accept the drug.

In addition, the decision stated, "The administrator reasonably accorded more weight to the opinions of the experts than to the laymen and doctors on which the petitioners relied."

In his 1993 book *Marihuana: The Forbidden Medicine,* the psychiatrist Dr. Lester Grinspoon assembled a group of anecdotes to justify the rescheduling of marijuana. Similar to the promarijuana lobby during rescheduling hearings, Grinspoon asserts that marijuana should be used to help relieve nausea (during cancer chemotherapy), glaucoma, wasting in AIDS, depression, menstrual cramps, pain, and virtually unlimited ailments. His anecdotes have no controls, no standardization of dose, no quality control, and no independent medical evaluation for efficacy or toxicity.

Only Anecdotes Prove Its Efficacy

The historical uses of marijuana in such cultures as India, Asia, the Middle East, South Africa, and South America are cited by Grinspoon as evidence of appropriate medical uses of the drug. One of Grinspoon's references is an 1860 assertion that marijuana had supposed beneficial effects "without interfering with the actions of the internal organs" (this is inaccurate). Let us not forget that medicine in earlier years was fraught with potions and remedies. Many of these were absolutely useless or even harmful to unsuspecting subjects. This is when our current FDA [Food and Drug Administration] and drug scheduling processes evolved, which should not be undermined.

The medical marijuana campaign gained momentum in February 1990, when a student project, initiated by Rick Doblin, published interpretations of a questionnaire that he had sent to oncologists. Doblin is closely associated with the Multidisciplinary Association for Psychedelic Studies, a drug-culture lobbying organization. This group strongly supports the legalization and medical uses of the street drugs LSD and MDMA (Ecstasy). Doblin's staff sponsor at Harvard, Mark Kleiman, voiced his support for the legalization of marijuana in his recent book *Against Excess.* Neither author has a medical background, nor do they disclose their intrinsic bias toward the legalization of marijuana.

By manipulation of the statistics, the authors contend that 48 percent of their respondents would prescribe marijuana if legal and 54 percent feel it should be available by prescription. But the researchers fail to relate that the respondents account for only 9 percent of practicing oncologists. Only 6 percent of those surveyed feel that marijuana was effective in 50 percent or more of their patients.

Only 18 percent of the surveyed group believe marijuana to be safe and efficacious. Five percent of those surveyed favor making marijuana available by prescription. These numbers become less significant if compared to the number of all practicing oncologists. Furthermore, this survey was conducted before the release for use of the medication ondansetron (Zofran®), which is extremely effective to relieve the nausea associated with chemotherapy.

Unfortunately, the "results" of this unscientific but well-publicized study incorrectly give the impression that oncologists want marijuana available as medicine. But researchers neither asked if the oncologists had systematically examined their patients for negative effects of marijuana use nor if the oncologists were familiar with the myriad of health consequences of marijuana use. Furthermore, they did not ask oncologists if their attitudes about marijuana were affected by their own current or past marijuana use.

Contrary to the findings of Doblin and Kleiman, Dr. Richard Schwartz determined through a survey of practicing oncologists that THC (the major active ingredient of marijuana) ranked ninth in their preference for the treatment of mild nausea and sixth for the treatment of severe nausea. Only 6 percent had prescribed THC (by prescription or marijuana) for more than 50 patients. It was found that nausea was relieved in only 50 percent of the patients who received THC and that 25 percent had adverse side effects.

Complications of Marijuana Use

According to the 1992 National Household Survey on Drug Abuse, 48 percent of young adults have used marijuana and 11 percent continue to use it. In 1992, 8.2 percent of young adults age 26 to 34 admitted having used marijuana in the last month, a figure that was up from 7.0 percent in 1991. Marijuana remains the most frequently used illegal drug. The chronic use of marijuana has now been demonstrated to lead to higher utilization of the health-care system, a long-suspected phenomenon.

Mental, affective, and behavioral changes are the most easily recognized consequences of marijuana use. Concentration, motor coordination, and memory are adversely impacted. For example, the ability to perform complex tasks such as flying is impaired even 24 hours after the acute intoxication phase. The association of marijuana use with trauma and intoxicated motor vehicle operation is also well established.

Memory is impaired for several months after cessation of use. After chronic use, marijuana addicts admit that their motivation to succeed lessens. Several biochemical models have demonstrated abnormal changes in brain cells, brain blood flow, and brain waves. Pathologic behavior such as psychosis is also associated with marijuana use. The more chronic the use, as would be necessary for treating diseases such as glaucoma, the higher the risk of mental problems.

Despite arguments from the drug culture to the contrary, marijuana is addictive. This addiction has been well described by users. It consists of both a physical dependence (tolerance and subsequent withdrawal) and a psychological habituation. Strangely, in the course of the rescheduling hearings, prodrug organizations admitted that "marijuana has a high potential for abuse and that abuse of the marijuana plant may lead to severe psychological or physical dependence," points that they now publicly deny. Unlike those addicted to many other drugs, the marijuana addict is exceptionally slow to recognize the addiction.

The gateway effect of marijuana is also well established in research. Use of alcohol, tobacco, and marijuana are major risk factors for subsequent addiction and more extensive drug use.

Smoked marijuana contains double to triple the concentrations of tar, carbon monoxide, and carcinogens found in cigarette smoke. Marijuana adversely impairs lung function by causing abnormalities in the cells lining the airways of the upper and lower respiratory tract and in the airspaces deep within the lung. It has been linked to head and neck cancer.

Contaminants of marijuana smoke include certain forms of bacteria and fungi. Users with impaired immunity are at particular risk for disease and infection when they inhale these substances.

Adverse effects of marijuana on the unborn were suspected after studies in Rhesus monkeys demonstrated spontaneous abortion. When exposed to marijuana during gestation, humans demonstrate changes in size and weight as well as neurologic abnormalities. A very alarming association also exists between maternal marijuana use and certain forms of cancer in offspring. Additionally, hormonal function in both male and female children is disrupted.

One of the earliest findings was the negative effect of marijuana on various immune functions, including cellular immunity and pulmonary immunity. Impaired ability to fight infection is now documented in humans who use marijuana. They have been shown to exhibit an inability to fight herpes infections and a blunted response to therapy for genital warts. The potential for these complications exists in all forms of administration of marijuana.

It should be clear that use of the drug bears substantial health risks. In populations at high risk for infection and immune suppression (AIDS and cancer chemotherapy patients), the risks are unacceptable.

Summary

The unfortunate reality is that the drug culture is exploiting the unwitting public and the suffering of patients with chronic illnesses for its own benefit. Under the false and dangerous claims that smoking marijuana is a harmless recreational activity and that it offers significant benefits to those suffering from a variety of tragic ailments, the drug culture seeks to use bogus information to gain public acceptance for the legalization of marijuana.

NO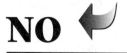

Ethan A. Nadelmann

Reefer Madness 1997: The New Bag of Scare Tactics

T he war on drugs is really a war on marijuana," says professor Lynn Zimmer, a sociologist at Queens College, in New York, who is widely regarded as one of the nation's leading analysts of drug policy. Marijuana, says Zimmer, is the leading justification for drug testing in the workplace, the main target of anti-drug efforts in the schools and the media, and the principal preoccupation of drug warriors in and out of government today. The drug warriors' tactics include—along with arrests, seizures, incarceration and the intimidation of doctors who would prescribe pot for the terminally ill—a more sinister approach. Spokesmen are quoted by journalists and appear on the evening news and on talk shows, making frightening claims about marijuana's harmful effects, spinning unproven theories and, in some cases, distorting the known truth in an effort to demonize even casual users of pot.

It's no wonder that the warriors find themselves in a quandary. They're essentially fighting a war against the 70 million Americans who have tried marijuana, including half of all Americans aged 18–35 and more than a quarter of everyone older than 35. Polls have indicated that a fourth of all adult Americans favor legalizing pot, which, after alcohol, tobacco and caffeine, is the fourth most popular psychoactive drug in the world.

"You can't scare middle-class parents with a war on heroin and cocaine," says Zimmer. "These drugs are too removed, too remote. Marijuana brings it home."

Bill Clinton's administration, desperate not to appear soft on drugs, has indulged in its share of scare tactics. Clinton's newly appointed drug czar, Gen. Barry McCaffrey, has set the tone for the federal government's new stance, threatening sanctions against medical doctors in California and Arizona (RS 750/751), where citizens voted in November to allow the medicinal use of cannabis. More typical, however, is the approach taken by Secretary of Health and Human Services Donna Shalala, who disingenuously told reporters last December [1996], "All available research has concluded that marijuana is dangerous to our health."

Is pot dangerous? Is there any scientific research to back up Shalala's claim? There are, of course, reasons to be concerned about marijuana. It is, like alcohol, a powerful psychoactive drug. Used irresponsibly, it contributes to accidents on the roads and in the workplace. During the period of intoxication, short-term memory is impaired. Heavy pot smokers face some of the same risks as cigarette smokers. And some people become dependent upon marijuana, using it as a crutch to avoid dealing with relationships and responsibilities.

Among kids, especially, it is the daily use of marijuana, not experimental or occasional use, that merits concern. According to the latest annual survey of drug use among high-school students, the percentage of eighth-graders who admit to daily pot smoking increased from 0.2 percent in 1991 to 1.5 percent in 1996. Among 10th-graders, there was an increase from 0.8 percent to 3.5 percent; among seniors, an increase from 2 percent to nearly 5 percent. Of course, smoking marijuana every day would contribute to a teenager's problems in school and socially, but more likely it is an indicator of something else that is basically wrong.

On the other hand, there is ample evidence that the majority of the 70 million Americans who have tried marijuana are doing just fine. Since the early 1970s, the government has funded studies that have ended up proving that pot is not harmful, then disavowed the findings. In 1988, following an extensive review of the scientific evidence on marijuana, the Drug Enforcement Administration's own administrative-law judge, Francis Young, concluded that marijuana "in its natural form is one of the safest therapeutically active substances known to man." Virtually every independent commission assigned to examine the evidence on marijuana and marijuana policy—including the Shafer Commission appointed by President Richard Nixon, a National Academy of Sciences committee in the early 1980s, and numerous others both in the U.S. and abroad—have concluded that marijuana poses fewer dangers to individuals and society than either alcohol or tobacco and should be decriminalized.

And there is little reason to expect anything different from the Clinton administration's January [1997] announcement that it will spend $1 million to review all the evidence on the medical benefits of marijuana. The problem is that no Congress or president has ever had the guts to follow through on the recommendations of independent commissions assigned to balance the risks and harms of marijuana with the risks and harms of marijuana policies. It's still impossible, for instance, for any government official to speak out publicly about the difference between responsible and irresponsible use of marijuana, as they would with alcohol. All marijuana use is defined as drug abuse—notwithstanding extensive evidence that most marijuana users suffer little if any harm. That position may be intellectually and scientifically indefensible, but those in government regard it as politically and legally obligatory.

So the government resorts to scare tactics and misinformation, relying increasingly on three claims: that today's marijuana is much more potent than the version that kids' parents smoked a decade or two ago; that new research has shown the drug to be more dangerous to our health than previously thought; and that marijuana use is a gateway to more dangerous drugs.

Are these claims true? Is today's marijuana much more potent? Is marijuana much more dangerous than previously believed? Is marijuana a "gateway drug"?

Most marijuana researchers depend on government grants to finance their studies. This poses two problems. First, the government tends to encourage and fund only those research proposals that seek to identify harmful effects of marijuana. There are few incentives to investigate the benefits of marijuana, medicinal or otherwise, and little interest in determining either the safety margins of occasional use or ways of reducing the harms of marijuana use. Studies that identify marijuana as harmful are well publicized by the government's public-affairs officers. Findings that fail to confirm any harms are ignored.

Second, few marijuana researchers dare publicly challenge the government's anti-marijuana campaign. Scientists know that the grant-review process can be both scientifically objective and politically subjective. If too many studies fail to identify and emphasize the harms of marijuana, subsequent research proposals may not fare well in grant competitions. It takes a lot of courage for a scientist—dependent upon government grants for his or her livelihood—to raise questions about government policies and statements regarding marijuana. Not many scientists are that brave.

Fortunately, there are a few researchers who maintain their independence. Zimmer, the sociologist at Queens College, and Dr. John P. Morgan, a physician and pharmacologist who teaches at the City University Medical School, in New York, don't rely on government funding. They have recently completed a book, *Marijuana Myths, Marijuana Facts: A Review of the Scientific Evidence,* that systematically analyzes and dissects hundreds of studies on marijuana, including virtually all of those cited by government officials and other anti-drug crusaders to justify the war on marijuana. The result is the most comprehensive and objective review of the scientific evidence on marijuana since the National Institute of Medicine's report in 1982—one that both debunks many of the myths propagated by drug warriors and tells the truth about what is actually known of marijuana's harms and margins of safety. What follows is drawn largely from their work.

The Potency Question

No claim has taken hold so well as the charge that marijuana is much more potent than in the past. "If people . . . confessing to marijuana use in the late '60s . . . sucked in on one of today's marijuana cigarettes, they'd fall down backward," said William Bennett, President George Bush's first drug czar, in 1990. "Marijuana is 40 times more potent today . . . than 10, 15, 20 years ago," another drug czar, Lee Brown, claimed, in 1995. And from the ranking Democrat of the Senate Judiciary Committee, Joseph Biden, in 1996: "It's like comparing buckshot in a shot-gun shell to a laser-guided missile."

Is any of this true? No. Although high-potency marijuana may be more available today than previously, the pharmacological experience of smoking marijuana today is the same as in the 1960s and 1970s. The only data on mari-

juana potency over time comes from the government-funded Potency Monitoring Project at the University of Mississippi. Since 1981, the average THC
(tetrahydrocannabinol, marijuana's principal psychoactive chemical) content
of PMP samples—all of which come from drug seizures by U.S. police agencies—
has fluctuated between 2.28 percent and 3.82 percent. The project's findings
during the 1970s were substantially lower, possibly because the samples were
improperly stored (which can cause degradation of THC) and partly due to an
overdependence on low-grade Mexican "kilobricks." Independent analyses of
marijuana during the 1970s, which included samples from sources other than
police agencies, reported much higher THC levels, ranging from 2 percent to 5
percent, with some samples as high as 14 percent.

Marijuana of less than 0.5 percent potency has almost no psychoactivity;
in fact, in laboratory studies, subjects are often unable to distinguish a placebo
from marijuana with less than 1 percent THC. It's not very likely that marijuana
would have become so popular during the 1970s if the average THC content
had been so low. Today, some regular marijuana users may have access to expensive, high-potency marijuana, often grown indoors under artificial light by
small-scale, low-volume growers. But the potency of the "commercial grade"
marijuana smoked by most Americans is not much different than it was 10, 15
or 20 years ago.

Even if marijuana potency had increased, that would not mean the drug
has necessarily become more dangerous. It is impossible to consume a lethal
dose of marijuana, regardless of its THC content. And in laboratory studies,
smokers often fail to distinguish variations in potency of up to 100 percent. Increases of 200 percent to 300 percent in potency result in only 35 percent to 40
percent increases in smokers' "subjective high" ratings. "Bad trips" and other
adverse psychoactive reactions typically have little to do with marijuana potency. Moreover, when potency increases, smokers tend to smoke less, thus
causing less damage to their lungs.

The bottom line is this: If parents want to know what their kids are smoking today, they need only recall their own experiences. Neither marijuana nor
the experience of smoking marijuana has changed much.

Sex, Health, and Memory

Claims of increased THC potency aside, much of the new war on marijuana relies on claims of new scientific research that shows marijuana to be far more
dangerous than previously thought.

There are tons of anecdotal reports that marijuana enhances sex. And
there are repeated claims that marijuana interferes with male and female sex
hormones, can cause infertility, and produces feminine characteristics in males
and masculine characteristics in females. Speaking at Framingham High
School, in Massachusetts, in late 1994, President Clinton spoke about "the danger of using marijuana, especially to young women, and what might happen to
their child-bearing capacity in the future."

What's the truth? Some animal studies indicate that high doses of THC diminish the production of some sex hormones and may impair reproduction. In human studies, however, scientists typically find no impact on sex-hormone levels. In the few studies that do show some impact, such as lower sperm counts and sperm motility, the effects are modest, temporary and of no apparent consequence for reproductive capacity. A real-life example: Jamaica's Rastafarians, who smoke large amounts of the sacred herb, appear to have no problem making babies.

In 1972, a letter to the *New England Journal of Medicine* described three cases of breast enlargement in men who had smoked marijuana. In 1980, a letter to the *Journal of Pediatrics* described a 16-year-old marijuana smoker who had failed to progress to puberty. Both reports received substantial publicity, but neither has been confirmed through research. But studies involving larger numbers of marijuana users and non-users have found no evidence that marijuana distorts or delays sexual development, masculinizes females or feminizes males. There may be good reasons for telling kids not to smoke marijuana, but the president's warnings were based on myth, not fact.

Now that thousands of people with AIDS are smoking marijuana to stimulate their appetites and promote weight gain, opponents keep insisting that marijuana's damaging effects on the immune system negate any potential benefits. Here again, the claims are based almost entirely on studies in which laboratory animals are given extremely large doses of THC. There's no evidence that marijuana users have higher rates of infectious disease than non-users. That's not to say that there are no dangers. For people with compromised immune systems, smoking can cause lung infections. There is also a risk for AIDS patients that they will contract a pulmonary disease called aspergillosis caused by fungal spores sometimes found on improperly stored marijuana. One solution to this problem would be careful screening of marijuana supplies, a role for the government or pharmaceutical companies. And that is another reason to prescribe legal, controlled marijuana to more than the eight Americans who are now entitled to receive it.

Everyone knows that marijuana—like other psychoactive drugs consumed in sufficient doses—screws up short-term memory. Kids who get high (or drunk) before going to class are less likely to learn what their teachers are trying to teach them. Their minds are more likely to wander. People under the influence of marijuana can remember things they learned previously, but their capacity to learn and recall new information is diminished. Although some find marijuana useful for problem solving and creative tasks, there is little question that marijuana is not conducive to learning in school and other highly structured environments.

The question of whether marijuana use permanently impairs memory and other cognitive functions is a separate issue. During the '70s, the U.S. government funded three comprehensive field studies in Jamaica, Greece and Costa Rica, in which long-term heavy cannabis users and non-users were subjected to a battery of standardized tests of their cognitive functions. The researchers found virtually no differences between the two groups.

More recently, two studies funded by the National Institute on Drug Abuse reported evidence of cognitive harm in high-dose marijuana users. The first, published in *Psychopharmacology,* in 1993, found that heavy marijuana users—who reported seven or more uses per week for an average of 6.5 years—scored lower than non-users on math and verbal tests. But the researchers also found that "intermediate" users—those smoking marijuana five to six times per week—were indistinguishable from non-users.

The second study, published in the *Journal of the American Medical Association,* in 1996, found differences between daily marijuana users and those who smoked fewer than 10 times per month, but the differences were minor. The light smokers performed slightly better on two memory tests and one card-sorting test—while no differences were found on tests of attention, verbal fluency and complex drawing.

What we know now, based on existing research, is that if heavy marijuana use produces cognitive impairment, it is relatively minor—and may have little or no practical significance.

Gateway Drugs?

The "gateway theory," formerly known as the "steppingstone hypothesis," has long been a staple of anti-marijuana campaigns. Marijuana use, it is claimed, leads inexorably to the use of more dangerous drugs like cocaine, heroin and LSD. If we can stop kids from trying marijuana, we can win the drug war.

The most recent, and oft-repeated, version of the gateway theory—an analysis conducted by the National Center on Addiction and Substance Abuse at Columbia University—asserts that youthful marijuana users are 85 times more likely than non-users to use cocaine. To obtain this figure, the proportion of marijuana users who had ever tried cocaine (17 percent) was divided by the proportion of cocaine users who had never used marijuana (0.2 percent). The "risk factor" is large not because so many marijuana users experiment with co-caine—only a minority actually do—but because people who use cocaine, a relatively unpopular drug, are likely to have also used the more popular drug marijuana. Similarly, marijuana users are more likely than non-users to have had previous experience with legal drugs like alcohol, tobacco and caffeine.

Alcohol, tobacco and caffeine do not cause people to use marijuana. And marijuana does not cause people to use cocaine, heroin or LSD. There is no pharmacological basis for the gateway theory, since marijuana does not change brain chemistry in a way that causes drug-seeking, drug-taking behavior. In fact, there is no theory here at all—just a description of the typical sequence in which people who use many drugs begin by using ones that are more common.

The relationship between marijuana use and the use of other drugs is constantly changing. In some societies, marijuana use follows, rather than precedes, use of heroin and other drugs. Among American high-school seniors, the proportion of marijuana users who have tried cocaine decreased from a high of 33 percent, in 1986, to 14 percent, in 1995. Americans who smoke pot may be more likely to try other illegal drugs than those who don't smoke it. But for a large majority of marijuana users, marijuana is a terminus rather than a gateway drug.

"Now we're putting the research into the hands of parents," Donna Shalala claimed at a recent press conference, renewing the government's war against marijuana. But if it's the truth that Shalala wants to distribute, Zimmer and Morgan's *Marijuana Myths, Marijuana Facts* is a better source.

POSTSCRIPT

Is Marijuana Dangerous and Addictive?

Recent initiatives in California and Arizona that bring marijuana closer to being legal are making many people nervous. The propositions in those states would allow the drug to be prescribed by physicians for medicinal purposes. The majority of Americans are against making marijuana completely legal. A compromise would be to decriminalize marijuana, making it neither strictly legal nor illegal. If decriminalized, there would be no penalty for personal or medical use or possession, although there would continue to be criminal penalties for sale for profit and distribution to minors. Marijuana has been decriminalized in a few states, but it is illegal in most of the country.

Decriminalization appeals to attorney Peter Riga, in "The Drug War Is a Crime: Let's Try Decriminalization," *Commonweal* (July 16, 1993); editor Marcia Angell, in "Alcohol and Other Drugs: Toward a More Rational and Consistent Policy," *The New England Journal of Medicine* (August 25, 1994); and journalist Robert Hough, in "Reefer Sadness," *Toronto Globe and Mail* (November 9, 1991). Eric Schlosser, in "Reefer Madness," *The Atlantic Monthly* (August 1994), argues that there are far too many people in jail for marijuana offenses.

In early 1992 the Drug Enforcement Administration published a document stating that the federal government was justified in its continued prohibition of marijuana for medicinal purposes. The report indicated that too many questions surrounded the effectiveness of medicinal marijuana. See "Medical Marijuana: To Prescribe or Not to Prescribe, That Is the Question," *Journal of Addictive Diseases* (vol. 14, 1995) and "The Right Not to Be in Pain: Using Marijuana for Pain Management," *The Nation* (February 3, 2003). The effectiveness of marijuana as therapy for cancer partients and AIDS patients continues to be debated, but the Center on Addiction and Substance Abuse of Columbia University maintains that recent research suggests that the drug is addictive and can wreck the lives of users, particularly teenagers. They argue that legalizing marijuana would undermine the impact of drug education and increase usage.

Other articles that debate the safety and legality of marijuana include "Does Heavy Marijuana Use Impair Human Cognition?" *JAMA* (February 21, 1996); "The Return of Reefer Madness," *The Progressive* (May 1996); "Smoke Alarm," *Reason* (May 1996); "Pot Luck," *National Review* (November 11, 1996); "The Battle for Medical Marijuana," *The Nation* (January 6, 1997); "Federal Foolishness and Marijuana," *The New England Journal of Medicine* (January 30, 1997); "The War Over Weed," *Newsweek* (February 3, 1997); "Prescription Drugs," *Reason* (February 1997); "Marijuana: Useful Medicine or Dangerous Drug?" *Consumers' Research Magazine* (May 1997); "Moving Marijuana," *Reason* (May 1998); "Bad News for Pot Smokers; Ounce for Ounce, a British Study Says, Marijuana

Does More Damage Than Tobacco," *The Report Newsmagazine* (December 16, 2002); "Cannabis Use Among Teens May Lead to Addiction," *Alcoholism & Drug Abuse Weekly* (April 14, 2003); "High Road: Is Marijuana a 'Gateway'?" *Reason* (March 2003). In the following article, marijuana is discussed in a risk versus benefit format: "Is Pot Good for You?" *Time* (November 4, 2002).

On the Internet . . .

American Dietetics Association

This official site of the American Dietetics Association offers FAQs, resources on nutrition and dieting, and a section on hot topics.

http://www.eatright.org/Public/

The Atkins Center

This is the official site of the Atkins Center for Complementary Medicine. This site includes information about Dr. Robert C. Atkins, the Atkins diet, and low-carbohydrate foods.

http://www.atkinscenter.com

Ask Dr. Weil

The Ask Dr. Weil Web site is a question-and-answer forum on a variety of medical topics.

http://www.drweil.com/app=cda/
drw_cda.html-command=Ask-pt=Ask

PART 6

Consumer Health

A *shift is occurring in medical care toward informed self-care. People are starting to reclaim their autonomy, and the relationship between doctor and patient is changing. Many patients are asking more questions of their physicians, considering a wider range of medical options, and becoming more educated about what determines their health. Although most physicians support dietary changes and moderate exercise, critics state that many people who follow diet and nutrition fads may actually develop nutritional deficiencies and increase their risk of physical complications from their diet. Many Americans, disillusioned with traditional medicine, are seeking alternative health providers and alternative health therapies. A debate on whether or not one should combine alternative and conventional medicines is included along with a discussion of multiple-chemical sensitivity, a disease that some assert is real and others state is psychological. This part debates some of the choices consumers may make regarding their health care and diets.*

- Does Multiple-Chemical Sensitivity Pose a Serious Health Threat?

- Is the Atkins Low-Carbohydrate Diet a Valid Weight-Loss Plan?

- Should Alternative Medicine Be Combined With Conventional Medicine?

ISSUE 19

Does Multiple-Chemical Sensitivity Pose a Serious Health Threat?

YES: Paul Yanick, Jr., from "Multiple Chemical Sensitivity: Understanding Causative Factors," *Townsend Letter for Doctors & Patients* (January 2001)

NO: Stephen Barrett, from "MCS: Mis-Concern Serious," *Priorities for Health* (vol. 11, no. 1, 1999)

ISSUE SUMMARY

YES: Journalist Paul Yanick, Jr. states that a condition known as multiple-chemical sensitivity is becoming one of our greatest health challenges.

NO: Psychiatrist Stephen Barrett argues that multiple-chemical sensitivity is an ill-defined problem and that no scientific test has ever provided evidence that it has an organic basis.

Multiple-chemical sensitivity (MCS) is a syndrome in which some individuals report having a wide range of symptoms due to exposure to various levels of chemical substances. The chemicals linked to their symptoms are ones that most people tolerate without any ill effects, and the condition itself cannot be explained in terms of any known medical or psychiatric disease. The development of MCS appears to be a two-stage process that begins with exposure to an environmental substance, such as a pesticide. The sufferer is then sensitized to the substance and begins to develop severe reactions to even tiny amounts of other ordinary chemicals, including air fresheners, perfumes, or aftershave lotion. The reported symptoms vary considerably but often include headaches, dizziness, fatigue, nausea, and muscle aches. These symptoms seem to develop within a fairly short time after some change in that person's environment. In some situations, sufferers are not able to identify the specific cause or trigger that could have led to the onset of the condition.

Mainstream researchers, however, are skeptical of the existence of MCS as a true medical condition. The American Medical Association, the American Academy of Allergy and Immunology, and the American College of Physicians do not accept MCS as an organic disease based on the fact that the syndrome does not generate any objective evidence of disease that can be observed and tested in a clinical setting. The major symptoms are mostly subjective and could be the result of hundreds of other causes. The condition is not associated with any specific substance or with any specific effect. There are also no data to explain how minute amounts of a variety of different substances could produce the many adverse health effects. Finally, most individuals with the condition appear to look perfectly healthy even though they self-report a broad range of symptoms that could lead to partial or total disability. Many patients state that they can no longer participate in their daily activities such as working, shopping, or eating in restaurants.

MCS has also become an economic, political, and social phenomenon. Many chemical manufacturing companies have become the target of groups supporting the sufferers of MCS. Multiple-chemical sensitivity has even been defined as a disability under the Americans With Disabilities Act, allowing those with the disease to receive special accommodations at school or in the workplace. Some states, under workers compensation laws, provide sufferers with free medical care and payment for lost wages.

Clearly, more research on MCS is needed. Whether more studies will confirm that MCS is or is not a disease remains to be seen. MCS patients, regardless of the findings, believe that they are the victims of a toxic, chemical environment.

In the following selections, Paul Yanick, Jr. contends that escalating levels of toxins build up in the body and can exceed the body's capability to detoxify them, resulting in MCS. Stephen Barrett argues that the symptoms of MCS most likely have an emotional basis and are not a response to single or multiple toxins.

Paul Yanick, Jr. 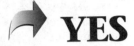 **YES**

Multiple Chemical Sensitivity: Understanding Causative Factors

Increasing worldwide pollution coupled with overcrowding, contaminated water and food, and indoor air contaminants gives a friendly welcome to a wide spectrum of serious and complex diseases. Escalating levels of these pollutants build up in the body and can exceed and incapacitate the body's natural detoxification capabilities, weakening immunity to the point where Multiple Chemical Sensitivity (MCS), chronic and fatal infections, and cancer are becoming our greatest health challenges. With the continual rise of cancer and the increase of many treatment-resistant syndromes, many professionals are challenged with multisystem, complex disorders that do not respond to their best clinical efforts.

Indoor air contaminants from the widespread use of synthetic cleaning agents and synthetic colognes, perfumes, body care products, and air fresheners wreck havoc with immune functions of the body. These pollutants infiltrate and damage delicate detoxification mechanisms of the body and rapidly deplete the body's nutrient reserves of precursors and co-factors needed by the liver to keep toxins from suppressing immunity and congesting the lymphatic system.

The prevalence of MCS is greater among individuals with a history of childhood allergies or who were not breast fed. Between 15 and 37% of the American population consider themselves sensitive or allergic to chemicals, car exhaust, tobacco smoke, air fresheners, and the scents of many common household cleaning agents and body care products. Only 5% of the these allergic individuals are actually diagnosed with MCS. Symptoms of MCS may include headaches, seizures, fainting, dizziness, extreme fatigue, muscle or joint pain, asthma, sinusitis, insomnia, irregular heartbeat, maldigestion, depression, anxiety or panic attacks, and skin disorders.

The best way to understand what MCS is—and what it is not—is to see how it affects the lives of people who have it. Many of the symptoms of MCS have serious implications and social effects that demand more public and professional understanding. Many MCS individuals experience personality changes—becoming angry, irritated, anxious, fearful, and lethargic—when exposed to certain chemicals. Most sufferers find it impossible to live a normal life. Shopping and the normal social routines of life can result in acute brain and nervous system reactions, an inability to breathe or a feeling of suffocation, intense headaches, dizziness, brain fog and short-term memory disorders, muscle spasms, and convulsions. Sadly, in an attempt to avoid these symptoms, MCS individuals experience isolation and withdrawal as they are often left with no choice but to avoid social situations where a given chemical could potentially trigger a serious or near fatal allergic reaction.

Problems with chemical sensitivity can occur at a number of different levels and in a number of different ways. Symptoms may be silent and internal, producing a symptom pattern that may be diagnosed as ADD [attention deficit disorder] or fibromylagia earlier in life. Indeed, many inflammatory disorders such as fibromylagia involve the excess storage of toxins in the joints and connective tissue. Many of these patients are resistant to treatment and continue to suffer because they and their doctors are not aware of the hidden and toxic effects of synthetic chemicals that are used in their body care and household products on a daily basis. When these irritating substances are eliminated from their body and home environment and other causative factors are corrected, many will respond in a positive manner to alternative health care approaches that previously yielded no results. Unknown to most consumers, 95% of most fragrances are synthetic compounds (acetone, camphor, benzene, ethanol, g-terpinene, propylene glycol, sodium lauryl sulfate, parabens) that deplete detoxification mechanisms and suppress immunity.

In the early stages of this illness, many patients with MCS are misdiagnosed with allergies, migraine headaches, sinusitis, asthma, while the real causes (indoor air pollution, dental foci and silent chronic infections, nutritional deficiencies and dietary factors, and toxicity) remain obscured and masked by antihistamines, decongestants, anti-inflammatory drugs, and cortisone. Taking a careful history of MCS patients along with energetic and biochemical testing may reveal clues as to why their body's detoxification are failing and why they can't disarm and excrete toxins in a healthy and natural way.

More and more practitioners are discovering that Native American medicine, Ayurvedic medicine, Chinese herbal medicine, homeopathy, nutrition, and Acupuncture have virtually little or no effect on counteracting these effects of MCS and repairing the resultant damage to the immune and neuroendocrine system in these cases. Treatment-resistant syndromes are increasing at an alarming rate as many traditional and natural methods fail to *stabilize* neuroendocrine balance, cellular physiology, and augment optimal detoxification of the kidneys, liver and lymphatic system. Clearly, natural health care practitioners of the 21st Century need to focus more on novel methods of nourishing and detoxifying patients that respond poorly or not at all to traditional or ancient healing systems. With immunomodulation and broad spectrum detoxification methods they will be able to free the body of trapped cellular and lymph toxins that cause MCS and immunosuppression.

With the view of an escalating toxic environment in mind, Quantum Medicine™ practitioners are being trained to assess the body's toxic stress factors and detoxification pathways to determine adjunctive support therapies/

supplements that permit deep detoxification of impregnated and layered toxins within the body's tissues and cells. By addressing specific patterns of biophysical and biomolecular dysfunction underlying an individual's illness along with traditional assessment, innovative methods of meridian stress measurement that emphasize the correct sequence of testing and interpretations of indicator drops and CRT thermography, practitioners can eliminate guesswork and make more intelligent decisions regarding ways to augment the body's innate ability to detoxify itself. In this quest for more accurate details regarding the effects of human toxicity, the dynamic equilibrium between the human energy system and the physical body makes the clinical picture clearer and gives both the patient and practitioner a deeper understanding of why and how the body becomes allergic or develops MCS.

For example, I have explained the importance of using novel detoxification approaches and emphasized how xenoestrogens can disrupt hormone functions or mimic hormones and wreak havoc by scrambling hormonal messages, inducing oxidative stress.[1-6] With this kind of chaos and disorganization in the body, toxins can sabotage fertility, weaken the immune system, accelerate aging, erode intelligence, and activate cytokine-driven inflammatory processes that lead to the onset of many high-profile diseases.

As the by-products from living in a highly industrialized world increase, it is critical that the body's internal regulation and communication system—involving hormones, neurotransmitters, hormone-like molecules, and energetic information—is assessed, stabilized, and balanced. This energetic connection to organ and glandular regulation have been elucidated by Dr. Omura who found hormones and neurotransmitters unique to each meridian within the boundary of most acupuncture points and on the surface of meridian lines.[7] Moreover, these energetic connections have been known to the Chinese for more than 4000 years. The energetic connections between the organs of detoxification and their allergic or MCS-related manifestations are caused, in part, by excess energy or inferior energy that is transported via acupuncture lines from the liver, pancreas, to the head and skin where they cause irritation and prolonged inflammation. Our clinical research and that of other practitioners has shown that the meridian connections to the teeth can trigger MCS symptoms by blocking detoxification functions of the liver and kidney and congesting the lymphatics with toxins or pleomorphic infections. The following dental factors may be involved as causative factors in MCS:

1. Tooth decay
2. Ostitis or jaw bone infections
3. Infected root canal teeth
4. Infected dental nerve
5. Gum infection
6. TMJ [temporomandibular joint] disorders
7. Dental material sensitivity
8. Dental material toxicity
9. Electrical current generation from metal fillings.

According to US government standards, silver fillings typically emit mercury vapor in the average mouth that is 80 times above the established safety limits for mercury vapor exposure. Moreover, these metal fillings can generate electrical currents that disturb and disrupt meridian-organ bioregulation. The interplay between dental foci and specific organs of the body is seriously underestimated by both traditional and holistic dentists. With the help of new electrodermal biofeedback procedures and CRT thermography, doctors are now able to locate and treat hidden dental foci and eliminate MCS symptoms whereas prior to dental treatment these patients did not respond to our best treatment efforts. It is important to note that in many of these cases, dental X-rays and exams were normal despite infection being obvious after laser surgery, laser root canals, or extractions. Acupuncture lines of energy flow influence the teeth-organ and teeth-sense organ connections and are commonly responsible for nasal reactions, headaches, and eye and ear symptoms of MCS and other immunological disorders.

The meridian stress measurement techniques described by the author are not to be confused with many similar, although not authentic, schools that teach electrodermal screening and assessment of the human energy system. Quantum medicine™ practitioners have discovered that many of these test methods are wrongly interpreted and fail to uncover sensitive and deep electromagnetic information in MCS and other chronically ill patients. Presently, board-certification and the standardization of quantum medical protocols will bring into sharp focus the patterns of energetic dysregulation that disturb organ functions, cause spinal segments, weaken endocrine glands, and induce inflammation and acute stress to the joints, muscles, and sense organs of the body. Quantum Medicine™ provides truly holistic, causal and individualized therapy in order to define dysregulation and then with the use of bioresonance, light beam photon generator therapies, meridian-matched resonant complexes (quantum nutrition) in order to slowly bring the body back into healthy patterns of bioregulation. It is only when bioregulation is restored that the body's innate, self-healing abilities can be activated more fully and with greater power. MCS is so complex that the assessment of disturbed oscillations from atoms, molecules, cells, tissues, organs and organ systems is necessary and this assessment yields extremely helpful information and helps a high percentage of treatment-resistant patients to re-regulate and activate their own self-healing mechanisms.

Computerized regulation thermography is helpful in revealing stagnant lymph flow, dental foci, and dysregulation of the extracellular matrix where many MCS patients seem to have high levels of toxicity. In many cases, lymph nodes become swollen and congested, losing their ability to protect the body against infection and other chemical stress factors. Since lymph capillaries, unlike the blood, are very permeable to proteins and foreign toxins, dental toxins and infections, these factors slowly find their way into lymph channels and clog and choke off the lymph-generated immune responses. Pleomorphic infections from dental factors, food, and airborne microbes can lead to serious incapacitating infections. Already, millions of Americans have infection with 1,500 people dying of septic shock every day. *Endotoxins,* the deadly agents of sepsis, can leak into the lymph system and organs from infected root canals or extraction sites with deep, hidden pockets of infection. These dental stressors can alter genetic expression and cause massive inflammation accompanied by blood clots in small blood vessels with concomitant damage of the lymphatic system and organs of the body. These proinflammatory states of abnormal physiology make the body extremely sensitive to chemicals and odors, leading to MCS and lifelong allergic symptoms that require seasonal or constant medication. And, in a high percentage of cases, these infections may lead to the virus proliferation, tumor formation and serious life-threatening illness.

There is chronic malnourishment in MCS patients and this is evident even when they take nutritional supplements and eat a healthy nutritional diet. The inefficient nutrient uptake by the villus cells in their stress-damaged gut interferes with the assimilation of co-factor/precursor nutrients used by the liver to detoxify the body, manufacture hormones, neurotransmitters, and immune factors. In these cases, the use of carriers and co-transporters to form whole complexes of nutrients improves the clinical outcome. Why? Nutrients can be transported via the villus cells to the cells of the body more efficiently with this nutrient delivery system. In addition, carrier proteins facilitate greater diffusion into the liver and immune system and can be used to help the immune system police the body and counteract potential toxic or allergic reactions in MCS patients.

Effective detoxification in MCS patients requires consideration of the fact that many carcinogens, transformed by normal enzyme activity, become strong *electrophiles* (electron-deficient molecules) and react with electron-rich molecules such as proteins and DNA. When an electrophile binds to DNA it becomes a powerful carcinogen that alters the structure of DNA causing mistranslations or DNA replication to be misread causing mutations and defective DNA repair mechanisms. In addition, this scenario depletes electrons. And, a deficiency of electrons creates less coherent RNA and DNA patterns. Our research and that of other practitioners using electromagnetic photon generator therapies demonstrates that electrophiles and protein clusters that trigger pain, inflammatory disorders, and many complex, multi-system illnesses can be effectively detoxified and excreted through lymphatic therapies and supplements that incorporate carrier proteins and co-transporters.

A wide array of bioactive compounds in plants, especially in medicinal mushrooms, have been shown to augment deficient immune functions and *modulate* powerful immune responses while specific phytochemicals can increase cellular levels of glutathione transferase and glucuronyl transferase to facilitate the destruction of reactive electrophiles and oxidants into innocuous, excretable metabolites.[8–16] Yet the increasing level of toxicity in supplements presents a serious challenge to the MCS patient in search of natural solutions for their disorder. We have uncovered that over 90% of natural supplements contain one or more toxic ingredients that trigger MCS symptoms. These toxic ingredients silently suppress immunity and slowly increase chemical sensitivities in these patients. Our research on the toxicity of supplements is confirmed by *in vitro* screening studies of 196 natural products that found 191 toxic or ineffective with only 5 or 2.5% non-toxic.[17]

In summary, most MCS patients have symptoms that are triggered by toxicity, cellular acidosis, dehydration and tissue hypoxia, and uncompensated dental disorders or silent chronic infections that lead to the functional impairment of immune cells, disorganization and chaos in the immune system, and chronic acidification and congestion of the lymphatic system. Most importantly, the integrity and balance of the acupuncture meridian system is crucial to detecting the causes of MCS and other treatment-resistant syndromes. Clinical methods need to be adapted to the increase in environmental toxicity that stresses patients and supplements must be chemically and energetically free of toxic resonances and effects. Clearly, the old practices of Traditional Chinese Medicine, although valid and beneficial, were developed thousands of years ago when the planet was not as polluted and food was not genetically-engineered, toxic or depleted in nutrients. The same holds true for ancient healing systems such as Native American medicine, Ayurvedic medicine, and even homeopathic medicine. Quantum medicine™ and quantum nutrition™ practitioners are being trained to use non-toxic, clinically-effective supplements that contain the correct resonances of healthy organs, glands and systems of the body along with the proper, pure and superior nourishment to support and strengthen weak physiology. The powerful synergism of using individualized and tested complexes of supplements to eliminate body stressors and upregulate nutrient uptake, allows the body to discharge toxins, eliminate opportunistic infections, and correct nutritional deficiency states in the shortest time possible.

References

1. Yanick P. Meridian/Organ Nutraceutic Resonant Complexes: New Hope for Chronically-Sick Individuals. *Townsend Letter for Doctors & Patients,* May, 2000, 136–39.
2. Yanick P. Lymphatic Therapy for Chronic Immune & Metabolic Disorders, Detoxification and Successful Pain Elimination. *Townsend Letter for Doctors,* January 1995, 34–40.
3. Yanick P. New Insights into Brain Fog, Memory & Learning Disorders, Insomnia, Anxiety, Depression and Immune Disorders. *Townsend Letter for Doctors & Patients,* June, 2000, 154–56.
4. Yanick P. Hormone Resistance and the Ground Regulation System. *Townsend Letter for Doctors & Patients,* January 1999, 88–90.
5. Yanick, P. *Quantum Medicine,* Writer Service Publications, Portland, Oregon, 2000.
6. Yanick, P. Boosting Nutrient Uptake in Chronic Illness, *Townsend Letter for Doctors & Patients,* December 2000.
7. Omura Y Connections found between each meridian & organ representation area of corresponding internal organs in each side of the cortex; release of common neurotransmitters and hormones unique to each meridian and corresponding organ point. *Acupuncture & Electro-therapeutics Research* 1989, 14:155–86.
8. Huang MT et al. *Food Phytochemicals for Cancer Prevention—American Chemical Society Symposium* 546, Washington DC: American Chemical Society 1994, 546.
9. *Cancer Causes, Occurrence and Control—IARC* Scientific Publication 2, 1991.
10. Borchers, AT et al. Mushrooms, tumors, and immunity *Proceedings of the Society of Experimental Biological Medicine,* 1999, 4:282–93.

11. Hamano K et al. The preoperative administration of lentinan ameliorated the impairment of NK activity after cardiopulmonary bypass. *International Journal of Immunopharmacology* 1999, 21(8)531–40.

12. Lin CY. Inhibition of activated human mesangial cell proliferation by the natural product Cordyceps sinensis: An implication for treatment of IgA mesangial nephropathy. *Journal of Laboratory & Clinical Medicine,* 1999, 133(1), 55–63.

13. Nakamura k. Activation of in vivo Kupffer cell function by oral administration of Cordyceps. *Japanese Journal of Pharmacology,* 1999; 79(3), 335–41.

14. Odani, S et al. The inhibitory properties and primary structure of a novel serine protienase inhibitor from the fruiting body of the basidiomycete, Lentinus edodes. *European Journal of Biochemistry,* 1999, 262 (3), 915–23.

15. Nanba H. Activity of maitake D-fraction to inhibit carncinogenesis and metastasis. *The Annals of NY Academy of Science,* 1995, 768: 243–5.

16. Zhu M et al. Triterpene antioxidants from ganoderma lucidum. *Phytotherapy Research* 1999, (6), 529–31.

17. See, D. *Journal of the American Nutraceutical Association,* 1996, Vol 2:1, 25–41.

MCS: Mis-Concern Serious

The notion of sensitivities to chemicals has broad appeal, even among persons who do not believe they have such a condition. Contributors to its appeal include environmental worries; concern about victimization; distrust of government, high technology, and standard medicine; and widespread interest in "alternative medicine."

"Multiple chemical sensitivity" [MCS] refers to an ill-defined problem whose sufferers misinterpret physical responses to irritants or to stress as allergies or "toxicities" and behave abnormally. Clinicians who advocate the MCS diagnosis assert that chemicals present in the environment at extremely low levels are to blame. But no scientific tests have ever yielded evidence that MCS has an organic basis. Moreover, no major medical organization has acknowledged MCS as a clinical (objective) disease. Advocates of the MCS diagnosis do not pursue well-designed research to test their claims. Rather, they propagandize their claims through publications, talk shows, "support groups," lawsuits, and political maneuvering.

Clinical diseases that the biomedical community has acknowledged—coronary heart disease, diabetes, and rheumatoid arthritis, for example—relate to clear-cut patient histories, physical findings, and lab tests. In contrast, with MCS the range of symptoms is virtually endless; the onset can be abrupt or gradual and may or may not be linked to any specific exposure or causal factor; and symptoms can vary in intensity, can "come and go," and typically do not correspond to objective physical findings and laboratory findings. For these reasons, standard medical textbooks do not list MCS as a diagnosis; nor does the standard reference book that classifies medical conditions (*International Classification of Diseases, Ninth Edition, Clinical Modification*).

Seconding That Emotion

Medical scholars realized more than a century ago that fatigue, pressure in the head, inability to concentrate, irritability, and many other common symptoms could have an emotional basis. One doctor who understood this was John Noland MacKenzie, M.D., an ear, nose and throat specialist in Baltimore, Mary-

From Stephen Barrett, "MCS: Mis-Concern Serious," *Priorities for Health*, vol. 11, no. 1 (1999). Copyright © 1999 by The American Council on Science and Health, 1995 Broadway, New York, NY 10023-5800. http://www.acsh.org and http://www.healthfactsandfears.com. Reprinted by permission.

land. In 1886 he wrote about a 32-year-old woman who believed she was sensitive to many environmental factors, especially the scent of roses. The woman had bouts of depression and numerous other complaints, including impairment of mental ability, irritability, malaise, and sneezing. MacKenzie did not believe that rose pollen was responsible for the woman's symptoms. So he obtained a realistic artificial rose and, to remove potential allergens from it, cleaned it carefully. During the woman's next visit, he found that she felt she was unusually well. Then he produced the artificial rose, which had been behind a screen, and kept it in his hand as they talked. Almost immediately, the woman's eyes began tearing and became red and itchy; her throat became itchy; her nose became runny and its membranes swelled; and she became hoarse and short of breath. When MacKenzie revealed the deception to his patient, she appeared amazed, but within a few days she could smell real roses uneventfully.

In the 1980s, in Denver, Colorado, allergist John Selner, M.D., and psychologist Herman Staudenmayer, Ph.D., tested many patients who believed they were hypersensitive to workplace and residential chemicals at low levels. In one experiment they used an environmental chamber that enabled exposing each of 20 such patients, unawares, to specific chemicals at specific levels. In preliminary tests, when the patients were made aware of the exposures beforehand, they consistently reported symptoms they had been associating with chemical exposures. Then the patients were randomly exposed to: (1) chemicals to which they considered themselves sensitive; (2) the same chemicals masked by the odor of anise oil, cinnamon oil, lemon oil, peppermint spirit, or another substance; (3) the odorous substance used to mask the suspect chemical; or (4) clean air. After each test period, the patients were asked whether they thought they had been exposed to a suspect chemical or to clean air. The patients were monitored for objective signs (such as skin reactions). They were also asked to report any symptoms experienced during testing and during the following three days. None of the 20 patients demonstrated a response pattern that implicated the chemicals they considered responsible for their symptoms. Nearly all reported an *absence* of symptoms at least once when the suspect chemical was present. Most reported symptoms at least once when the suspect chemical was absent. It became clear that many of the subjects had been reacting not to the chemicals they considered at fault but to their own feelings about the test. Informing the patients of this helped recovery in some cases.

What Isn't MCS?

About 50 years ago allergist Theron G. Randolph, M.D., concluded that patients had become ill from exposures to substances at levels far below those that experts consider safe. He asserted that humankind's failure to adapt to modern manmade chemicals had resulted in a new form of chemical sensitivity. Over the years the condition he posited has been called "allergic toxemia," "cerebral allergy," "chemical sensitivity," "ecologic illness," "environmental illness," "immune system dysregulation," "total allergy syndrome," "20th century disease," "universal allergy," and other names that suggest various physical causal factors. "Multiple chemical sensitivity" is the favorite.

The complaints associated with these labels include chest pain, constipation, diarrhea, depression, dizziness, drowsiness, fatigue, forgetfulness, frequency of urination, headache, inability to concentrate or to think clearly, irritability, itchiness of the eyes and nose, lightheadedness, mental exhaustion (also called "brain fog" or "brain fag"), mood swings, muscle and joint pain, muscle incoordination, nasal stuffiness, rashes, sneezing, wheezing, stomach upset, swelling of various parts of the body, and tingling of fingers and toes. William J. Rea, M.D., who says he has treated more than 20,000 environmentally ill patients, has stated that such persons "may manifest any symptom in the textbook of medicine."

Most physicians who "diagnose" and treat MCS call themselves "clinical ecologists" or "specialists in environmental medicine." About 400 such doctors belong to the American Academy of Environmental Medicine, which Randolph founded in 1965 as the Society for Clinical Ecology. Most of its members are M.D.s and osteopaths. Clinical ecologists also figure in the American Academy of Otolaryngic Allergy, which Randolph helped to found in 1941. Clinical ecology has never been established as a medical specialty, is not advocated in any standard medical textbook, and is not a component of medical-school or specialty training programs. Environmental medicine is a component of the specialty of preventive medicine (public health) but does not embrace the theories and practices of clinical ecology. To avoid confusion, I refer to all self-styled "specialists in environmental medicine" who advocate such theories and practices as "clinical ecologists."

What Doesn't Trigger MCS?

Many proponents of the MCS concept depict the immune system as a barrel that continually fills with chemicals and overflows, whereupon symptoms arise. Some further claim that just one serious episode of infection, psychological stress, or chemical exposure can trigger "immune system dysregulation." Possible MCS-related stressors supposedly include practically any substance common in industrialized areas, for example: building materials; cedar closets; certain plastics; diesel exhaust; felt-tip pens; fragrances; fresh paint or tar; gas for cooking and heating; household cleansers; medications; newsprint; organic solvents and pesticides; permanent press and synthetic textiles; rubbing alcohol; tap water; tobacco smoke; urban air; and even electromagnetic forces. Proponents of the MCS diagnosis also assert:

- that a substance may be an adverse factor even if it has no effect alone, because different substances at low levels can augment or multiply one another's effects;
- that hypersensitivity develops when the "total body load" of physical and psychologic stresses exceeds one's tolerance; and
- that once the process of chemical sensitivity begins, new sensitivities can develop rapidly and from diminishingly low exposures.

These speculations clash with what is known in the fields of human physiology, pathology, toxicology, clinical medicine, and allergy and immunology. No known mechanism explains how chemicals at low levels, or how widely assorted chemicals, might interact adversely with numerous organ systems. Moreover, if the "total body load" concept were valid, low-level exposure to many unrelated chemicals (as well as infections and psychological stress) would have the same effects as high-level exposure to a single chemical—which is not so. The physiologic effects of chemicals are specific, and levels of exposure fix the development and severity of these effects.

Dubious Diagnosis

Clinical ecologists typically "diagnose" MCS in a large proportion of their patients. Their diagnostic evaluation usually involves taking an "ecological oriented history," performing a physical, and ordering lab tests. The history-taking procedure may include the patient's filling out a long questionnaire that focuses on dietary habits and exposure to environmental chemicals. The relevance of findings from physical exams to MCS is unclear, as no combination of such findings can validate a diagnosis of MCS. And findings from standard allergy tests are often normal in MCS patients.

The test clinical ecologists consider paramount is called "provocation–neutralization." During this procedure, the patient is asked to report any symptoms that develop after various substances under suspicion have been placed under the tongue or injected into the skin. If the patient reports symptoms, the test is considered positive, and the substance considered causal is administered in various concentrations until the symptoms are "neutralized." In addition, the clinical ecologist may prescribe other substances, such as hormones and food extracts, as "neutralizing" agents. "Neutralization" superficially resembles the desensitization process that allergists use. But allergists test for—and treat their patients with substances that can elicit—measurable allergic reactions. In contrast, clinical ecologists base their diagnostic and treatment decisions on subjective responses. Many use tests related to immune function or to exposure to specific chemicals. Samples of blood, urine, body fat, and hair may be tested for various environmental chemicals. Blood may be tested to determine levels of immunoglobulins, other immune complexes, lymphocytes, and "antipollutant enzymes." Some of these tests lack both standardization and a protocol that has proved reliable. Moreover, it has not been demonstrated that any of these tests yields data that enable distinguishing persons with MCS.

Some treatments are based on blood tests that enable detecting chemicals in concentrations of parts per billion. Thus, clinically insignificant levels may be misinterpreted as evidence of unusual and harmful exposure. If any "toxin" level is deemed abnormal, the clinical ecologist may prescribe a "detoxification" or "purification" regimen to remove undesirable chemicals from the body. Such regimens may include exercise, "herbal wraps," massage, saunas, showers, megavitamin therapy, self-injection of "neutralizing" agents, and the use of devices for purifying air and water.

Researchers at the University of California conclusively debunked provocation– neutralization in the early 1980s. The test sites were the offices of the clinical ecologists who had been treating the subjects. During three-hour sessions, the patients received three injections of suspect food extracts and nine injections of normal saline (dilute salt water). Sixteen patients were tested once, and two were tested twice. In "nonblinded" trials, the patients reported symptoms whenever food extracts were injected, and they consistently reported an absence of symptoms when normal saline was injected. In double-blind trials, however, they developed symptoms with 16 (27%) of the 60 food-extract injections and with 44 (24%) of the 180 saline injections. The symptoms that accompanied the food-extract injections and those that accompanied the saline injections were identical and included: abdominal discomfort; aches in the legs; breathing difficulty; burning or watering of the eyes; chills; coughing; depression; disorientation; dizziness; dryness of the mouth; a feeling of fullness in or plugging of the ears; a feeling of tightness or pressure in the head; headache; intestinal gassiness or rumbling; nasal itching; nausea; nervousness; an odd taste; ringing of the ears; scratchiness of the throat; tingling of the face or scalp; and tiredness. The researchers thus demonstrated that the patients' symptoms were placebo effects; i.e., that the symptoms resulted from undergoing the experiment rather than from any chemical exposure.

They also debunked the claim that administering the offending substances at "neutralizing" doses can relieve the patient's symptoms: The responses to food-extract injections of each of the seven patients who had been "treated" during the experiment had been equivalent to their responses to saline injections.

Questionable Treatment

How clinical ecologists treat illness is as questionable as how they diagnose it. They usually emphasize avoidance of suspect substances and prescribe lifestyle changes that range from small alterations to sweeping transformations. For example, they generally instruct their patients to modify their diets and to avoid such items as aftershave; automobile exhaust; cigarette smoke; deodorants; scented shampoos; and carpets, clothing, and furniture that contain synthetic fibers. More extreme restrictions that clinical ecologists prescribe include wearing a charcoal-filter mask, using a portable oxygen device, staying home for months, relocating, quitting a job, and avoiding physical contact with members of one's family. Clinical ecologists also advise many patients to take vitamin, mineral, and other supplements. "Neutralization therapy," which is based on provocation–neutralization findings, may include the administration of extracts under the tongue or by injection.

Many experts have concluded that the basis of MCS is psychologic rather than physical. Many MCS patients suffer from an emotional problem termed "somatization disorder." This is characterized by persistent symptoms that no known medical condition can fully explain but that may require medical treatment. Some MCS patients are paranoids, who are prone to believe that their problems have external causes. Others suffer from agoraphobia, depression, panic disorder, or other anxiety states that induce physical reactions. Many patients are relieved when a clinical ecologist offers what they think they need and encourages them to participate actively in their recovery. But the "treatment" MCS patients receive may do them much more harm than good. ACSH scientific advisor Ronald E. Gots, M.D., Ph.D., president of the International Center for Toxicology and Medicine, in Rockville, Maryland, reviewed the medical records of more than a hundred MCS patients and concluded:

> Unlike many alternative medical practices, the diagnosis of MCS begins a downward spiral of fruitless treatments, culminating in . . . withdrawal from society and condemning the sufferer to a life of misery and disability. . . . The diagnosis is far more disabling than the symptoms.

Political Action

To mandate that public places be designed or redesigned to accommodate variable and unpredictable individual responses is unfair. Yet MCS support groups have lobbied to persuade employers and government agencies to adopt policies that "accommodate employees and members of the public disabled by chemical barriers." Such groups have demanded:

- better ventilation systems;
- purchase of only the "least toxic/allergenic" building materials and office furniture, equipment, and supplies;
- prenotifying employees of any construction or remodeling in which an adhesive, carpet shampoo, floor wax, paint, or a solvent will be applied; and
- the proscribing of (a) air fresheners, (b) smoking in or near workplaces, (c) synthetic lawn chemicals near workplaces, and (d) except in emergencies, pesticides indoors.

Many MCS patients would have their workplaces completely odorless—without, for example, the scents of colognes and fragrant hygiene products. But attempts to accommodate persons who consider themselves sensitive to chemicals are often futile. The most publicized example of such futility is Ecology House, an eight-unit "safe house" in San Rafael, California. The U.S. Department of Housing and Urban Development (HUD) contributed $1.2 million toward the project's total cost of $1.8 million. A lottery decided which of 100 applicants around the U.S. would become tenants. Although the building was designed to be "free" of synthetic chemicals, most of the initial tenants said it sickened them.

Legal Mischief

Many people who say they have MCS have filed lawsuits claiming that exposure to environmental chemicals and particular foods has made them ill. Many of these suits allege that chemical exposures cause disease by injuring the immune system. This notion is maintained by professionals who misinterpret laboratory data so that the data look like evidence of a correlation between virtually any symptom and exposure to almost anything. Some plaintiffs have not complained of physical ills but rather have alleged that low-level exposure to environmental chemicals affected their immune systems and may eventually predispose them to cancer or to other diseases. Some plaintiffs have even sought damages for emotional distress that they've ascribed to an alleged toxic exposure.

Claims and lawsuits have also been filed to obtain workers' compensation and Social Security Disability benefits. Some courts have accepted MCS as a compensable occupational disease or a disability. But even a court that does not regard MCS as such may neglect causation and award benefits to a plaintiff it considers disabled by a somatization disorder or by another psychologic impairment.

Cumulative or high-level exposure to toxic chemicals can, of course, injure persons. But many MCS–related lawsuits rest on laboratory detection of insignificant traces of chemicals or on a small deviation from normal in some measure of immune function.

A 1993 U.S. Supreme Court decision strengthened the ability of judges to exclude unscientific testimony. Rule 702 of the Federal Rules of Evidence states that "expert testimony" is admissible if it is relevant and the witness is qualified by knowledge, skill, experience, training, or education. In *Daubert v Merrell Dow* the court upheld this rule and stated:

> The trial judge must determine at the outset. . . . whether the expert is proposing to testify to (1) scientific knowledge that (2) will assist the trier of fact to understand or determine a fact in issue. This entails a preliminary assessment of whether the reasoning or methodology underlying the testimony is scientifically valid and of whether the reasoning or methodology properly can be applied to the facts in issue.

Since 1993 many judges have, on this basis, not permitted advocates of the MCS diagnosis to testify as experts.

Public Protection Is Needed

Meaningful research on the prevalence of a condition cannot be performed without clear-cut criteria for diagnosing it. None of the proposed definitions of "multiple chemical sensitivity" and its synonyms meets this standard. Yet hundreds of thousands of tax dollars have been wasted on such studies.

Meanwhile, clinical ecologists are emotionally and financially exploiting persons who think they have MCS. Moreover, dubious claims for disability benefits and damages burden insurance companies, employers, educational facilities, homeowners, other taxpayers, and, ultimately, all citizens.

These problems can be reduced by establishing comprehensive, government-supported treatment programs that include environmental-chamber testing for chemical sensitivities. Whenever no chemical sensitivities are found, the psychologic nature of the problem can be clarified and the patient treated accordingly.

To protect the public, state licensing boards should scrutinize the practices of clinical ecologists and decide whether the overall quality of their patient care warrants permitting them to practice medicine. I believe that most of them should be delicensed.

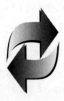

POSTSCRIPT

Does Multiple-Chemical Sensitivity Pose a Serious Health Threat?

Hundreds of personal injury lawsuits have been filed against the manufacturers of carpets, paints, and household cleaners stating that the products have triggered multiple-chemical sensitivities. While many of these suits have been dismissed or settled out of court, cases continue to be filed. See "Carpet Politics and Alternatives: Chemicals Given Off by Carpeting Found to Cause Health Problems," *Townsend Letter for Doctors and Patients* (August 2001).

In 1998 the federal government convened a panel to evaluate and review the scientific literature on MCS and to develop recommendations on policy and technical issues. The interagency work group called for additional research that would focus on the condition's mechanism of action. The group also demanded more education and information to raise understanding and awareness of the problem by doctors.

More recently, a delegation from the Chemical Injury Information Network (CIIN) met with congressional representatives in Washington in an effort to create a definitive definition of multiple-chemical sensitivity. According to CIIN, MCS affects approximately 15 percent of the population—3 percent to 4 percent so severely that lifestyle changes are mandatory for survival—and thousands have been placed on permanent or long-term disability. MCS can arise from long-term, low-level exposure or short, significant exposure. Symptoms involving multiple organ systems flare up with re-exposure and subside only when exposure ceases. See "Task Force Seeks Definition for Multiple Chemical Sensitivity," *Occupational Hazards* (October 2002).

While the CIIN and sufferers of the syndrome declare a multitude of symptoms, doctors remain skeptical. For scientists' perceptions on the disease, see "Multiple Chemical Sensitivities: An Iatrogenically Perpetuated Disorder and Example of the Placebo Effect," *Scientific Review of Alternative Medicine* (Winter 2001). Other readings that address the issue of MCS include "Multiple Chemical Sensitivities," *Psychiatric Times* (January 1, 2003); "Reported Chemical Sensitivities in a Health Survey of United Kingdom Military Personnel," *Occupational and Environmental Medicine* (March 2002); "Multiple Chemical Sensitivity: Discriminant Validity of Case Definitions," *Archives of Environmental Health* (September–October 2001); "Multiple Chemical Sensitivity May Be a Psychophysiological Condition," *Clinical Psychiatry News* (July 2001); "Illness May Have Genetic Link to Panic Disorder: Multiple Chemical Sensitivity," *Genomics & Genetics Weekly* (June 22, 2001); "A Multiple Center Study of Multiple Chemical Sensitivity Syndrome," *Archives of Environmental Health* (May 2001); and "Are There Risk Populations For 'Environmental Illness'?" *Journal of Toxicology: Clinical Toxicology* (April 2001).

ISSUE 20

Is the Atkins Low-Carbohydrate Diet a Valid Weight-Loss Plan?

YES: Gary Taubes, from "What If It's All Been a Big Fat Lie?" *The New York Times Magazine* (July 7, 2002)

NO: Michael Fumento, from "Big Fat Fake: The Atkins Diet Controversy and the Sorry State of Science Journalism," *Reason* (March 2003)

ISSUE SUMMARY

YES: Journalist Gary Taubes asserts that eating fatty meats, cheeses, cream, and butter is the key to a long, healthy life.

NO: Michael Fumento, senior fellow at the Hudson Institute, argues that there are ample studies that dispute the benefits of a high-fat, low-carbohydrate diet.

Close to 50 million Americans are currently dieting. However, most will not lose as much weight as they want, and many will not keep off the weight they have lost despite the millions of dollars spent on diet books and programs.

The number of Americans who are overweight and obese has been steadily climbing. Obesity has been linked with increased risks for certain diseases, including diabetes, heart disease, and some cancers. In addition, there are social and economic implications related to obesity. Many contend that overweight individuals are less likely to marry, earn less money, and are less likely to be accepted to elite colleges.

It has been shown that most diets fail regardless of the way people attempt to lose weight. Many dieters try one diet after another in an effort to find the one plan that works. Many of the weight-loss diets that have come and gone have been based on altering the usual proportion of the three basic type of nutrients—protein, fat, and carbohydrate. The high-fat, low-fat, high-carbohydrate, low-carbohydrate, high-protein, and low-protein diets have all been popular at one time. The one plan that has had considerable staying power has been the diet developed by the late Dr. Robert Atkins who published the best seller *Dr. Atkins Diet Revolution* in the late 1960s, followed by *Dr. Atkins New Diet Revolution* in the late 1990s. The diet developed by Atkins, a cardiologist, restricts carbohydrate foods, such as bread, potatoes, fruits, vegetables, and milk and allows unlimited meat, fish, poultry, eggs, and butter. Dieters are attracted to this diet because it promises rapid weight loss and still permits an "all you can eat" program of protein and fat. The diet is effective in the beginning because much of the weight loss is from the burning of water and fat, causing a condition called *ketosis*. Ketosis is an abnormal body process that occurs during starvation due to lack of carbohydrate. Ketosis can cause fatigue, constipation, nausea, and vomiting. Potential long-term side effects of ketosis include heart disease, bone loss, and kidney damage. In addition to ketosis, some maintain that long-term use of the Atkins diet can cause health problems, including calcium and nutrient loss. Atkins advocates taking advantage of ketosis to accelerate weight loss.

Some physicians and nutritionists are concerned about the potential high intake of saturated fats found in animal products by those on the Atkins diet. Saturated fats are linked to the elevation of serum cholesterol, a risk factor in heart disease. The diet's lack of fruits and vegetables can also be a cause for unease since these foods offer vitamins, minerals, and fiber and may also contain cancer-fighting compounds known as *phyto-chemicals*. Meats, which are high in saturated fats, are associated with colorectal and other cancers. Some health and nutrition professionals are strongly opposed to the Atkins diet and encourage their patients and clients to consume diets that are high in unrefined carbohydrates, especially fruits and vegetables, and low in saturated fats.

To complicate the diet picture, in the 1990s some nutritionists started promoting high-carbohydrate, low-fat diets. Advocates of reducing total fat assert that it helps to control weight since fat contains more calories per ounce than carbohydrates or protein. Consumers embraced the high-carbohydrate, low-fat diet, and many consumed large amounts of pasta, breads, and fat-free baked goods, which in many cases resulted in weight gain instead of weight loss.

In the following selections, Gary Taubes maintains that the low-fat diets of the 1990s have been responsible for the rise in obesity and that, for many people, the Atkins diet is beneficial. Michael Fumento counters that the Atkins diet has been proven in countless studies to be harmful, and that it fails to produce significant, long-lasting weight loss.

Gary Taubes 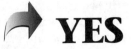 **YES**

What If It's All Been a Big Fat Lie?

If the members of the American medical establishment were to have a collective find-yourself-standing-naked-in-Times-Square-type nightmare, this might be it. They spend 30 years ridiculing Robert Atkins, author of the phenomenally-best-selling "Dr. Atkins' Diet Revolution" and "Dr. Atkins' New Diet Revolution," accusing the Manhattan doctor of quackery and fraud, only to discover that the unrepentant Atkins was right all along. Or maybe it's this: they find that their very own dietary recommendations—eat less fat and more carbohydrates—are the cause of the rampaging epidemic of obesity in America. Or, just possibly this: they find out both of the above are true.

When Atkins first published his "Diet Revolution" in 1972, Americans were just coming to terms with the proposition that fat—particularly the saturated fat of meat and dairy products—was the primary nutritional evil in the American diet. Atkins managed to sell millions of copies of a book promising that we would lose weight eating steak, eggs and butter to our heart's desire, because it was the carbohydrates, the pasta, rice, bagels and sugar, that caused obesity and even heart disease. Fat, he said, was harmless.

Atkins allowed his readers to eat "truly luxurious foods without limit," as he put it, "lobster with butter sauce, steak with bearnaise sauce ... *bacon* cheeseburgers," but allowed no starches or refined carbohydrates, which means no sugars or anything made from flour. Atkins banned even fruit juices, and permitted only a modicum of vegetables, although the latter were negotiable as the diet progressed.

Atkins was by no means the first to get rich pushing a high-fat diet that restricted carbohydrates, but he popularized it to an extent that the American Medical Association considered it a potential threat to our health. The A.M.A. attacked Atkins's diet as a "bizarre regimen" that advocated "an unlimited intake of saturated fats and cholesterol-rich foods," and Atkins even had to defend his diet in Congressional hearings.

Thirty years later, America has become weirdly polarized on the subject of weight. On the one hand, we've been told with almost religious certainty by everyone from the surgeon general on down, and we have come to believe with almost religious certainty, that obesity is caused by the excessive consumption of fat, and that if we eat less fat we will lose weight and live longer. On the other, we have the ever-resilient message of Atkins and decades' worth of best-selling diet books, including "The Zone," "Sugar Busters" and "Protein Power" to name a few. All push some variation of what scientists would call the alternative hypothesis: it's not the fat that makes us fat, but the carbohydrates, and if we eat less carbohydrates we will lose weight and live longer.

The perversity of this alternative hypothesis is that it identifies the cause of obesity as precisely those refined carbohydrates at the base of the famous Food Guide Pyramid—the pasta, rice and bread—that we are told should be the staple of our healthy low-fat diet, and then on the sugar or corn syrup in the soft drinks, fruit juices and sports drinks that we have taken to consuming in quantity if for no other reason than that they are fat free and so appear intrinsically healthy. While the low-fat-is-good-health dogma represents reality as we have come to know it, and the government has spent hundreds of millions of dollars in research trying to prove its worth, the low-carbohydrate message has been relegated to the realm of unscientific fantasy.

Over the past five years, however, there has been a subtle shift in the scientific consensus. It used to be that even considering the possibility of the alternative hypothesis, let alone researching it, was tantamount to quackery by association. Now a small but growing minority of establishment researchers have come to take seriously what the low-carb-diet doctors have been saying all along. Walter Willett, chairman of the department of nutrition at the Harvard School of Public Health, may be the most visible proponent of testing this heretic hypothesis. Willett is the de facto spokesman of the longest-running, most comprehensive diet and health studies ever performed, which have already cost upward of $100 million and include data on nearly 300,000 individuals. Those data, says Willett, clearly contradict the low-fat-is-good-health message "and the idea that all fat is bad for you; the exclusive focus on adverse effects of fat may have contributed to the obesity epidemic."

These researchers point out that there are plenty of reasons to suggest that the low-fat-is-good-health hypothesis has now effectively failed the test of time. In particular, that we are in the midst of an obesity epidemic that started around the early 1980's, and that this was coincident with the rise of the low-fat dogma. (Type 2 diabetes, the most common form of the disease, also rose significantly through this period.) They say that low-fat weight-loss diets have proved in clinical trials and real life to be dismal failures, and that on top of it all, the percentage of fat in the American diet has been decreasing for two decades. Our cholesterol levels have been declining, and we have been smoking less, and yet the incidence of heart disease has not declined as would be expected. "That is very disconcerting," Willett says. "It suggests that something else bad is happening."

The science behind the alternative hypothesis can be called Endocrinology 101, which is how it's referred to by David Ludwig, a researcher at Harvard Medical School who runs the pediatric obesity clinic at Children's Hospital Boston, and who prescribes his own version of a carbohydrate-restricted diet to his patients. Endocrinology 101 requires an understanding of how carbohydrates affect insulin and blood sugar and in turn fat metabolism and appetite. This is basic endocrinology, Ludwig says, which is the study of hormones, and it is still considered radical because the low-fat dietary wisdom emerged in the 1960's from researchers almost exclusively concerned with the effect of fat on cholesterol and heart disease. At the time, Endocrinology 101 was still underdeveloped, and so it was ignored. Now that this science is becoming clear, it has to fight a quarter century of anti-fat prejudice.

The alternative hypothesis also comes with an implication that is worth considering for a moment, because it's a whopper, and it may indeed be an obstacle to its acceptance. If the alternative hypothesis is right—still a big "if"— then it strongly suggests that the ongoing epidemic of obesity in America and elsewhere is not, as we are constantly told, due simply to a collective lack of will power and a failure to exercise. Rather it occurred, as Atkins has been saying (along with Barry Sears, author of "The Zone"), because the public health authorities told us unwittingly, but with the best of intentions, to eat precisely those foods that would make us fat, and we did. We ate more fat-free carbohydrates, which, in turn, made us hungrier and then heavier. Put simply, if the alternative hypothesis is right, then a low-fat diet is not by definition a healthy diet. In practice, such a diet cannot help being high in carbohydrates, and that can lead to obesity, and perhaps even heart disease. "For a large percentage of the population, perhaps 30 to 40 percent, low-fat diets are counterproductive," says Eleftheria Maratos-Flier, director of obesity research at Harvard's prestigious Joslin Diabetes Center. "They have the paradoxical effect of making people gain weight."

⋅⟨◉⟩⋅

Scientists are still arguing about fat, despite a century of research, because the regulation of appetite and weight in the human body happens to be almost inconceivably complex, and the experimental tools we have to study it are still remarkably inadequate. This combination leaves researchers in an awkward position. To study the entire physiological system involves feeding real food to real human subjects for months or years on end, which is prohibitively expensive, ethically questionable (if you're trying to measure the effects of foods that might cause heart disease) and virtually impossible to do in any kind of rigorously controlled scientific manner. But if researchers seek to study something less costly and more controllable, they end up studying experimental situations so oversimplified that their results may have nothing to do with reality. This then leads to a research literature so vast that it's possible to find at least some published research to support virtually any theory. The result is a balkanized community—"splintered, very opinionated and in many instances, intransigent," says Kurt Isselbacher, a former chairman of the Food and Nutrition Board of the National Academy of Science—in which researchers seem easily convinced that their preconceived notions are correct and thoroughly uninterested in testing any other hypotheses but their own.

What's more, the number of misconceptions propagated about the most basic research can be staggering. Researchers will be suitably scientific describing the limitations of their own experiments, and then will cite something as gospel truth because they read it in a magazine. The classic example is the statement heard repeatedly that 95 percent of all dieters never lose weight, and 95 percent of those who do will not keep it off. This will be correctly attributed to the University of Pennsylvania psychiatrist Albert Stunkard, but it will go unmentioned that this statement is based on 100 patients who passed through Stunkard's obesity clinic during the Eisenhower administration.

With these caveats, one of the few reasonably reliable facts about the obesity epidemic is that it started around the early 1980's. According to Katherine Flegal, an epidemiologist at the National Center for Health Statistics, the percentage of obese Americans stayed relatively constant through the 1960's and 1970's at 13 percent to 14 percent and then shot up by 8 percentage points in the 1980's. By the end of that decade, nearly one in four Americans was obese. That steep rise, which is consistent through all segments of American society and which continued unabated through the 1990's, is the singular feature of the epidemic. Any theory that tries to explain obesity in America has to account for that. Meanwhile, overweight children nearly tripled in number. And for the first time, physicians began diagnosing Type 2 diabetes in adolescents. Type 2 diabetes often accompanies obesity. It used to be called adult-onset diabetes and now, for the obvious reason, is not.

So how did this happen? The orthodox and ubiquitous explanation is that we live in what Kelly Brownell, a Yale psychologist, has called a "toxic food environment" of cheap fatty food, large portions, pervasive food advertising and sedentary lives. By this theory, we are at the Pavlovian mercy of the food industry, which spends nearly $10 billion a year advertising unwholesome junk food and fast food. And because these foods, especially fast food, are so filled with fat, they are both irresistible and uniquely fattening. On top of this, so the theory goes, our modern society has successfully eliminated physical activity from our daily lives. We no longer exercise or walk up stairs, nor do our children bike to school or play outside, because they would prefer to play video games and watch television. And because some of us are obviously predisposed to gain weight while others are not, this explanation also has a genetic component—the thrifty gene. It suggests that storing extra calories as fat was an evolutionary advantage to our Paleolithic ancestors, who had to survive frequent famine. We then inherited these "thrifty" genes, despite their liability in today's toxic environment.

This theory makes perfect sense and plays to our puritanical prejudice that fat, fast food and television are innately damaging to our humanity. But there are two catches. First, to buy this logic is to accept that the copious negative reinforcement that accompanies obesity—both socially and physically—is easily overcome by the constant bombardment of food advertising and the lure of a supersize bargain meal. And second, as Flegal points out, little data exist to support any of this. Certainly none of it explains what changed so significantly to start the epidemic. Fast-food consumption, for example, continued to grow steadily through the 70's and 80's, but it did not take a sudden leap, as obesity did.

As far as exercise and physical activity go, there are no reliable data before the mid-80's, according to William Dietz, who runs the division of nutrition and physical activity at the Centers for Disease Control; the 1990's data show obesity rates continuing to climb, while exercise activity remained unchanged.

Figure 1

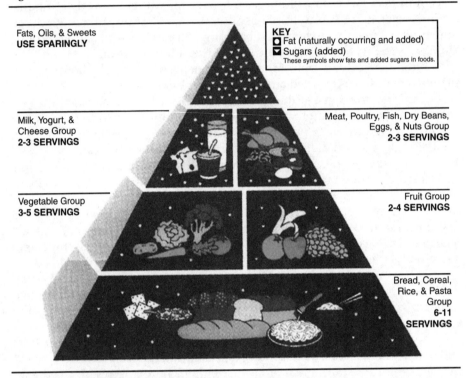

Source: U.S. Department of Agriculture/U.S. Department of Health and Human Services

From pyramid to pear: The Agriculture Department's recommendations may be partly responsible for America's increasing obesity rates.

This suggests the two have little in common. Dietz also acknowledged that a culture of physical exercise began in the United States in the 70's—the "leisure exercise mania," as Robert Levy, director of the National Heart, Lung and Blood Institute, described it in 1981—and has continued through the present day.

As for the thrifty gene, it provides the kind of evolutionary rationale for human behavior that scientists find comforting but that simply cannot be tested. In other words, if we were living through an anorexia epidemic, the experts would be discussing the equally untestable "spendthrift gene" theory, touting evolutionary advantages of losing weight effortlessly. An overweight homo erectus, they'd say, would have been easy prey for predators.

It is also undeniable, note students of Endocrinology 101, that mankind never evolved to eat a diet high in starches or sugars. "Grain products and concentrated sugars were essentially absent from human nutrition until the invention of agriculture," Ludwig says, "which was only 10,000 years ago." This is discussed frequently in the anthropology texts but is mostly absent from the obesity literature, with the prominent exception of the low-carbohydrate-diet books.

What's forgotten in the current controversy is that the low-fat dogma itself is only about 25 years old. Until the late 70's, the accepted wisdom was that fat and protein protected against overeating by making you sated, and that carbohydrates made you fat. In "The Physiology of Taste," for instance, an 1825 discourse considered among the most famous books ever written about food, the French gastronome Jean Anthelme Brillat-Savarin says that he could easily identify the causes of obesity after 30 years of listening to one "stout party" after another proclaiming the joys of bread, rice and (from a "particularly stout party") potatoes. Brillat-Savarin described the roots of obesity as a natural predisposition conjuncted with the "floury and feculent substances which man makes the prime ingredients of his daily nourishment." He added that the effects of this fecula—i.e., "potatoes, grain or any kind of flour"—were seen sooner when sugar was added to the diet.

This is what my mother taught me 40 years ago, backed up by the vague observation that Italians tended toward corpulence because they ate so much pasta. This observation was actually documented by Ancel Keys, a University of Minnesota physician who noted that fats "have good staying power," by which he meant they are slow to be digested and so lead to satiation, and that Italians were among the heaviest populations he had studied. According to Keys, the Neapolitans, for instance, ate only a little lean meat once or twice a week, but ate bread and pasta every day for lunch and dinner. "There was no evidence of nutritional deficiency," he wrote, "but the working-class women were fat."

By the 70's, you could still find articles in the journals describing high rates of obesity in Africa and the Caribbean where diets contained almost exclusively carbohydrates. The common thinking, wrote a former director of the Nutrition Division of the United Nations, was that the ideal diet, one that prevented obesity, snacking and excessive sugar consumption, was a diet "with plenty of eggs, beef, mutton, chicken, butter and well-cooked vegetables." This was the identical prescription Brillat-Savarin put forth in 1825.

It was Ancel Keys, paradoxically, who introduced the low-fat-is-good-health dogma in the 50's with his theory that dietary fat raises cholesterol levels and gives you heart disease. Over the next two decades, however, the scientific evidence supporting this theory remained stubbornly ambiguous. The case was eventually settled not by new science but by politics. It began in January 1977, when a Senate committee led by George McGovern published its "Dietary Goals for the United States," advising that Americans significantly curb their fat intake to abate an epidemic of "killer diseases" supposedly sweeping the country. It peaked in late 1984, when the National Institutes of Health officially recommended that all Americans over the age of 2 eat less fat. By that time, fat had become "this greasy killer" in the memorable words of the Center for Science in the Public Interest, and the model American breakfast of eggs and bacon was well on its way to becoming a bowl of Special K with low-fat milk, a glass of orange juice and toast, hold the butter—a dubious feast of refined carbohydrates.

In the intervening years, the N.I.H. spent several hundred million dollars trying to demonstrate a connection between eating fat and getting heart disease and, despite what we might think, it failed. Five major studies revealed no such link. A sixth, however, costing well over $100 million alone, concluded that reducing cholesterol by drug therapy could prevent heart disease. The N.I.H. administrators then made a leap of faith. Basil Rifkind, who oversaw the relevant trials for the N.I.H., described their logic this way: they had failed to demonstrate at great expense that eating less fat had any health benefits. But if a cholesterol-lowering drug could prevent heart attacks, then a low-fat, cholesterol-lowering diet should do the same. "It's an imperfect world," Rifkind told me. "The data that would be definitive is ungettable, so you do your best with what is available."

Some of the best scientists disagreed with this low-fat logic, suggesting that good science was incompatible with such leaps of faith, but they were effectively ignored. Pete Ahrens, whose Rockefeller University laboratory had done the seminal research on cholesterol metabolism, testified to McGovern's committee that everyone responds differently to low-fat diets. It was not a scientific matter who might benefit and who might be harmed, he said, but "a betting matter." Phil Handler, then president of the National Academy of Sciences, testified in Congress to the same effect in 1980. "What right," Handler asked, "has the federal government to propose that the American people conduct a vast nutritional experiment, with themselves as subjects, on the strength of so very little evidence that it will do them any good?"

Nonetheless, once the N.I.H. signed off on the low-fat doctrine, societal forces took over. The food industry quickly began producing thousands of reduced-fat food products to meet the new recommendations. Fat was removed from foods like cookies, chips and yogurt. The problem was, it had to be replaced with something as tasty and pleasurable to the palate, which meant some form of sugar, often high-fructose corn syrup. Meanwhile, an entire industry emerged to create fat substitutes, of which Procter & Gamble's olestra was first. And because these reduced-fat meats, cheeses, snacks and cookies had to compete with a few hundred thousand other food products marketed in America, the industry dedicated considerable advertising effort to reinforcing the less-fat-is-good-health message. Helping the cause was what Walter Willett calls the "huge forces" of dietitians, health organizations, consumer groups, health reporters and even cookbook writers, all well-intended missionaries of healthful eating.

⋖◈⋗

Few experts now deny that the low-fat message is radically oversimplified. If nothing else, it effectively ignores the fact that unsaturated fats, like olive oil, are relatively good for you: they tend to elevate your good cholesterol, high-density lipoprotein (H.D.L.), and lower your bad cholesterol, low-density lipoprotein (L.D.L.), at least in comparison to the effect of carbohydrates. While higher L.D.L. raises your heart-disease risk, higher H.D.L. reduces it.

What this means is that even saturated fats—a.k.a., the bad fats—are not nearly as deleterious as you would think. True, they will elevate your bad cholesterol, but they will also elevate your good cholesterol. In other words, it's a virtual wash. As Willett explained to me, you will gain little to no health benefit by giving up milk, butter and cheese and eating bagels instead.

But it gets even weirder than that. Foods considered more or less deadly under the low-fat dogma turn out to be comparatively benign if you actually look at their fat content. More than two-thirds of the fat in a porterhouse steak, for instance, will definitely improve your cholesterol profile (at least in comparison with the baked potato next to it); it's true that the remainder will raise your L.D.L., the bad stuff, but it will also boost your H.D.L. The same is true for lard. If you work out the numbers, you come to the surreal conclusion that you can eat lard straight from the can and conceivably reduce your risk of heart disease.

The crucial example of how the low-fat recommendations were oversimplified is shown by the impact—potentially lethal, in fact—of low-fat diets on triglycerides, which are the component molecules of fat. By the late 60's, researchers had shown that high triglyceride levels were at least as common in heart-disease patients as high L.D.L. cholesterol, and that eating a low-fat, high-carbohydrate diet would, for many people, raise their triglyceride levels, lower their H.D.L. levels and accentuate what Gerry Reaven, an endocrinologist at Stanford University, called Syndrome X. This is a cluster of conditions that can lead to heart disease and Type 2 diabetes.

It took Reaven a decade to convince his peers that Syndrome X was a legitimate health concern, in part because to accept its reality is to accept that low-fat diets will increase the risk of heart disease in a third of the population. "Sometimes we wish it would go away because nobody knows how to deal with it," said Robert Silverman, an N.I.H. researcher, at a 1987 N.I.H. conference. "High protein levels can be bad for the kidneys. High fat is bad for your heart. Now Reaven is saying not to eat high carbohydrates. We have to eat something."

Surely, everyone involved in drafting the various dietary guidelines wanted Americans simply to eat less junk food, however you define it, and eat more the way they do in Berkeley, Calif. But we didn't go along. Instead we ate more starches and refined carbohydrates, because calorie for calorie, these are the cheapest nutrients for the food industry to produce, and they can be sold at the highest profit. It's also what we like to eat. Rare is the person under the age of 50 who doesn't prefer a cookie or heavily sweetened yogurt to a head of broccoli.

"All reformers would do well to be conscious of the law of unintended consequences," says Alan Stone, who was staff director for McGovern's Senate committee. Stone told me he had an inkling about how the food industry would respond to the new dietary goals back when the hearings were first held. An economist pulled him aside, he said, and gave him a lesson on market disincentives to healthy eating: "He said if you create a new market with a brand-new manufactured food, give it a brand-new fancy name, put a big advertising budget behind it, you can have a market all to yourself and force your competitors to catch up. You can't do that with fruits and vegetables. It's harder to differentiate an apple from an apple."

Nutrition researchers also played a role by trying to feed science into the idea that carbohydrates are the ideal nutrient. It had been known, for almost a century, and considered mostly irrelevant to the etiology of obesity, that fat has nine calories per gram compared with four for carbohydrates and protein. Now it became the fail-safe position of the low-fat recommendations: reduce the densest source of calories in the diet and you will lose weight. Then in 1982, J.P. Flatt, a University of Massachusetts biochemist, published his research demonstrating that, in any normal diet, it is extremely rare for the human body to convert carbohydrates into body fat. This was then misinterpreted by the media and quite a few scientists to mean that eating carbohydrates, even to excess, could not make you fat—which is not the case, Flatt says. But the misinterpretation developed a vigorous life of its own because it resonated with the notion that fat makes you fat and carbohydrates are harmless.

As a result, the major trends in American diets since the late 70's, according to the U.S.D.A. agricultural economist Judith Putnam, have been a decrease in the percentage of fat calories and a "greatly increased consumption of carbohydrates." To be precise, annual grain consumption has increased almost 60 pounds per person, and caloric sweeteners (primarily high-fructose corn syrup) by 30 pounds. At the same time, we suddenly began consuming more total calories: now up to 400 more each day since the government started recommending low-fat diets.

If these trends are correct, then the obesity epidemic can certainly be explained by Americans' eating more calories than ever—excess calories, after all, are what causes us to gain weight—and, specifically, more carbohydrates. The question is why?

The answer provided by Endocrinology 101 is that we are simply hungrier than we were in the 70's, and the reason is physiological more than psychological. In this case, the salient factor—ignored in the pursuit of fat and its effect on cholesterol—is how carbohydrates affect blood sugar and insulin. In fact, these were obvious culprits all along, which is why Atkins and the low-carb-diet doctors pounced on them early.

The primary role of insulin is to regulate blood-sugar levels. After you eat carbohydrates, they will be broken down into their component sugar molecules and transported into the bloodstream. Your pancreas then secretes insulin, which shunts the blood sugar into muscles and the liver as fuel for the next few hours. This is why carbohydrates have a significant impact on insulin and fat does not. And because juvenile diabetes is caused by a lack of insulin, physicians believed since the 20's that the only evil with insulin is not having enough.

But insulin also regulates fat metabolism. We cannot store body fat without it. Think of insulin as a switch. When it's on, in the few hours after eating, you burn carbohydrates for energy and store excess calories as fat. When it's off, after the insulin has been depleted, you burn fat as fuel. So when insulin levels are low, you will burn your own fat, but not when they're high.

This is where it gets unavoidably complicated. The fatter you are, the more insulin your pancreas will pump out per meal, and the more likely you'll develop what's called "insulin resistance," which is the underlying cause of Syndrome X. In effect, your cells become insensitive to the action of insulin, and so you need ever greater amounts to keep your blood sugar in check. So as you gain weight, insulin makes it easier to store fat and harder to lose it. But the insulin resistance in turn may make it harder to store fat—your weight is being kept in check, as it should be. But now the insulin resistance might prompt your pancreas to produce even more insulin, potentially starting a vicious cycle. Which comes first—the obesity, the elevated insulin, known as hyperinsulinemia, or the insulin resistance—is a chicken-and-egg problem that hasn't been resolved. One endocrinologist described this to me as "the Nobel-prize winning question."

Insulin also profoundly affects hunger, although to what end is another point of controversy. On the one hand, insulin can indirectly cause hunger by lowering your blood sugar, but how low does blood sugar have to drop before hunger kicks in? That's unresolved. Meanwhile, insulin works in the brain to suppress hunger. The theory, as explained to me by Michael Schwartz, an endocrinologist at the University of Washington, is that insulin's ability to inhibit appetite would normally counteract its propensity to generate body fat. In other words, as you gained weight, your body would generate more insulin after every meal, and that in turn would suppress your appetite; you'd eat less and lose the weight.

Schwartz, however, can imagine a simple mechanism that would throw this "homeostatic" system off balance: if your brain were to lose its sensitivity to insulin, just as your fat and muscles do when they are flooded with it. Now the higher insulin production that comes with getting fatter would no longer compensate by suppressing your appetite, because your brain would no longer register the rise in insulin. The end result would be a physiologic state in which obesity is almost preordained, and one in which the carbohydrate-insulin connection could play a major role. Schwartz says he believes this could indeed be happening, but research hasn't progressed far enough to prove it. "It is just a hypothesis," he says. "It still needs to be sorted out."

David Ludwig, the Harvard endocrinologist, says that it's the direct effect of insulin on blood sugar that does the trick. He notes that when diabetics get too much insulin, their blood sugar drops and they get ravenously hungry. They gain weight because they eat more, and the insulin promotes fat deposition. The same happens with lab animals. This, he says, is effectively what happens when we eat carbohydrates—in particular sugar and starches like potatoes and rice, or anything made from flour, like a slice of white bread. These are known in the jargon as high-glycemic-index carbohydrates, which means they are absorbed quickly into the blood. As a result, they cause a spike of blood sugar and a surge of insulin within minutes. The resulting rush of insulin stores the blood sugar away and a few hours later, your blood sugar is lower than it was before you ate. As Ludwig explains, your body effectively thinks it has run out of fuel, but the insulin is still high enough to prevent you from burning your own fat. The result is hunger and a craving for more carbohydrates. It's another vicious circle, and another situation ripe for obesity.

The glycemic-index concept and the idea that starches can be absorbed into the blood even faster than sugar emerged in the late 70's, but again had no influence on public health recommendations, because of the attendant controversies. To wit: if you bought the glycemic-index concept, then you had to accept that the starches we were supposed to be eating 6 to 11 times a day were, once swallowed, physiologically indistinguishable from sugars. This made them seem considerably less than wholesome. Rather than accept this possibility, the policy makers simply allowed sugar and corn syrup to elude the vilification that befell dietary fat. After all, they are fat-free.

Sugar and corn syrup from soft drinks, juices and the copious teas and sports drinks now supply more than 10 percent of our total calories; the 80's saw the introduction of Big Gulps and 32-ounce cups of Coca-Cola, blasted through with sugar, but 100 percent fat free. When it comes to insulin and blood sugar, these soft drinks and fruit juices—what the scientists call "wet carbohydrates"—might indeed be worst of all. (Diet soda accounts for less than a quarter of the soda market.)

The gist of the glycemic-index idea is that the longer it takes the carbohydrates to be digested, the lesser the impact on blood sugar and insulin and the healthier the food. Those foods with the highest rating on the glycemic index are some simple sugars, starches and anything made from flour. Green vegetables, beans and whole grains cause a much slower rise in blood sugar because they have fiber, a nondigestible carbohydrate, which slows down digestion and lowers the glycemic index. Protein and fat serve the same purpose, which implies that eating fat can be beneficial, a notion that is still unacceptable. And the glycemic-index concept implies that a primary cause of Syndrome X, heart disease, Type 2 diabetes and obesity is the long-term damage caused by the repeated surges of insulin that come from eating starches and refined carbohydrates. This suggests a kind of unified field theory for these chronic diseases, but not one that coexists easily with the low-fat doctrine.

At Ludwig's pediatric obesity clinic, he has been prescribing low-glycemic-index diets to children and adolescents for five years now. He does not recommend the Atkins diet because he says he believes such a very low carbohydrate approach is unnecessarily restrictive; instead, he tells his patients to effectively replace refined carbohydrates and starches with vegetables, legumes and fruit. This makes a low-glycemic-index diet consistent with dietary common sense, albeit in a higher-fat kind of way. His clinic now has a nine-month waiting list. Only recently has Ludwig managed to convince the N.I.H. that such diets are worthy of study. His first three grant proposals were summarily rejected, which may explain why much of the relevant research has been done in Canada and in Australia. In April, however, Ludwig received $1.2 million from the N.I.H. to test his low-glycemic-index diet against a traditional low-fat-low-calorie regime. That might help resolve some of the controversy over the role of insulin in obesity, although the redoubtable Robert Atkins might get there first.

⚬⟨◉⟩⚬

The 71-year-old Atkins, a graduate of Cornell medical school, says he first tried a very low carbohydrate diet in 1963 after reading about one in the Journal of the American Medical Association. He lost weight effortlessly, had his epiphany and turned a fledgling Manhattan cardiology practice into a thriving obesity clinic. He then alienated the entire medical community by telling his readers to eat as much fat and protein as they wanted, as long as they ate little to no carbohydrates. They would lose weight, he said, because they would keep their insulin down; they wouldn't be hungry; and they would have less resistance to burning their own fat. Atkins also noted that starches and sugar were harmful in any event because they raised triglyceride levels and that this was a greater risk factor for heart disease than cholesterol.

Atkins's diet is both the ultimate manifestation of the alternative hypothesis as well as the battleground on which the fat-versus-carbohydrates controversy is likely to be fought scientifically over the next few years. After insisting Atkins was a quack for three decades, obesity experts are now finding it difficult to ignore the copious anecdotal evidence that his diet does just what he has claimed. Take Albert Stunkard, for instance. Stunkard has been trying to treat obesity for half a century, but he told me he had his epiphany about Atkins and maybe about obesity as well just recently when he discovered that the chief of radiology in his hospital had lost 60 pounds on Atkins's diet. "Well, apparently all the young guys in the hospital are doing it," he said. "So we decided to do a study." When I asked Stunkard if he or any of his colleagues considered testing Atkins's diet 30 years ago, he said they hadn't because they thought Atkins was "a jerk" who was just out to make money: this "turned people off, and so nobody took him seriously enough to do what we're finally doing."

In fact, when the American Medical Association released its scathing critique of Atkins's diet in March 1973, it acknowledged that the diet probably worked, but expressed little interest in why. Through the 60's, this had been a subject of considerable research, with the conclusion that Atkins-like diets were low-calorie diets in disguise; that when you cut out pasta, bread and potatoes, you'll have a hard time eating enough meat, vegetables and cheese to replace the calories.

That, however, raised the question of why such a low-calorie regimen would also suppress hunger, which Atkins insisted was the signature characteristic of the diet. One possibility was Endocrinology 101: that fat and protein make you sated and, lacking carbohydrates and the ensuing swings of blood sugar and insulin, you stay sated. The other possibility arose from the fact that Atkins's diet is "ketogenic." This means that insulin falls so low that you enter a state called ketosis, which is what happens during fasting and starvation. Your muscles and tissues burn body fat for energy, as does your brain in the form of fat molecules produced by the liver called ketones. Atkins saw ketosis as the obvious way to kick-start weight loss. He also liked to say that ketosis was so energizing that it was better than sex, which set him up for some ridicule. An inevitable criticism of Atkins's diet has been that ketosis is dangerous and to be avoided at all costs.

When I interviewed ketosis experts, however, they universally sided with Atkins, and suggested that maybe the medical community and the media confuse ketosis with ketoacidosis, a variant of ketosis that occurs in untreated diabetics and can be fatal. "Doctors are scared of ketosis," says Richard Veech, an N.I.H. researcher who studied medicine at Harvard and then got his doctorate at Oxford University with the Nobel Laureate Hans Krebs. "They're always worried about diabetic ketoacidosis. But ketosis is a normal physiologic state. I would argue it is the normal state of man. It's not normal to have McDonald's and a delicatessen around every corner. It's normal to starve."

Simply put, ketosis is evolution's answer to the thrifty gene. We may have evolved to efficiently store fat for times of famine, says Veech, but we also evolved ketosis to efficiently live off that fat when necessary. Rather than being poison, which is how the press often refers to ketones, they make the body run more efficiently and provide a backup fuel source for the brain. Veech calls ketones "magic" and has shown that both the heart and brain run 25 percent more efficiently on ketones than on blood sugar.

The bottom line is that for the better part of 30 years Atkins insisted his diet worked and was safe, Americans apparently tried it by the tens of millions, while nutritionists, physicians, public-health authorities and anyone concerned with heart disease insisted it could kill them, and expressed little or no desire to find out who was right. During that period, only two groups of U.S. researchers tested the diet, or at least published their results. In the early 70's, J.P. Flatt and Harvard's George Blackburn pioneered the "protein-sparing modified fast" to treat postsurgical patients, and they tested it on obese volunteers. Blackburn, who later became president of the American Society of Clinical Nutrition, describes his regime as "an Atkins diet without excess fat" and says he had to give it a fancy name or nobody would take him seriously. The diet was "lean meat, fish and fowl" supplemented by vitamins and minerals. "People loved it," Blackburn recalls. "Great weight loss. We couldn't run them off with a baseball bat." Blackburn successfully treated hundreds of obese patients over the next decade and published a series of papers that were ignored. When obese New Englanders turned to appetite-control drugs in the mid-80's, he says, he let it drop. He then applied to the N.I.H. for a grant to do a clinical trial of popular diets but was rejected.

The second trial, published in September 1980, was done at the George Washington University Medical Center. Two dozen obese volunteers agreed to follow Atkins's diet for eight weeks and lost an average of 17 pounds each, with no apparent ill effects, although their L.D.L. cholesterol did go up. The researchers, led by John LaRosa, now president of the State University of New York Downstate Medical Center in Brooklyn, concluded that the 17-pound weight loss in eight weeks would likely have happened with any diet under "the novelty of trying something under experimental conditions" and never pursued it further.

Now researchers have finally decided that Atkins's diet and other low-carb diets have to be tested, and are doing so against traditional low-calorie-low-fat diets as recommended by the American Heart Association. To explain their motivation, they inevitably tell one of two stories: some, like Stunkard, told me that someone they knew—a patient, a friend, a fellow physician—lost considerable weight on Atkins's diet and, despite all their preconceptions to the contrary, kept it off. Others say they were frustrated with their inability to help their obese patients, looked into the low-carb diets and decided that Endocrinology 101 was compelling. "As a trained physician, I was trained to mock anything like the Atkins diet," says Linda Stern, an internist at the Philadelphia Veterans Administration Hospital, "but I put myself on the diet. I did great. And I thought maybe this is something I can offer my patients."

None of these studies have been financed by the N.I.H., and none have yet been published. But the results have been reported at conferences—by researchers at Schneider Children's Hospital on Long Island, Duke University and the University of Cincinnati, and by Stern's group at the Philadelphia V.A. Hospital. And then there's the study Stunkard had mentioned, led by Gary Foster at the University of Pennsylvania, Sam Klein, director of the Center for Human Nutrition at Washington University in St. Louis, and Jim Hill, who runs the University of Colorado Center for Human Nutrition in Denver. The results of all five of these studies are remarkably consistent. Subjects on some form of the Atkins diet—whether overweight adolescents on the diet for 12 weeks as at Schneider, or obese adults averaging 295 pounds on the diet for six months, as at the Philadelphia V.A.—lost twice the weight as the subjects on the low-fat, low-calorie diets.

In all five studies, cholesterol levels improved similarly with both diets, but triglyceride levels were considerably lower with the Atkins diet. Though researchers are hesitant to agree with this, it does suggest that heart-disease risk *could* actually be reduced when fat is added back into the diet and starches and refined carbohydrates are removed. "I think when this stuff gets to be recognized," Stunkard says, "it's going to really shake up a lot of thinking about obesity and metabolism."

All of this could be settled sooner rather than later, and with it, perhaps, we might have some long-awaited answers as to why we grow fat and whether it is indeed preordained by societal forces or by our choice of foods. For the first time, the N.I.H. is now actually financing comparative studies of popular diets. Foster, Klein and Hill, for instance, have now received more than $2.5 million from N.I.H. to do a five-year trial of the Atkins diet with 360 obese individuals. At Harvard, Willett, Blackburn and Penelope Greene have money, albeit from Atkins's nonprofit foundation, to do a comparative trial as well.

Should these clinical trials also find for Atkins and his high-fat, low-carbohydrate diet, then the public-health authorities may indeed have a problem on their hands. Once they took their leap of faith and settled on the low-fat dietary dogma 25 years ago, they left little room for contradictory evidence or a change of opinion, should such a change be necessary to keep up with the science. In this light Sam Klein's experience is noteworthy. Klein is president-elect of the North American Association for the Study of Obesity, which suggests that he is a highly respected member of his community. And yet, he described his recent experience discussing the Atkins diet at medical conferences as a learning experience. "I have been impressed," he said, "with the anger of academicians in the audience. Their response is 'How dare you even present data on the Atkins diet!'"

This hostility stems primarily from their anxiety that Americans, given a glimmer of hope about their weight, will rush off en masse to try a diet that simply seems intuitively dangerous and on which there is still no long-term data on whether it works and whether it is safe. It's a justifiable fear. In the course of my research, I have spent my mornings at my local diner, staring down at a plate of scrambled eggs and sausage, convinced that somehow, some way, they must be working to clog my arteries and do me in.

After 20 years steeped in a low-fat paradigm, I find it hard to see the nutritional world any other way. I have learned that low-fat diets fail in clinical trials and in real life, and they certainly have failed in my life. I have read the papers suggesting that 20 years of low-fat recommendations have not managed to lower the incidence of heart disease in this country, and may have led instead to the steep increase in obesity and Type 2 diabetes. I have interviewed researchers whose computer models have calculated that cutting back on the saturated fats in my diet to the levels recommended by the American Heart Association would not add more than a few months to my life, if that. I have even lost considerable weight with relative ease by giving up carbohydrates on my test diet, and yet I can look down at my eggs and sausage and still imagine the imminent onset of heart disease and obesity, the latter assuredly to be caused by some bizarre rebound phenomenon the likes of which science has not yet begun to describe. The fact that Atkins himself has had heart trouble recently does not ease my anxiety, despite his assurance that it is not diet-related.

This is the state of mind I imagine that mainstream nutritionists, researchers and physicians must inevitably take to the fat-versus-carbohydrate controversy. They may come around, but the evidence will have to be exceptionally compelling. Although this kind of conversion may be happening at the moment to John Farquhar, who is a professor of health research and policy at Stanford University and has worked in this field for more than 40 years. When I interviewed Farquhar in April, he explained why low-fat diets might lead to weight gain and low-carbohydrate diets might lead to weight loss, but he made me promise not to say he believed they did. He attributed the cause of the obesity epidemic to the "force-feeding of a nation." Three weeks later, after reading an article on Endocrinology 101 by David Ludwig in the Journal of the American Medical Association, he sent me an e-mail message asking the not-entirely-rhetorical question, "Can we get the low-fat proponents to apologize?"

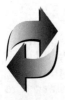

NO ↵

Michael Fumento

Big Fat Fake: The Atkins Diet Controversy and the Sorry State of Science Journalism

It was exactly what millions of obese Americans wanted to hear: Diet guru Robert Atkins has been right all along; conversely, the "medical establishment" that has routinely *criticized him has been entirely wrong. Unlimited-calorie,* high-fat meals are the key to low-fat bodies. So claimed award-winning science writer Gary Taubes in an 8,000-word *New York Times Magazine* blockbuster that appeared last July, "What If It's All Been a Big Fat Lie?"

The magazine's cover was even juicier than the title: It featured a slab of steak topped with butter and asked, "What If Fat Doesn't Make You Fat?" In fact, Taubes declared in his article, the consumption of *too little* fat could explain the explosion in obesity.

Atkins quickly wrote an editorial for his Web site claiming the article "validated" his work. Gushingly favorable follow-up stories appeared on NBC's *Dateline,* CBS' *48 Hours,* and ABC's *20/20. Dr. Atkins' New Diet Revolution,* with 11 million copies already in print, shot up from No. 5 to the top spot on the *New York Times* paperback bestseller list for "Advice, How-To, and Miscellaneous" books. It went from No. 178 to No. 5 in Amazon's rankings. Taubes himself landed a book contract from publisher Alfred A. Knopf for a big fat $700,000.

But there were serious problems with this revolutionary argument about one of our nation's most serious health problems. For example, Taubes omitted any reference to hundreds of refereed scientific studies published during the last three decades that contradicted his position. Researchers from whom he could not pull even a single useful quote supportive of his thesis were banished from the piece, while many of those whom Taubes did end up quoting now complain that he twisted their words.

"I was greatly offended by how Gary Taubes tricked us all into coming across as supporters of the Atkins diet," says one such source, Stanford University cardiologist John Farquhar. "I think he's a dangerous man. I'm sorry I ever talked to him."

Upon closer examination, Taubes' "What If It's All Been a Big Fat Lie?" turns into a big fat mess. The misguided hoopla over the *New York Times*

Magazine article and the Atkins Diet is a short study in the sorry state of scientific and medical reporting, not to mention a diet industry that routinely panders to people's worst impulses.

The Fat Shall Set Ye Free?

In *Dr. Atkins' New Diet Revolution,* Robert Atkins claims that by simply minimizing your carbohydrate intake you can quickly lose massive amounts of weight, even while pigging out daily on fatback, pork rinds, and lard. He also claims his diet will relieve "fatigue, irritability, depression, trouble concentrating, headaches, insomnia, dizziness, joint and muscle aches, heartburn, colitis, premenstrual syndrome, and water retention and bloating."

Claims like those should make anyone suspicious, even those who have barely scraped through high school biology. Gary Taubes has gone well beyond that level. He's a contributing correspondent to America's preeminent scientific journal, *Science.* He has won the National Association of Science Writers' Science in Society Journalism Award three times—the maximum allowed. Only one other writer has ever achieved that status.

Nonetheless, at the very outset of his piece (viewable in its entirety at www.atkinsdiet.com) Taubes set forth the proposition that Atkins was crucified by the "American medical establishment," which claimed his diet was ineffective and possibly dangerous and in so doing encouraged the "rampaging epidemic of obesity in America."

There is a nugget of truth in Taubes' criticisms of establishment dietary fat advice. Well-meaning but misguided health officials and health reporters, joined by opportunistic anti-fat diet book gurus, have convinced much of the public that the major culprit—perhaps the *only* culprit—in obesity is dietary fat. Avoid fat, we were told, and you won't get fat. Given license to eat as many calories as we wanted from the other nutrient groups, many of us have done exactly that. This goes far to explain why almost one-third of us are obese and almost two-thirds of us are overweight. But even here Taubes is no pioneer; the damage caused by fat-free fanaticism was pointed out long before. (See, for example, my own 1997 book, *The Fat of the Land.*)

Moreover, the Atkins-Taubes thesis of "fat won't make you fat" encourages obesity in a similar way: It offers carte blanche for consuming limitless calories, only this time swapping carbohydrates for fat. Taubes made that swap while presenting a far less scientific case than is presented in an Atkins infomercial.

Ask Stanford endocrinologist Gerald Reaven. He's best known for calling attention to "Syndrome X," a cluster of conditions that may indicate a predisposition to diabetes, hypertension, and heart disease. Among Reaven's recommendations for lowering the risk of that syndrome is to reduce consumption of highly refined carbohydrates such as those present in soft drinks and table sugar. But that's where the overlap with Atkins ends.

"I thought [Taubes'] article was outrageous," Reaven says. "I saw my name in it and all that was quoted to me was not wrong. But in the context it looked like I was buying the rest of that crap." He adds, "I tried to be helpful and a good citizen, and I ended up being embarrassed as hell. He sort of set me up." When I first contacted Reaven, he was so angry he wouldn't even let me interview him.

But his position on Atkins was all over the Internet in interviews posted long before Taubes talked to him. Do "low-carb diets like *The Zone* [by Barry Sears] and Atkins work?" one asked. Answer: "One can lose weight on a low-calorie diet if it is primarily composed of fat calories or carbohydrate calories or protein calories. It makes no difference!"

The very person with whom Taubes chose to end his article, Stanford's John Farquhar, was as livid as Reaven. Taubes said that Farquhar had sent Taubes "an e-mail message asking the not-entirely-rhetorical question, 'Can we get the low-fat proponents to apologize?'" On this powerful note, the article ended.

But it's Taubes whom Farquhar wants to apologize. "I was greatly offended by how Gary Taubes tricked us all into coming across as supporters of the Atkins diet," he wrote in an e-mail he broadcast to reporters and to colleagues who were stunned that Farquhar might actually hold the beliefs Taubes attributed to him. "We are against the Atkins Diet," he wrote, speaking for himself and Reaven. "I told him [Taubes] there is the minor degree of merit" to the idea that "people are getting fatter because too much emphasis is being placed on just cutting fats," Farquhar told me. But "once I gave him that opening—bingo—he was off and running, even though I said about six times that this is *not* the cause of the obesity epidemic."

Diets and Data

Taubes proved as adept at clipping data as at clipping quotes. Thus he claimed that one of the "reasons to suggest that the low-fat-is-good-health hypothesis has now effectively failed the test of time" is "that the *percentage* of fat in the American diet has been decreasing for two decades." (Emphasis added.)

That's true, but irrelevant. The *amount* of fat consumed has been steadily climbing, as has consumption of all calories. Individual caloric consumption jumped from 3,300 calories per day in 1970–79 to 3,900 in 1997, an 18 percent increase. Per-person consumption of fat grams increased from 149 to 156, a 4.5 percent increase. "We're eating just too darned much of everything," says Farquhar.

Taubes also shoved aside decades of published, controlled, randomized clinical trials comparing nutrient intake and weight loss. His apparent justification in the article was that the "research literature [is] so vast that it's possible to find at least some published research to support virtually any theory." But that's sheer nihilism. Good science is cautious and skeptical, not permanently open-ended. That's why terms like *weight of the evidence* are used. And the evidence against Atkins-like low-carbohydrate diets is crushing.

In April 2002, for example, the *Journal of the American Dietetic Association* (*JADA*) published a review of "all studies identified" that looked at diet nutrient composition and weight loss. It found over 200, with "no studies of the health and nutrition effects of popular diets in the published literature" excluded. In some, subjects were put on "ad libitum" diets, meaning they were allowed to eat as much as they wanted as long as they consumed fat, protein, and carbohydrates in the directed proportions. In others, subjects were put on controlled-calorie diets that also had directed nutrient proportions. The conclusion: Those who *ate* the least fat *carried* the least fat.

An alternative method of comparing diets is a meta-analysis, which means not looking at the sum of the whole but actually combining the data. One such meta-analysis, covering 16 ad libitum studies and almost 2,000 people, appeared in the *International Journal of Obesity and Related Metabolic Disorders* in December 2000. The conclusion: Those on low-fat diets had "a greater reduction in energy intake" and a "greater weight loss than control groups."

"Aren't all these studies highly relevant to the issue of whether an Atkins-like diet works, and don't they indicate that it does not?" I ask Dr. Louis Aronne, director of the Comprehensive Weight Control Program at New York's Weill Cornell Medical Center. "I agree completely," he says. "You're absolutely right."

This wasn't the first time Taubes had published a lengthy article on fat while leaving out this vital information. He also did so in one of his award-winning pieces, a precursor to the "Big Fat Lie" article called "The Soft Science of Dietary Fat" that appeared in *Science* in March 2001. In a subsequent letter to the journal, three obesity research co-authors, including James Hill, director of the University of Colorado Center for Human Nutrition in Denver, noted, "What Taubes does not mention are the meta-analyses of intervention studies comparing ad libitum intakes of higher fat diets with low-fat diets that clearly show reduced caloric intake and weight loss on the low-fat diet." Taubes responded to the letter but again refused to address these studies.

Why? "They're not worth mentioning," he told me in a telephone interview. They weren't done correctly. None of them? None. The one meta-analysis Taubes thinks was properly conducted appeared in 2002 in *The Cochrane Library*. Yet it, too, found no advantage to low-carbohydrate diets, merely that "fat-restricted diets are no better than calorie restricted" ones.

Where, I ask Taubes, did all these researchers go wrong? The problem is inherent to an intervention study, he says. "When you counsel people you change their behavior." But doesn't that apply to all the groups in a study? Yes, he grants. "But the idea is to make the intervention effect equal for everyone, whichever diet they happen to be on," he says. "If the interventions aren't the same, then you just don't know how to interpret the results." That may be true, but it's also irrelevant. There's no reason to think persons on either low-fat or high-fat diets got more or less intervention in these myriad studies. Indeed, in some of them virtually all the intervention emphasis was on *exercise*, with little nutrition counseling one way or the other.

Finally, the comprehensive *JADA* review published last April [2002] also looked at persons who weren't in intervention studies at all but rather were part of the U.S. Department of Agriculture's Continuing Survey of Food Intake by Individuals. An updated report on the survey appeared [in] June in the *Journal of the American College of Nutrition*. Both survey reports came to the same conclusion as the intervention studies.

Dr. Aronne is quick to point out that this wealth of data supporting lower-fat diets "is not an endorsement for eating unlimited amounts of nonfat muffins and soda simply because they're fat-free." All carbohydrate sources are not equal. For example, fiber appears to play a powerful role in weight control, but there is no more fiber in a soda than there is in a steak. That said, a high-fat diet does carry an inherent metabolic disadvantage in that fat has nine calories per gram, while carbohydrates and protein each have four.

Abstract Weight Loss

Having circumvented this mass of peer-reviewed literature readily open to public scrutiny in libraries and often online, Taubes instead tried to make his case with a mere *five* studies. All five were (and are) available only in abstract form. That is, they are summaries of about 300 words each that have been presented at various obesity conferences. "The results of all five of these studies are remarkably consistent," Taubes averred. "Subjects on some form of the Atkins diet ... . lost twice the weight as the subjects on the low-fat, low-calorie diets."

One of the five studies, conducted at the Durham Veterans Administration Medical Center in North Carolina, was funded by the Atkins Center. Those researchers repeatedly have publicized their interpretation of their findings and unsurprisingly have conferred their full blessings on the diet. They did so most recently in late November, garnering tremendous favorable media attention. (See "Hold the Lard" at www.reason.com/hod/mf120502.shtml.) The authors of the other four studies, however, have been reticent about releasing their data, in part because pre-publicity in the lay press makes it more difficult to get published in medical journals. But when I interviewed researchers for two of the other studies, they all insisted Taubes grossly mischaracterized their findings.

"The Atkins diet produces weight loss, as does the grapefruit diet, the rotation diet, and every other fad diet out there," says one of the researchers, Colorado's James Hill. "I haven't seen any data anywhere saying Atkins is better than these other diets for weight loss. Taubes is trying to fly in the face of the scientific evidence." Referring to the book deal, he says, "Taubes sold out."

Hill's co-researcher, Gary Foster of the University of Pennsylvania, says "the probable explanation for the greater weight loss in the groups on the Atkins regimen" is that it "gives people a framework to eat fewer calories, since most of the choices in this culture are carbohydrate driven. . . . You're left eating a lot of fat, and you get tired of that. Over time people eat fewer calories." That would make the Atkins plan nothing more than a low-calorie diet in disguise.

Another of the abstracts came from the University of Cincinnati. The Atkins-like group "did have twice as much weight loss, and to completely lose that point would be unfair," says one of the co-authors, Randy Seeley of the university's Obesity Research Center. But his explanation is similar to Foster's, if more colorful. "If you're only allowed to shop in two aisles of the grocery store, does it matter which two they are?" he asks.

All the researchers I interviewed also insisted the studies weren't long enough to be conclusive, with none lasting more than a year. And the kicker is that all five were *intervention studies,* conducted using the same methodology that Taubes cites to dismiss the mountain of published material that undercuts his position.

Seeley and co-researcher David D'Alessio were also upset that Taubes made use of their material at all and not just because it hurt their chances of publication. "One of the things I object to most in the Taubes article is the idea that we're going to carry out this scientific debate in the lay press with data that's unavailable for scientists to review," says Seeley. "I believe in the peer-review process." Indeed, one "danger of trying to conduct this out in the lay press," he says, is that "you have a guy like Taubes going through it and just picking up the pieces that support his opinion."

3,000 MIAS

Taubes also ignored the approximately 3,000 members of a database called the National Weight Control Registry. For 10 years, the registry has tracked people who have lost at least 30 pounds and kept it off for at least a year. The average member has maintained a loss of about 60 pounds for about five years.

Co-administered by Hill in Denver and Rena Wing of the University of Pittsburgh, the registry is aimed at finding out what works and what doesn't. According to its members, what *doesn't* work is a high-fat diet. On average, they consume only 23 percent of calories from fat. "Almost nobody's on a low-carbohydrate diet," Hill says. Another important lesson that may be drawn from the registry is that the importance of *any* type of diet in weight control may be overemphasized. Ninety-one percent of the subjects said they regularly exercised.

While relying on self-interpretation of unpublished abstracts is valid methodology to Taubes, he insists the registry is so unscientific as to be worthless. One problem, he told me, is that it represents only a tiny fraction of all those who have succeeded at weight loss. Further, the sample is entirely self-selected rather than randomized. "Its method of recruiting could bias the selection toward those who use low-fat diets," he says.

Yet the registry data have been considered valid and important enough to have been written up in such peer-reviewed medical publications as the *American Journal of Clinical Nutrition,* the *Journal of the American Dietetic Association,* the *International Journal of Obesity, Health Psychology,* and *Obesity Research.*

"You can't get around" the problem of self-selection, says Suzanne Phelan, a co-investigator of the registry at Brown University Medical School. "But why would non-Atkins people select in and Atkins ones stay out?" Atkins dieters, she notes, "seem to be very dedicated." (Other researchers have described them as having an almost religious fervor.) Originally, recruits were selected "based on a random-digit dialing procedure," she says. But that proved onerous, and "as media such as *USA Today* and *CNN* began talking about the registry, we just let them take over" the recruiting process. "There's no reason to think that people who see those media are more likely to have a certain diet," Phelan says.

Oh, and there's another place where joining the registry has been promoted: the Atkins Web site. So we're left wondering why successful low-fat eaters would be especially likely to select into the registry or why the purchasers of over 11 million Atkins diet books consistently opt out.

Feeling Full

For all its 8,000 words, there were few actual data in the Taubes piece. It was rather like reading a treatise explaining how the Chicago Cubs may well be the best team in baseball history without being informed they haven't won a pennant since 1945. Instead readers were regaled with explanations of physiological mechanisms—the basis for which, Taubes wrote, is "Endocrinology 101"—that might explain how dieters shed pounds and inches. *Endocrinology 101* is a term popularized by Dr. David Ludwig, who runs the pediatric obesity clinic at Children's Hospital Boston.

According to Taubes, Endocrinology 101 "requires an understanding of how carbohydrates affect insulin and blood sugar and in turn fat metabolism and appetite." In brief, it says there are aspects of a high- or low-carbohydrate diet that affect both how much we want to eat (referred to as "satiety") and how efficiently the body converts the various nutrients into body fat. And the theory says an Atkins-like diet is both more satiating and less efficient in converting calories to fat.

Yet the published literature that Taubes ignored says otherwise. The aforementioned review of over 200 studies in the *Journal of the American Dietetic Association* expressly nixed the idea that any type of food converts less efficiently to body fat. "None of the popular diet research we reviewed suggests a metabolic advantage with respect to weight loss," it declared.

Nor can Taubes fall back on his five studies, according to Seeley. "Ultimately our data do not support *any* of the mechanisms" for why a low-carbohydrate diet might be especially effective in inducing weight loss "that Atkins and proponents of the diet have [suggested]," he told me. Indeed, each explanation that Taubes presents for how an Atkins diet *might* cause weight loss collapses under the weight of the published research he ignores.

Consider the matter of satiety. How, Taubes wondered, could a low-calorie regimen "suppress hunger, which Atkins insisted was the signature characteristic of the diet." One possibility, he said, was, yes, "Endocrinology 101: that fat and protein make you sated and, lacking carbohydrates and the ensuing swings of blood sugar and insulin, you stay sated."

But is there any empirical support for this? No, according to an April 2002 review of studies in the *Journal of the American College of Nutrition* that summarized "high and low fat treatments when subjects were allowed to eat ad libitum." It found "energy intake on the low-fat diets ranged from 16 percent to 24 percent less than those on high fat diets."

"We've done masses of studies on fat and satiety," says Barbara Rolls, professor of nutrition at Pennsylvania State University, where she has authored four books and written about 60 medical journal articles on human food intake.

She's widely considered the nation's top authority on satiety. Some of her experiments involved ingestion; in others, "We directly infused pure fat and pure carbohydrates both directly into [human] veins and directly into stomachs." Says Rolls, "We found very little difference between fats and carbohydrates."

Rolls does say there is some evidence that high-protein diets may be more satiating, but Atkins isn't really high protein; it's just high fat. According to an analysis in the journal *Circulation,* Atkins starts off at 36 percent protein from calories and declines to 24 percent in the "maintenance" stage.

What really counts when it comes to satisfying hunger, Rolls says, is "foods that give big portions without a lot of calories. We call these low-energy-density foods." She adds, "The Atkins diet would not be a good way to reduce energy density at all, especially with the restrictions on fruits and vegetables that are really the keys to a low-energy diet." Further, because fat contains more than twice the energy per ounce as either carbohydrates or protein, "high-fat foods are so energy-dense that it's really easy to eat excessive portions."

Rolls says she sent a big pile of her material on satiety to Taubes, but he "just brushed it aside." She says he also interviewed her for over six hours, but every last sentence disappeared into a black hole. Likewise for the interviews Taubes conducted with James Hill and at least five other top obesity researchers from whom he apparently couldn't extract even a single useful line: Dr. F. Xavier Pi-Sunyer of St. Luke's-Roosevelt Hospital in New York; Marion Nestle, chairwoman of the Department of Nutrition and Food Studies at New York University; Dr. Arne Astrup of Denmark; and Dr. Jules Hirsch, whom Taubes interviewed in his office at Rockefeller University in New York. "I just kept telling him, it doesn't matter what kind of calories you eat," says Hirsch.

Taubes is "very selective in what he chooses to include because he's trying to sell a specific line," Rolls says. "He is a good writer; that's the thing that scares me. This is such a good example of how you can pick and choose your facts to present the story you want. But that's not how science should be done. You can't interview everybody and simply ignore the people you don't want to hear." She means that rhetorically, of course.

Gorging on Theory

Stacking theory atop theory, Taubes roared on. Something called "hyperinsulinemia" could also favor the Atkins dieter, he insisted. When carbohydrates are ingested they are broken down in the intestine into glucose and other sugars. Glucose then stimulates cells in the pancreas to secrete insulin to remove that glucose and take it into tissues to be used as fuel or stored. Protein and fat consumption don't have nearly the same impact on insulin production because the whole point of insulin is to maintain the stability of the sugar level.

The Atkins hyperinsulinemia theory, explained Taubes, is that carbohydrates can "cause a spike of blood sugar and a surge of insulin within minutes. The resulting rush of insulin stores the blood sugar away and a few hours later, your blood sugar is lower than it was before you ate." The brain receives a signal that the body needs more food, and the vicious circle repeats itself. Carbohydrates at the top of what's called the "hypoglycemic index" are the most evil of the evil, since they cause blood sugar to rise the fastest. The index ranks potatoes as slightly worse than jelly beans.

For support, Taubes once again fell back on "Endocrinology 101." David Ludwig "notes that when diabetics get too much insulin, their blood sugar drops and they get ravenously hungry," wrote Taubes. "They gain weight because they eat more, and the insulin promotes fat deposition." But according to Seeley, this applies to diabetics injecting massive amounts of insulin into the bloodstream, not to carbohydrate consumers.

"Yes," Seeley says, "if you give people a big wallop of insulin they do eat a lot, but do people under normal circumstances ever get close to that by *eating?* No. Is it possible that *some* people are that reactive? Yes. Is it likely that lots of people fall into that category? No."

Taubes presented University of Washington endocrinologist Michael Schwartz, whom he had interviewed, as a proponent of the idea that blood insulin levels as altered by carbohydrates could be a significant contributor to weight gain. But a commentary in the same magazine Taubes writes for, *Science,* sharply contradicted that position. "Although the concept that insulin triggers weight gain has little scientific merit, it remains a key selling point for advocates of diets that are low in carbohydrate and high in protein and fat," it read. "If hyperinsulinemia has adverse consequences, obesity does not appear to be among them," it concluded. Who wrote that? Michael Schwartz.

Indeed, Schwartz was also the primary author of a study concluding that obese people whose systems secrete insulin at high levels may be *protected* against further weight gain. "Relatively reduced insulin secretion," he concluded, "is a significant and independent predictor of the tendency to gain weight and adiposity in Pima Indians.

The Pima in Arizona have been the focus of a tremendous amount of research because even by American standards they are incredibly obese and suffer horrific rates of diabetes and heart disease. Comparisons of the Arizona Pima with genetically similar Pima in Mexico find that the Arizonans eat about twice as much fat (although the Mexicans also do far more manual labor) and are almost 60 pounds heavier on average. A National Institutes of Health evaluation of the traditional Pima diet (that is, back when they were thin and healthy) found that it was extremely high in carbohydrates, from 70 percent to 80 percent.

Schwartz says it's not that he believes insulin *can't* play a role in promoting weight gain, but he rejects "Endocrinology 101" based on what he calls "Scientific Methodology 101." "Before you draw conclusions you need data," he says. "There is no compelling evidence that in normal individuals day-to-day fluctuations of the blood glucose level are an important determinant of how much food is consumed."

The Diet Revolution That Isn't

Two distinct controversies have always swirled around the Atkins diet. First, is it effective for long-term weight loss? Second, could those using it be harming themselves by raising their blood lipids (cholesterol and trigylcerides)? The five unpublished abstracts do seem to indicate that for people who manage to stick to a high-fat Atkins diet, it may not be as harmful as was once generally believed. But this finding is quite preliminary and in any case certainly must depend greatly on which types of fat are consumed.

This is a distinction Taubes decided to lose.

Thus he quoted or invoked the name of the chairman of the Department of Nutrition at the Harvard School of Public Health, Walter Willett, seven times during his piece. Willett protests, however, that "I told Taubes several times that red meat is associated with higher risk of colon and possibly prostate cancer, but he left that out." And don't forget the illustration on the cover of *The New York Times Magazine;* that wasn't a flounder with heart-healthy flaxseed oil sitting on top of it.

Taubes also told readers that a metabolic process called ketosis, often invoked to show the Atkins diet could be dangerous, was quite harmless, providing reassuring words from National Institutes of Health researcher Richard Veech that "ketosis is a normal physiologic state." Veech told me by e-mail that the quote was correct, but that Taubes "omitted to say that I strongly urged people to not use the Atkins diet without the supervision of a physician because of the likely elevation of blood cholesterol and lipid on a high fat diet." But you don't have an impact if you insist that a fad diet be supervised by a doctor.

There's nothing "revolutionary" about the Atkins diet. A similar diet appeared in an 1863 booklet by a British undertaker named William Banting, who got the idea from a surgeon. It has popped up in various guises ever since, including a 1946 book extolling the virtues of eating whale blubber, and a 1958 book, *Eat Fat and Grow Slim,* written by a psychiatrist.

Likewise, there has long been convincing evidence that the diet fails to live up to its claims. Taubes wrote that "when the American Medical Association (AMA) released its scathing critique of Atkins' diet in March 1973, it acknowledged that the diet probably worked but expressed little interest in why."

The heavily endnoted document, which appeared in the June 4, 1973, issue of *The Journal of the American Medical Association* but unfortunately is not available on the Internet even in abstract form, was indeed scathing. But the rest of Taubes' description is false.

"The notion that sedentary persons, without malabsorption or hyperthyroidism, can lose weight on a diet containing 5,000 calories a day is incredible," the article says. Statements such as "No scientific evidence exists to suggest that the low-carbohydrate ketogenic diet has a metabolic advantage over more conventional diets for weight reduction," and "there is no reason to associate a diet rich in carbohydrate with obesity" hardly seem to acknowledge "that the diet probably worked." Other terms the AMA used to described Atkins' theories included "naive," "biochemically incorrect," "inaccurate," and "without scientific merit."

It also explained *why* the diet didn't work, mocking Atkins' basic thesis that fat and protein cannot cause weight gain in the absence of carbohydrate consumption as a "thermodynamic miracle."

Three additional decades of research have merely played "pile on" with the AMA's findings. The explanation for weight loss on Atkins given by Foster and Seeley was right there. "When obese patients reduce their carbohydrate intake drastically, they are apparently unable to make up the ensuing deficit by means of an appreciable increase in protein and diet," said the AMA.

Girth of a Nation

What *has* changed drastically in the last three decades is the girth of a nation. American obesity is increasing at a terrifying rate.

Since the publication of Taubes' article, numerous doctors, scientists, and health writers have picked apart various pieces of his argument. A fatlash has formed against Taubes, *The New York Times Magazine,* and Knopf. Originally riding an adulatory wave, Taubes complained bitterly to the weekly *New York Observer* in November that he was "being attacked by sleazebags."

The New York Times Magazine has printed no clarification or retraction of any kind. Yet not only should the magazine's editors have known there were serious problems with the piece, but Farquhar says he told them so outright, based on what he had gleaned from two fact checkers. He says he told those checkers that if Taubes "tries to make it look like I'm saying that I was supporting the idea that the obesity epidemic was from overloading on carbohydrates that this was so far off the mark that I would have to vomit."

At Knopf, Taubes' acquisitions editor, Scott Segal, has wrapped himself in the flag, telling the *Observer,* "It's a free country: First Amendment," as if he believes the Constitution requires publishers to hand out $700,000 checks to all authors. Equally bizarre is his effort to distance the book acquisition from the article. They "chose to put a certain picture on the cover and to use a certain approach to the subject in 5,000 [*sic*] words, but that's not the book,' he said. Critics "are reacting to a magazine piece I had nothing to do with." Yet Taubes told me that his article had barely hit the stands when Knopf's offer dropped in his lap, as did an even larger offer from another publisher that he says he rejected because it's the publisher of Atkins' book and it might hurt his credibility.

But obesity and the millions of individual tragedies it has produced are ultimately far more important than this skirmish over a single story. Louis Aronne says, "I think people are getting increasingly confused about what to do. I'm afraid they'll just give up." Randy Seeley says journalism like Taubes' "just makes people confused and frustrated."

Taubes "gave his readers what they wanted to hear," says James Hill. "But what people want to hear is killing them."

POSTSCRIPT

Is the Atkins Low-Carbohydrate Diet a Valid Weight-Loss Plan?

American weight gain has increased despite the fact that millions are dieting on any given day. Many experts argue that the fat content of a diet is not a good gauge of nutritional quality. It is also asserted that it is not correct to abandon a varied diet in order to consume more pasta, white rice, and fat-free baked goods. On the other hand, the Atkins diet, with its ample protein and fat, reduces the consumption of fruits, vegetables, whole grains, and low-fat dairy products that are essential for health. These foods are naturally low in fat and calories, and they are high in fiber and other nutrients. Although most experts believe that a low-fat, high-fiber diet is better for health, it is unclear what is the best way to permanently lose weight.

In "Atkins Diet: What's Wrong With It?" *Consumer Reports* (June 2002), the authors contend that only healthy dieters with low cholesterol should go on the Atkins diet and only for a short time They maintain that the diet should not be part of a sustainable eating regimen. This belief is echoed in "Eat Fat, Get Thin?" *Berkeley Wellness Letter* (April 2000). In "Fad Diets: What You May Be Missing," *Journal of the American Dietetic Association* (February 2000), it is stated that weight-loss advice comes in literally hundreds of disguises. Most often the "new" and "revolutionary" diets are really old fad diets making an encore appearance. Examples of fad diets include those that tout or ban a specific food or food group. Food-specific diets rely on the myth that some foods have special properties that can cause weight loss or gain. But this is not necessarily true. These diets do not teach healthful eating habits; therefore, most people are not able to stick with them. Sooner or later, they will have a taste for something else—anything that is not among the foods "allowed" on the diet.

The popular high-protein, low-carbohydrate diets, including the Atkins diet, are based on the idea that carbohydrates are unhealthy. Proponents of these diets assert that many people are "allergic" to carbohydrates or are insulin-resistant and therefore gain weight when they eat carbohydrate-rich foods. The truth is that people are eating more total calories and performing less physical activity, and that, according to many, is the real reason that people are gaining weight. See also "The Truth About the Atkins Diet," *Nutrition Action Healthletter* (November 2002); "Persons Successful at Long-Term Weight Loss and Maintenance Continue to Consume a Low-Energy, Low-Fat Diet," *Journal of the American Dietetics Association* (April 1998); "Read My Lipids," *Nutrition Action Healthletter* (October 2001); and "Popular Diets: Correlation to Health, Nutrition, and Obesity," *Journal of the American Dietetic Association* (April 2001).

ISSUE 21

Should Alternative Medicine Be Combined With Conventional Medicine?

YES: Andrew Weil, from "Is Integrative Medicine the Medicine of the Future?" A Debate Between Arnold S. Relman, MD, and Andrew Weil, MD, *Archives of Internal Medicine* (October 11, 1999)

NO: Arnold S. Relman, from "Is Integrative Medicine the Medicine of the Future?" A Debate Between Arnold S. Relman, MD, and Andrew Weil, MD, *Archives of Internal Medicine* (October 11, 1999)

ISSUE SUMMARY

YES: Andrew Weil, director of the University of Arizona Program on Integrative Medicine, asserts that alternative medicine helps patients and should be incorporated into conventional medical practices.

NO: Physician and editor Arnold S. Relman argues that integrating alternative healing with conventional medicine would be a step backward and would not improve medical care.

Alternative medicine can be categorized into four divisions: spiritual (faith-based) treatment, nutritional therapies, physical therapies, and yoga. The term *alternative* usually refers to medicines that are meant to be substituted for traditional medical care, while *integrated* medicine is an attempt to unite the best of both worlds; joining, for example, herbal formulas and therapies with conventional drug treatment. While mainstream physicians and health providers may not completely support integrated medicine, many consumers have endorsed these treatments. From 1990 to 1997 the use of herbal remedies increased by nearly 400 percent. In the late 1990s over one-third of Americans used herbs, spending nearly $4 billion for these products. In addition to the use of herbs, studies have shown that as many as a third of Americans have visited an alternative practitioner. It seems that many patients are dissatisfied with traditional medicine. These consumers may even be distrustful of conventional health providers, whom they may perceive as profit-motivated, too technological, and lacking in warmth and bedside manner. For Americans without health insurance, alternative treatments may offer treatment at a lower cost.

Some maintain that alternative therapies offer a more natural approach to treatment with fewer side effects. Some promoters of natural treatments assert that their products are natural and therefore, safer than traditional medicines. These promoters may also argue that their products have been used for hundreds or thousands of years.

Many conventional practitioners are concerned about the shift by some patients to favoring alternative medicines over traditional medicines. They argue that many alternative therapies are unproven, therefore not a good substitution for traditional drugs and treatments. Another potentially dangerous practice is when people take alternative drugs to assist them as they go through serious medical procedures. Some herbs taken prior to surgery may prolong blood coagulation, which can lead to severe bleeding. Finally, there is concern over the lack of rigorous testing of alternative drug therapies. Many lack scientific validation and are supported more by testimonials than by the regulation and testing that is required of traditional drugs.

In 1998 the National Institutes of Health (NIH) created the National Center for Complementary and Alternative Medicine, which is designed to sort the beneficial from the worthless alternative treatments. To some, this move means that scientific rigor will be upheld. However, many took this recognition as a legitimization of the entire field. This includes the more accepted chiropractic and acupuncture treatments along with less accepted treatments and remedies.

In the following selections, Andrew Weil supports both conventional and alternative therapies. He states that physicians are doing their patients a disservice by withholding information on the benefits of some alternative treatments. Andrew S. Relman counters that untested alternative therapies do not advance medicine, instead they undermine the many achievements accomplished by modern scientists and practitioners.

Andrew Weil 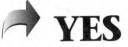 **YES**

Is Integrative Medicine the
Medicine of the Future? Yes

In this country and throughout the world, patients in unprecedented numbers are going outside of conventional medicine to look for help. This is a movement that has been building since the late 1960s, and it's now reached the point that visits to alternative practitioners exceed visits to primary care providers and the amount of money spent on these visits exceeds that spent on visits to primary care providers, so this is a very powerful social and cultural force that we're witnessing. Now, why are people doing this? Clearly, there is dissatisfaction with conventional medicine. I don't think it is simply with the recent impersonality and time constraints that have come with managed care, because this movement began long before that. In my experience—and I know this is a phrase that Dr [Arnold S.] Relman doesn't like, but I consider experience to be one valuable source of data—in my experience, many patients use alternative methods because they work. If a patient has tried a method and found that it works, that patient needs no further proof, does not need to read the reports of a randomized double-blind controlled trial in a medical journal to be convinced of the efficacy of treatment. So, I think large numbers of patients have found that there are treatments out there that their conventional physicians did not know about, did not advise them about, that have worked for them in some cases after conventional medicine has failed. One of the arguments that I hear from opponents of this movement is that patients in going this route are refusing or delaying real treatment from conventional medicine. That also goes against my experience of many years as a practitioner of this kind of medicine. The vast majority of patients who have come to me and the vast majority of patients who now come to the integrative medicine clinic in this institution are patients who have been through conventional medicine, often many times over, have been tested to death, have tried many conventional therapies, and have found that they haven't worked or have caused harm or both, and it is that which motivates them now to look for other kinds of treatments. We have to take this consumer movement seriously. It is not just that consumers want it. I think there are valid reasons why they want it and have found it to be useful, and furthermore, it is not just consumers who want a change in medical education. Significant numbers of medical students today are asking for this kind of instruction, as are physicians in training and physicians in practice. There is a large and growing gulf in this country between what patients expect of doctors and what medical schools are training them to do. Patients want physicians who have the time to sit down with them and listen and explain to them in language they can understand the nature of their problems, who are aware of nutritional influences on health, who will not just push drugs and surgery as the only approach to treating illness, who can intelligently answer questions about dietary supplements, who are sensitive to mind-body interactions, who will not laugh in your face if you ask questions about Chinese medicine, who are willing to look at you as more than just a physical body. I think those are reasonable requests, but that's not what we're training physicians to do. It is that widening gulf between patient expectations and physician realities that is leading so many patients to go elsewhere for treatment. One of the reasons that I feel passionate about bringing this kind of training into our medical schools is that I feel a very strong commitment to my profession, and I would like to see it better answer the needs of people. My impression is that many patients now going to alternative practitioners, if given a choice, would prefer to go to a physician who had basic medical training and was also knowledgeable about and open-minded about other treatment options, who could act as a guide or an advisor in making difficult treatment decisions. For example, our integrative medicine clinic has seen an enormous number of cancer patients over the past year and a half, and I must say I feel very sorry for many of them. I think they're left out in the cold. Their conventional oncologists give them standard treatments and tell them that there's nothing else to be done. They know that there are other things to be done, that there are remedies that can mitigate the toxicity of the standard therapies, can protect their immune systems from those therapies, can enhance general health. They go to alternative practitioners who tell them that if they use the conventional therapies they may as well not bother with the alternative treatments. So, it's the patient that suffers. How much better it would be if there were physicians trained to advise patients about the intelligent combination of the available therapies. This is what patients want, but they can't find that kind of service. By the way, I think it is interesting that some of our critics who don't really know what we do have accused us of taking all cancer patients off chemotherapy and putting them on herbs. We went back and looked at the records of cancer patients we have seen over the past year and a half. Of the first 60, none was taken off any kind of conventional therapy, and 11 who said that they would not do conventional therapies were persuaded by our integrative medicine fellows to do them in combination with other supportive measures.

I would like to say something about the issue of science-based medicine and evidence-based medicine. I consider myself a scientist. The word *science* comes from the root of a verb *to know*. There are various ways of knowing. One is paying attention to one's own experiences, as I have said. Another way is from the collective experience of other cultures. Here is an example from my own field of ethnobotany. If you are a pharmaceutical company looking for new drugs in the rain forest, you have a choice as to how you can go about the search. You can go into a geographical area, take every plant that grows in the area, bring it back, and screen it for biological activity, or you can target a particular plant family. But there is another way you can do things. You can go to the shamans in the cultures who live there, and you can ask them to show you the plants that they have learned work for certain conditions and take those back for testing. When you compare those 2 approaches, there is a significantly higher percentage of hits if you take the plants that have been brought into use by people over thousands of years of experimentation. Another aspect of this issue is the claim that conventional medicine is science supported by evidence. The Office of Technology Assessment of the US Congress has estimated that fewer than 30% of procedures currently used in conventional medicine have been rigorously tested, and I think there are many, many examples of procedures in common use today that are not backed up by the kind of evidence that Dr Relman would like to see. That includes the use of open heart surgery in general and coronary artery bypass grafting in patients where the evidence does not support its use. I am all for refining our medical practice and making it more consistent with scientific evidence, but as Dr Relman himself has pointed out in an editorial in the *New England Journal of Medicine,* medicine constantly operates in areas of uncertainty where the evidence has not yet come in. There is a great difference between being a researcher and being a practitioner. As a researcher, you have the luxury of insisting on rigorous scientific testing and you have the leisure to wait for results to come in. As a practitioner, you are in the trenches working with patients who have medical needs and you often have to guess to use your best medical judgment in the absence of definitive evidence. What do you do then? It seems to me that you do the best you can, and the first principle from which you operate, or should operate, is that you do no harm. That was Hippocrates' most famous teaching, and I fear that it is not sufficiently stressed in medical education today. As an example of what I mean, I would cite a lead article that was published in the *Journal of the American Medical Association* exactly a year ago entitled "The Incidence of Adverse Drug Reactions in Hospitalized Patients" that estimated that there are now 100 000 deaths a year in US hospitals directly caused by pharmaceutical drugs. In contrast to the few disasters that happen with herbal medication, these are the correct drugs, correctly prescribed for the correct condition. In herbal medicine, often a misidentified plant has gotten into commerce and caused a problem, but this article concerned the right drugs and the right doses being given to the right patients killing 100 000 patients a year, and this is now estimated to rank between the fourth and sixth leading cause of death in hospitals in this country. These drugs have come through the process of rigorous testing. They have come through the FDA's regulatory mechanisms, and nonetheless, they are producing this degree of harm. If integrative medicine did nothing other than reduce the incidence of this direct kind of iatrogenic harm, I think it would be very worth incorporating into our medical schools and teaching.

I would also like to comment on the kinds of bias that exist in conventional science, especially in medical journals, against the acceptance of novel ideas, and here again, let me just cite one example that also appeared a year ago.

An article that was published in the *Proceedings of the National Academy of Sciences* described excellent research that used MRI [magnetic resonance imaging] scans of the living brain to show that stimulation of acupuncture points on the lateral aspect of the foot, points associated with vision in traditional Chinese medicine, caused activation of the visual cortex identical to the activation caused by stimulation of the retina by light. Stimulation of points a few centimeters off from these traditional acupuncture points did not cause visual cortex activation. That paper was rejected by the *New England Journal of Medicine,* and it was rejected by the *Journal of the American Medical Association* before it finally found a home in the *Proceedings of the National Academy of Sciences.* Despite what Dr Relman says, there is very strong prejudice against accepting ideas that run counter to preconceptions such as Chinese medicine being superstitious and on the face of it absurd; such attitudes lead journal editors and heads of medical institutions to ignore or at worst to suppress evidence that comes in contrary to expectations. I don't think you can have it both ways. You can't demand evidence, and then when evidence is presented that contradicts your preconceptions, say you aren't going to look at it. I am not so optimistic about resolving our differences because, while we do have common ground, I think there is a real difference in world view here. I feel strongly that integrative medicine is the future, not only because people want it, but because very powerful forces operating both within science and outside of science are moving us in this direction. Demand for it is not just coming from the customers. It is now beginning to come very strongly from practitioners and members of the profession. Large numbers of physicians in practice realize that they did not get the training required of them to satisfy the needs of patients today, and increasing numbers of medical students are asking why they aren't learning about botanicals, why they aren't learning about the role of phytoestrogens in flax and, say, as possible preventives of breast cancer, for example. So I think it is inevitable that we move in this direction. I feel very fortunate to be at a medical institution that recognizes this reality and supports the development of new curriculum as well as the studies that I strongly agree with Dr Relman are required to produce the kind of evidence that will lead to changes in how we practice medicine. Thank you.

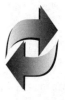

Arnold S. Relman

← **NO**

Is Integrative Medicine the Medicine of the Future? No

So-called alternative medicine, and its challenge to conventional medicine, is a large subject that cannot be adequately explored in a relatively brief debate . . . Instead, Dr [Andrew] Weil and I have agreed to concentrate primarily on the question of whether alternative medicine can and should be combined with conventional medicine to create a new entity called integrative medicine. He thinks such a step would be a major advance. He says, "Integrative medicine is the future and our healthcare institutions will not survive without it." I think he is seriously mistaken. In my view, integrating alternative medicine with mainstream medicine would not be an advance but a return to the past, an interruption of the remarkable progress achieved by science-based medicine over the past century. I can't see how such integration, even if it were possible, would improve medical care or further the cause of human health. What is more, considering all the dubious and disparate theories and practices gathered under the banner of alternative medicine, I don't see how our medical schools could make sense of such a hodgepodge, much less unify it with conventional medicine. Most alternative systems of treatment are based on irrational or fanciful thinking and false or unproven factual claims. Their theories often violate basic scientific principles and are at odds not only with each other, but with current knowledge of the structure and function of the human body as now taught in our medical schools. They could not be woven into the fabric of the medical curriculum without confusion, contradiction, and an undermining of the scientific foundation upon which modern medicine rests. Future advances in clinical practice will depend on the application of new developments in science, biotechnology, molecular pharmacology, and on the use of clinical epidemiology based on the analysis of objective clinical data. Indeed, it is hard to imagine any progress at all in the prevention, diagnosis, or treatment of disease without continued, even closer cooperation between modern science and evidence-based medical practice. With the promise of so many new breakthroughs in the offing, why on earth should we now want to drive a wedge between medicine and science? Alternative medicine stands apart from modern science, challenging many of its assumptions and methods and depending for its verification largely on personal belief and subjective experience. In sharp contrast to mainstream medicine, alternative medicine makes no distinction between objective phenomena and subjective experience or between the external world and human consciousness. This allows the practitioners of alternative medicine to believe in the power of mind and thought to change physical matter and heal organic diseases—a concept that basically contradicts the laws of physics in the modern scientific view of nature. Furthermore, since alternative practitioners also are convinced that individual subjective experience is the ultimate verification of truth, most of them do not see the need to obtain objective statistically significant data in order to test whether their methods really work. Medical science teaches practitioners to look for objective evidence before adopting a clinical method. But alternative medicine teaches that faith in a method will make it effective and that the strongest kind of evidence is the patient's belief that a treatment is working. How would the proposed new integrated curriculum deal with this wide philosophical gulf between alternative and conventional medicine? Dr Weil seems to be of two minds: On the one hand, he says that "good medicine must be consistent with good science" and he believes in basing clinical practice on clinical trials and other objective evidence. On the other hand, he often ignores medical science by supporting the concept of healing through the physical action of nonphysical forces, and by advocating the superiority of alternative treatments and herbs over conventional treatments and standard pharmaceuticals, based on little more than his own opinions and undocumented experience, or on the stories of others.

Here is just a very small but representative sample of the many unproven and often highly unlikely claims made by Dr Weil in his book:

1. Improper breathing is a common cause of ill health and breathing exercises will cure disease and promote good health.
2. Massive doses of intravenous vitamin C speed the healing of surgical wounds.
3. Guided imagery, meditation, or hypnotherapy will reduce the frequency of recurrent attacks of herpes simplex.
4. Topical application of human urine is effective treatment for athlete's foot.
5. Two tablespoons of ground flaxseed daily reduces the risk of breast cancer.
6. Cutting down on sugar intake decreases the frequency of urinary tract infections in nondiabetic women.
7. Therapeutic touch and other forms of so-called energy medicine can heal disease through the manual transmission or adjustment of types of so-called energy that are simply too subtle to be detectable by instruments.
8. Belief alone, without any physical intervention, can cure organic disease as "proven" by visits to miracle shrines, faith healers, and Christian Science practitioners. (Here, I might note in passing that, with respect to the investigation of claims of miraculous cures, the Catholic church

lately seems to be doing a more thorough job than the apostles of alternative medicine.)

Would such teaching become part of Dr Weil's new curriculum?

When challenged about the scientific implausibility of many of his methods, particularly those based on the alleged healing power of thought, Dr Weil sometimes invokes quantum mechanics and other recent developments in theoretical physics. Like other gurus of alternative medicine (Deepak Chopra, for example), he apparently believes that quantum physics proves that human consciousness can change and even create external reality. Thus, he believes that the mind may be able to heal serious physical illnesses through mechanisms that classical physics can't explain or even test. This presumably is why he believes a new integrated medical curriculum should include recent developments in physics.

This idea cannot be taken seriously. It reflects a basic misunderstanding of science in general and of quantum theory in particular. As clearly stated by every distinguished physicist who has ever written about these matters, all physical theories, new or old, must be validated by objective data. Advocates of alternative medicine cannot avoid the need to test their methods simply by their vague allusions to "new scientific paradigms." Without objectively verifiable evidence, there is no reason to believe the claims of alternative medicine, particularly when there is no plausible biological mechanism by which many of its methods might work. Furthermore, as several leading physicists have written, quantum theory says nothing about human consciousness or its possible effects on the physical world, and it provides no support for the belief in so-called paranormal phenomena. Quantum theory is simply a mathematical tool for describing and predicting subatomic phenomena. It is not permission to believe in the kinds of magical cures claimed by Dr Weil in his books.

Before completing my argument, I want to say something very briefly about herbal therapy, which would be an important feature of Dr Weil's proposed new curriculum. In one sense, herbal therapy should not be in fundamental conflict with the conventional medical curriculum, because many plant-derived materials have important biological effects. We all know that many pharmaceuticals now in use were derived from plants, and doubtless many more will be discovered.

Unfortunately, however, herbal products are not regulated by the FDA [Food and Drug Administration], and so commercially marketed herbal preparations are highly variable in content, purity, and potency. What is more, they have passed no tests for therapeutic effectiveness or safety. Despite these facts, drugstore and supermarket shelves are filled with all kinds of herbal products and dietary supplements, and consumers are increasingly being bombarded by a confusing and misleading advertising blitz from the manufacturers.

Dr Weil says that the FDA "needs to create a new division of natural therapeutics to regulate herbs, vitamins, minerals, and other dietary supplements," but he hasn't said, that I am aware of, what kind of regulation he has in mind or whether and why the regulation should be different from the FDA's existing oversight of prescription pharmaceuticals. He ought to tell us what is special about these "natural" therapeutic substances that might require a different regulatory approach, if that is what he believes. Is it the fact that natural plant preparations contain many different kinds of active molecules rather than a single active molecule as in most prescription drugs? If so, these can and should be identified and tested, singly or in combination, for effectiveness and safety. We need to see many more controlled studies comparing standardized herbal preparations with conventional pharmaceuticals before concluding that herbs have any special advantage over conventional drugs and that herbal therapy should be taught in medical schools. The March 1990 issue, the last issue of *Consumer Reports,* has an excellent article on this subject that explains why today's over-the-counter herbals are not ready for prime-time medical use.

The paucity of good clinical studies of alternative methods and herbal therapy in the peer-reviewed medical literature is said by some to be explained by the biases of medical journal editors against such studies. As a former editor, I know that claim to be untrue. The fact is that there have been relatively few rigorous clinical studies of alternative methods submitted to the leading peer-reviewed journals. As Dr Weil correctly argues, this is partly due to lack of funds to support such studies, but I believe that the main explanation is that alternative practitioners, so far, have had very little use for the conventional scientific approach, preferring instead their own "person-friendly" version of "alternative science," which depends more on subjective experience and intuition than on objective quantitative evidence.

A new interest in alternative medicine is now generating support from government agencies and foundations for clinical trials of alternative methods, and that is all to the good. We should certainly reserve final judgment about the alternative methods presently undergoing, or slated soon to undergo, clinical trial. But why, in the name of common sense, should we now rush to bring most of what is called alternative medicine into the mainstream of medical education and practice, when the existing evidence to support its claims and theories is so weak and the probabilities of the validity so small?

If any alternative methods prove to be effective in treating disease, they should be integrated into the medical curriculum, and they will be. All clinical biases and preconceptions, whether in alternative medicine or conventional medical practice, must fall before the objective evidence, and we should all be assiduous in seeking such evidence to improve our practices. However, in the absence of evidence, it makes no sense to remodel our clinical training programs to include alternative medicine simply because many "customers," to use Dr Weil's term, seem to want it. If alternative medicine is considered a business, I suppose that would be sufficient reason, but I hold to the old-fashioned view that medicine is a profession and that physicians owe their patients something more than simply offering services that are currently popular. At the least, they owe patients their best professional advice, based on the most reliable information. By that standard, alternative medicine does not qualify for admission to the medical mainstream.

POSTSCRIPT

Should Alternative Medicine Be Combined With Conventional Medicine?

Some alternative medicines, such as acupuncture and herbal remedies, have been used for thousands of years. Other alternative medicines, such as chiropractic treatments and homeopathy, are more recent and were developed, in part, as an alternative to the severe practices of conventional medicine in the eighteenth and nineteenth centuries. During those times, patients' bodies were purged of illness through the use of a variety of irritants. Blood-letting, leeches, and enemas were all used by legitimate doctors to treat illnesses of which they had no real understanding. These therapies generally damaged the patient and negatively affected the outcome of the disease.

Today, patients with chronic diseases and pain still explore alternative treatments that offer a cure for the disease and/or relief from pain. With the widespread availability of herbal remedies, alternative practitioners, and various unconventional treatments, the consumer's problem is determining what alternative therapies might be beneficial and safe. Unfortunately, there is little monitoring of these therapies, and there is also limited research on efficacy and overall safety.

While many consumers are satisfied with the care that they receive from modern medicine, others continue to explore alternative medicines to supplement or replace conventional treatment. Further reading on the subject includes "Patient's Sense of Increased Control Correlates With Alternative Medicine Use," *Cancer Weekly* (March 25, 2003); "Listening to the Consumers— The Integration of Conventional and Alternative Medicine," *Healthcare Review* (March 18, 2003); "Alternative Medicine Ain't Disco: What Nostrums Are Your Patients Taking? If You Don't Know, You Won't Be Able to Help Them," *Medical Economics* (March 7, 2003); "A Critical Overview of Homeopathy," *Annals of Internal Medicine* (March 4, 2003); "Alternative Prescribing and Negligence," *British Medical Journal* (February 22, 2003); and "Complementary and Alternative Medical Therapies: Implications for Medical Education," *Annals of Internal Medicine* (February 4, 2003).

Contributors to This Volume

EDITOR

EILEEN L. DANIEL, a registered dietitian and licensed nutritionist, is an associate professor in the Department of Health Science at the State University of New York College at Brockport. She received a B.S. in nutrition and dietetics from the Rochester Institute of Technology in 1977, an M.S. in community health education from SUNY College at Brockport in 1978, and a Ph.D. in health education from the University of Oregon in 1986. A member of the Eta Sigma Gamma National Health Honor Society, the American Dietetics Association, the New York State Dietetics Society, and other professional and community organizations, she has published over 35 articles on issues of health, nutrition, and health education. She is the author of *A Guidebook for Nutrition* (Morton, 1998).

STAFF

Jeffrey L. Hahn   Vice President/Publisher
Theodore Knight   Managing Editor
David Brackley   Senior Developmental Editor
Juliana Gribbins   Developmental Editor
Rose Gleich   Permissions Assistant
Brenda S. Filley   Director of Production/Manufacturing
Julie Marsh   Project Editor
Juliana Arbo   Typesetting Supervisor
Richard Tietjen   Publishing Systems Manager
Charles Vitelli   Designer

AUTHORS

GEORGE J. ANNAS is the Edward R. Utley Professor of Law and Medicine at Boston University's Schools of Medicine and Public Health in Boston, Massachusetts. He is also director of Boston University's Law, Medicine, and Ethics Program and chair of the Department of Health Law. His publications include *Standard of Care: The Law of American Bioethics* (Oxford University Press, 1993) and *Some Choice: Law, Medicine, and the Market* (Oxford University Press, 1998).

JOYCE ARTHUR is the editor of the Canadian newsletter *Pro-Choice Press* and an abortion rights activist.

RONALD BAILEY is a science correspondent for *Reason* magazine.

STEPHEN BARRETT is a retired psychiatrist and a nationally renowned author, editor, and consumer health advocate. He is a board member of the National Council Against Health Fraud and a scientific and editorial adviser to the American Council on Science and Health. In 1986 he was awarded honorary life membership in the American Dietetic Association. He has written more than 36 books.

HERBERT BENSON is a physician and associate professor of medicine at Harvard Medical School and the Deaconess Hospital. He is also president and founder of their Mind/Body Institute.

PATRICIA LANOIE BLANCHETTE is a professor of medicine and public health in the John A. Burns School of Medicine at the University of Hawaii, Honolulu. She is also the director of their geriatric medicine program.

ESTEBAN GONZÁLEZ BURCHARD is a physician in the Division of General Internal Medicine at the San Francisco General Hospital. He is also on the faculty of the University of California, San Francisco. Burchard is director of the UCSF/SFGH DNA Banking Facility.

CHRISTOPHER CALDWELL is a senior writer for *The Weekly Standard.*

RICHARD S. COOPER is a physician with the Department of Preventive Medicine and Epidemiology at the Loyola Stritch School of Medicine in Maywood, Illinois.

MICHELLE COTTLE is senior editor of *The New Republic.*

WILLIAM F. CURRENT is president of WFC & Associates, a national consulting firm specializing in drug-free workplace policies.

WILLIAM S. CUSTER is an associate professor in the Department of Risk Management and Insurance in the College of Business Administration at Georgia State University.

GAYLE FELDMAN is a writer living in New York City.

BARBARA LOE FISHER is coauthor of *DPT: A Shot in the Dark* (Warner Books, 1986), and she is also cofounder and president of the National Vaccine Information Center.

MICHAEL FUMENTO, a former AIDS analyst and attorney for the U.S. Commission on Civil Rights, is a senior fellow at the Hudson Institute and the author of *The Fat of the Land: The American Obesity Epidemic and How Overweight Americans Can Help Themselves* (Viking Press, 1997).

RONALD J. GLASSER is a pediatrician in Minneapolis, Minnesota, and the author of *The Greatest Battle* (Random House, 1976) and *The Light in the Skull: An Odyssey of Medical Discovery* (Faber & Faber, 1997).

RICHARD T. HULL is professor emeritus of philosophy at the State University of New York at Buffalo.

DAVID JACOBSEN is a surgeon with Harvard Pilgrim Health Care in Boston. He is coauthor, with Eric D. Jacobsen, of *Doctors Are Gods: Corruption and Unethical Practices in the Medical Profession* (Thunder's Mouth Press, 1994).

MICHAEL F. JACOBSON is executive director of the Center for Science in the Public Interest.

CHARLES N. KAHN III is president of the American Federation of Hospitals. He is also chairman of the University of Michigan's Economic Research Initiative on the Uninsured and writes about health care financing.

MARTIJN B. KATAN is a professor of human nutrition at the Agricultural University in Wageningen, the Netherlands.

DON B. KATES is a civil liberties lawyer and criminologist based in San Francisco, California. He has authored or coauthored a number of books, including *Handgun Prohibition and the Original Meaning of the Second Amendment* (Second Amendment Foundation, 1984) and *The Great American Gun Debate: Essays on Firearms and Violence* (Pacific Research Institute for Public Policy, 1997).

JAY S. KAUFMAN is an epidemiologist with the University of North Carolina School of Public Health in Chapel Hill.

CHRISTOPHER F. KOLLER is CEO of Neighborhood Health Plan of Rhode Island.

ALAN I. LESHNER is director of the National Institute on Drug Abuse at the National Institutes of Health.

WILLIAM B. LINDLEY is an associate editor of *Truth Seeker* magazine.

ETHAN A. NADELMANN is director of the Lindesmith Center, a New York drug-policy research institute, and an assistant professor of politics and public affairs in the Woodrow Wilson School of Public and International Affairs at Princeton University in Princeton, New Jersey. He was the founding coordinator of the Harvard Study Group on Organized Crime, and he has been a consultant to the Department of State's Bureau of International Narcotics Matters.

MARION NESTLE is professor and chair of the Department of Nutrition, Food Studies, and Public Health at New York University.

DAYN PERRY is a freelance writer.

UWE E. REINHARDT is James Madison Professor of Political Economy at Princeton University. He recently edited *Regulating Managed Care: Theory, Practice, and Future Options* (Jossey-Bass, 1999).

ARNOLD RELMAN is editor-in-chief emeritus of *The New England Journal of Medicine* and is also a physician.

JOHN A. ROBERTSON is a professor in and the Vinson and Elkins Chair of the University of Texas School of Law in Austin, Texas. He earned his B.A. from Dartmouth College in 1964 and his J.D. from Harvard University in 1968.

SALLY L. SATEL is a practicing psychiatrist in Washington, DC, and a lecturer in psychiatry at Yale University School of Medicine.

HENRY E. SCHAFFER is a professor of genetics and biomathematics at North Carolina State University in Raleigh, North Carolina. He is coauthor, with Lawrence E. Mettler and Thomas G. Gregg, of *Population Genetics and Evolution* (Prentice Hall, 1988).

STEVEN P. SHELOV is chairman of the Department of Pediatrics at the Babies' and Children's Hospital of Brooklyn at the Maimonides Medical Center in New York City.

MARGARET SOMERVILLE is Samuel Gale Professor of Law and professor in the Faculty of Medicine at McGill University Centre for Medicine, Ethics, and Law in Montreal, Canada.

MARG STARK is a freelance journalist specializing in medical news and features and the author of *What No One Tells the Bride* (Hyperion, 1998).

JOSH SUGARMANN is the executive director of the Violence Policy Center, an educational foundation that researches firearm violence and advocates gun control. The former communications director of the National Coalition to Ban Handguns, he is the author of *National Rifle Association: Money, Firepower and Fear* (National Press Books, 1992).

JACOB SULLUM is a senior editor at *Reason* magazine. He writes on several public policy issues, including freedom of speech, criminal justice, and education. His work has appeared in the *Wall Street Journal*, the *New York Times*, and the *Los Angeles Times*.

GARY TAUBES is a freelance journalist in New York City.

STEVEN UNGERLEIDER is a clinical psychologist and an adjunct professor at the University of Oregon.

ERIC A. VOTH is chairman of the International Drug Strategy Institute and clinical assistant professor with the Department of Medicine at the University of Kansas School of Medicine. He is also the medical director of Chemical Dependency Services at St. Francis Hospital in Topeka, Kansas. He has testified for the Drug Enforcement Administration in opposition to legalizing marijuana, and he is recognized as an international authority on drug abuse.

RYK WARD is a researcher with the Department of Biological Anthropology at Oxford University in the United Kingdom.

WILLIAM C. WATERS IV practices medicine in Atlanta, Georgia.

ANDREW WEIL is director of the University of Arizona Program on Integrative Medicine. He is the author of eight books and many scientific and popular articles on the incorporation of complementary interventions into modern medical practice.

THOMAS F. WILDSMITH IV is a policy research actuary for the Health Insurance Association of America.

ALAN WILLIAMS is with the Department of Social Work at the University of Manchester, England.

PAUL YANICK, JR., is a physician and the author of *Quantum Medicine: A Guide to the New Medicine of the 21st Century* (Basic Health Publications, 2003).

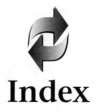

Index